T0177205

Handbook of Service User Involvement in Mental Health Research

World Psychiatric Association *Evidence and Experience in Psychiatry* Series

Series Editor: Helen Herrman (2005 -   )
WPA Secretary for Publications, University of Melbourne, Australia

The *Evidence & Experience in Psychiatry* series, launched in 1999, offers unique insights into both investigation and practice in mental health. Developed and commissioned by the World Psychiatric Association, the books address controversial issues in clinical psychiatry and integrate research evidence and clinical experience to provide a stimulating overview of the field.

Focused on common psychiatric disorders, each volume follows the same format: systematic review of the available research evidence followed by multiple commentaries written by clinicians of different orientations and from different countries. Each includes coverage of diagnosis, management, pharma and psycho- therapies, and social and economic issues. The series provides insights that will prove invaluable to psychiatrists, psychologists, mental health nurses and policy makers.

Depressive Disorders, 3e

Edited by Helen Herrman, Mario Maj and Norman Sartorius
ISBN: 9780470987209

Substance Abuse

Edited by Hamid Ghodse, Helen Herrman, Mario Maj and Norman Sartorius
ISBN: 9780470745106

Schizophrenia 2e

Edited by Mario Maj, Norman Sartorius
ISBN: 9780470849644

Dementia 2e

Edited by Mario Maj, Norman Sartorius
ISBN: 9780470849637

Obsessive-Compulsive Disorders 2e

Edited by Mario Maj, Norman Sartorius, Ahmed Okasha, Joseph Zohar
ISBN: 9780470849668

Bipolar Disorders

Edited by Mario Maj, Hagop S Akiskal, Juan José López-Ibor, Norman Sartorius
ISBN: 9780471560371

Eating Disorders

Edited by Mario Maj, Kathrine Halmi, Juan José López-Ibor, Norman Sartorius
ISBN: 9780470848654

Phobias

Edited by Mario Maj, Hagop S Akiskal, Juan José López-Ibor, Ahmed Okasha
ISBN: 9780470858332

Personality Disorders

Edited by Mario Maj, Hagop S Akiskal, Juan E Mezzich
ISBN: 9780470090367

Somatoform Disorders

Edited by Mario Maj, Hagop S Akiskal, Juan E. Mezzich, Ahmed Okasha
ISBN: 9780470016121

Other World Psychiatric Association titles

Series Editor (2005 -): Helen Herrman, WPA Secretary for Publications, University of Melbourne, Australia

Special Populations

The Mental Health of Children and Adolescents: an area of global neglect

Edited by Helmut Remschmidt, Barry Nurcombe, Myron L. Belfer, Norman Sartorius and Ahmed Okasha
ISBN: 9780470512456

Contemporary Topics in Women's Mental Health: global perspectives in a changing society

Edited by Prabha S. Chandra, Helen Herrman, Marianne Kastrup, Marta Rondon, Unaiza Niaz, Ahmed Okasha and Jane Fisher
ISBN: 9780470754115

Families and Mental Disorders

Edited by Norman Sartorius, Julian Leff, Juan José López-Ibor, Mario Maj, Ahmed Okasha
ISBN: 9780470023822

Disasters and Mental Health

Edited by Juan José López-Ibor, George Christodoulou, Mario Maj, Norman Sartorius, Ahmed Okasha
ISBN: 9780470021231

Approaches to Practice and Research

Psychiatric Diagnosis: challenges and prospects

Edited by Ihsan M. Salloum and Juan E. Mezzich
ISBN: 9780470725696

Recovery in Mental Health: reshaping scientific and clinical responsibilities

By Michaela Amering and Margit Schmolke
ISBN: 9780470997963

Psychiatry and Religion: beyond boundaries

Edited by Peter J Verhagen, Herman M van Praag, Juan José López-Ibor, John Cox, Driss Moussaoui
ISBN: 9780470694718

Psychiatrists and Traditional Healers: unwitting partners in global mental health

Edited by Mario Incayawar, Ronald Wintrob and Lise Bouchard,
ISBN: 9780470516836

Psychiatric Diagnosis and Classification

Edited by Mario Maj, Wolfgang Gaebel, Juan José López-Ibor, Norman Sartorius
ISBN: 9780471496816

Psychiatry in Society

Edited by Norman Sartorius, Wolfgang Gaebel, Juan José López-Ibor, Mario Maj
ISBN: 9780471496823

Psychiatry as a Neuroscience

Edited by Juan José López-Ibor, Mario Maj, Norman Sartorius
ISBN: 9780471496564

Early Detection and Management of Mental Disorders

Edited by Mario Maj, Juan José López-Ibor, Norman Sartorius, Mitsumoto Sato, Ahmed Okasha
ISBN: 9780470010839

Handbook of Service User Involvement in Mental Health Research

Edited by

Jan Wallcraft, Beate Schrank and Michaela Amering

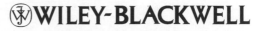

A John Wiley & Sons, Ltd., Publication

This edition first published 2009 © 2009, John Wiley & Sons

Wiley-Blackwell is an imprint of John Wiley & Sons, formed by the merger of Wiley's global Scientific, Technical and Medical business with Blackwell Publishing.

Registered office:
John Wiley & Sons Ltd, The Atrium, Southern Gate, Chichester, West Sussex, PO19 8SQ, UK

Other Editorial Offices:
9600 Garsington Road, Oxford, OX4 2DQ, UK
111 River Street, Hoboken, NJ 07030-5774, USA

For details of our global editorial offices, for customer services and for information about how to apply for permission to reuse the copyright material in this book please see our website at www.wiley.com/wiley-blackwell

The right of the author to be identified as the author of this work has been asserted in accordance with the Copyright, Designs and Patents Act 1988.

All rights reserved. No part of this publication may be reproduced, stored in a retrieval system, or transmitted, in any form or by any means, electronic, mechanical, photocopying, recording or otherwise, except as permitted by the UK Copyright, Designs and Patents Act 1988, without the prior permission of the publisher.

Wiley also publishes its books in a variety of electronic formats. Some content that appears in print may not be available in electronic books.

Designations used by companies to distinguish their products are often claimed as trademarks. All brand names and product names used in this book are trade names, service marks, trademarks or registered trademarks of their respective owners. The publisher is not associated with any product or vendor mentioned in this book. This publication is designed to provide accurate and authoritative information in regard to the subject matter covered. It is sold on the understanding that the publisher is not engaged in rendering professional services. If professional advice or other expert assistance is required, the services of a competent professional should be sought.

The contents of this work are intended to further general scientific research, understanding, and discussion only and are not intended and should not be relied upon as recommending or promoting a specific method, diagnosis, or treatment by physicians for any particular patient. The publisher and the author make no representations or warranties with respect to the accuracy or completeness of the contents of this work and specifically disclaim all warranties, including without limitation any implied warranties of fitness for a particular purpose. In view of ongoing research, equipment modifications, changes in governmental regulations, and the constant flow of information relating to the use of medicines, equipment, and devices, the reader is urged to review and evaluate the information provided in the package insert or instructions for each medicine, equipment, or device for, among other things, any changes in the instructions or indication of usage and for added warnings and precautions. Readers should consult with a specialist where appropriate. The fact that an organization or Website is referred to in this work as a citation and/or a potential source of further information does not mean that the author or the publisher endorses the information the organization or Website may provide or recommendations it may make. Further, readers should be aware that Internet Websites listed in this work may have changed or disappeared between when this work was written and when it is read. No warranty may be created or extended by any promotional statements for this work. Neither the publisher nor the author shall be liable for any damages arising herefrom.

Library of Congress Cataloguing-in-Publication Data

Handbook of service user involvement in mental health research

Edited by Jan Wallcraft, Beate Schrank, and Michaela Amering
Includes bibliographical references and index.
ISBN 978-0-470-99795-6
1. Psychiatry–Research–Handbooks, manuals, etc. 2. Mental health services–Citizen participation–Handbooks, manuals, etc. 3. Human experimentation in psychology–Handbooks, manuals, etc. I. Wallcraft, Jan. II. Schrank, Beate. III. Amering, Michaela. [DNLM: 1. Mental Health. 2. Research. 3. Consumer Participation. 4. Mentally Ill Persons. 5. Researcher-Subject Relations. WM 20 H236 2009]
RC337.H367 2009
616.89–dc22   2008044456

ISBN: 978-0-470-99795-6

Cover design by Sara Wallcraft

A catalogue record for this book is available from the British Library.
Set in 10/12pt Times by Thomson Digital, Noida, India
Printed in Singapore by Markono Print Media Pte Ltd
First Impression   2009

Contents

Foreword   ix

Preface   xi

About the Editors   xiii

About the Authors   xiv

Chapter 1   **History, Context and Language**   1
            Jan Wallcraft and Mary Nettle

Chapter 2   **Principles and Motives**   13
            Alison Faulkner

Chapter 3   **Levels and Stages**   25
            Angela Sweeney and Louise Morgan

Chapter 4   **Values**   37
            Bill (KWM) Fulford and Jan Wallcraft

Chapter 5   **Roles**   61
            Jasna Russo and Peter Stastny

Chapter 6   **Capacity-building**   73
            Kim Hopper and Alisa Lincoln

Chapter 7   **Purposes and Goals**   87
            *Larry Davidson, Priscilla Ridgway, Timothy Schmutte
            and Maria O'Connell*

Chapter 8   **Topics**   99
            Paulo Del vecchio and Crystal R. Blyler

Chapter 9   **Methods**   113
            Jean Campbell

Chapter 10   Service Users as Paid Researchers   **139**
               Jonathan Delman and Alisa Lincoln

Chapter 11   Consultation   **153**
               Virginia Minogue

Chapter 12   Collaboration   **169**
               Diana Rose

Chapter 13   Control   **181**
               Peter Beresford

Chapter 14   Power   **199**
               *Paddy McGowan, Líam Mac Gabhann, Chris Stevenson
               and Jim Walsh*

Chapter 15   Money   **213**
               Sarah Hamilton

Chapter 16   Politics   **227**
               Daniel B. Fisher

Chapter 17   Good Practice Guidance   **243**
               Beate Schrank and Jan Wallcraft

Index   **249**

Foreword

Mental health science should aspire to being a 'well-ordered' science. For this, the full engagement of service users is crucial.

The concept of a 'well-ordered' science was developed by Kitcher in *Science, Truth and Democracy* (2003).[1] Its key aspect is how a research agenda is to be determined. Conventionally, what is to be researched, and how, has been determined by 'elites' – either by communities of scientists engaged in a particular field, or by scientists in association with a privileged group of outsiders, predominantly the funders of research. Some paymasters, such as government departments or research councils, are seen as representing society, though rarely is that representation wide; others, such as charities, represent narrower interest groups, perhaps restricted to a particular disease. Another paymaster, industry, has a central interest in making a profit.

Kitcher argues that elitism is not a sound basis for setting a research agenda for a society. Science has the potential to improve the lives of many and their voices need to be heard. However, 'vulgar democracy' as a means for setting the agenda, Kitcher warns, leads to a 'tyranny of the ignorant' – an emphasis being placed on what is currently fashionable or a 'hot topic' and with a short-term focus. The ideal basis for a 'well-ordered' science is what he terms 'enlightened democracy'. Decisions are made on the basis of 'tutored preferences'. Groups representing as broad a range of interests as practicable are 'tutored' by scientists about what is known, how we know it and the prospects for knowing more about a particular problem. They are exposed to the conflicts within science, as well as its successes. Non-scientist deliberators will then understand the goals, methods and limitations of a particular research approach as a means for solving a particular problem. They thus become deliberators with 'tutored preferences' who engage in discussions with the scientists, funders, government and each other about what research is best for the common good. But deliberations involve a two-way 'tutoring' process; non-scientist deliberators also tutor the scientists about the personal meanings, social value and political implications of their knowledge. Tutored preferences will lead to a science which is 'ordered' – that is, with an agenda constructed by informed deliberators who will balance competing interests and who will agree on the problems to be researched, the kinds of science required to solve them and the constraints that need to be imposed (such as ethical and budgetary ones).

This is clearly a description of an ideal and is regarded as such by Kitcher. An 'enlightened democracy' along the lines described above is unlikely to be realised, at least in the foreseeable future. There are many critics who argue that self-interest is impossible to set aside and that the ideal community of tutored deliberators cannot exist.

---

[1]Kitcher, P (2003) *Science, Truth and Democracy*. New York: Oxford University Press.

However, I believe that in the recent history of service user involvement in research, we can see processes and practices that move us in that direction. A modest achievement, perhaps, in terms of the grand ideal but, in mental health research terms, not a small one. Of course one can point to the obstacles – the difficulties in hearing or understanding each other's viewpoints. For service users, the science can be hugely difficult to understand, as can be the convoluted and sometimes alarmingly competitive workings of the academic world, while for the scientist, the lived experience of mental illness in all of its complexity and implications can be difficult to grasp or even acknowledge.

One might argue that progress towards a 'well-ordered science' in mental health is the most important in the medical or human sciences. This is because 'values' are so much more clearly at issue than, say, in cardiovascular disease. So much is contested in mental health – even the idea of 'illness' itself, and thus the value of entire domains of science as applied to the problems of mental health. If progress can be made in establishing 'tutored preferences' for all parties in this arena – researchers, service users, funders, government – then it surely can be achieved in any area of health research.

Looking at the contributions in this book, it very much looks as though more progress has been made in mental health than in any other area of healthcare. Within that community whose interest is mental health, deliberations have exceeded, in some respects, what Kitcher has proposed. In some places, the research agenda is now significantly influenced by service users; studies adopted for research have increasing service user involvement – ranging from 'consultation' and 'collaboration' to 'control'; service users are increasingly effective in determining the aims, methods and design of studies; and they regularly serve as members on project management or steering committees. Furthermore, service users are increasingly themselves becoming researchers and instigators of research. Some projects could not be carried out without their involvement. In the UK, topic-specific (disease-specific) research networks funded by the Department of Health to enhance the quality of research look to the Mental Health Research Network for ideas about service user involvement.

Of course this is only a start. There is a long way to go and there are many tensions. But let us remember that the notion of user involvement in research is very recent. In fact, I am now less troubled by the progress in deliberations between the 'tutored' partners within the mental health research community, than by the state of its relationship with the larger community. Mental health is grossly underfunded in relation to the disability for which it accounts, while government and industry often pursue interests that are far from 'tutored preferences'. Often they fit, rather aptly, Kitcher's description of 'vulgar' democracy and 'tyranny of ignorance'. Governments tend to respond to 'hot-topics' or 'moral panics', seeking quick fixes to short-term concerns. 'Epistemic significance' – what it is important to know because it will provide the means of solving important problems – is, in our society, always at risk. Strong partnerships between tutored scientists and tutored service users may be the only means of shifting policies from 'vulgar' to 'enlightened'.

Professor George Szmukler

Professor of Psychiatry and Society at the Institute
of Psychiatry, King's College London

Preface

We have set out to produce an international textbook on the involvement of mental health 'service users', 'consumers', 'survivors', 'patients' and 'ex-patients' in mental health research. This book will be a practical tool for all those who want to (or need to) establish service user involvement in their research projects as well as for service users who intend to become involved in research.

We begin the work of consensus-building by bringing together a wide range of expertise from people who are acknowledged pioneers in this field, and drawing out from their writings some common issues, such as values, methods, desired outcomes, common problems encountered and examples of successful resolution of some of these problems. We also set out some fundamental challenges to the knowledge base and philosophical underpinning of conventional mental health research. Service users have long been conducting their own research independently, as individuals, groups or partnerships with professional allies in voluntary and statutory organisations. This work has often been ignored for being too small-scale, classified with the so-called 'grey literature' and placed on the bottom rungs of the hierarchy of evidence. In spite of this, service users have developed skills and confidence as researchers and their work has often challenged and inspired professionals and the public, and influenced policy-makers.

'Service user' or 'consumer' involvement in mental health research is now on the political agenda in many countries. Service users/survivors/(ex-)patients are increasingly striving to introduce their lived experience of mental illness and service use into the research scene in order to improve the relevance and utility of what is being researched. Traditional academic researchers have begun to realise the potential benefits of such involvement. Last but not least, funding bodies in various countries demand such involvement as a prerequisite for obtaining grants.

Despite greater acceptance by policy-makers of the principles of involvement, service user participation in mainstream mental health research as a truly collaborative enterprise between researchers with and without lived experience is still in its infancy. Much confusion still surrounds the concept of service user involvement, as do unrealistic or even false expectations and a lack of practical knowledge on how to embark on this promising enterprise, potentially leading to difficulties and frustration on the part of all groups concerned (service users, researchers and funders).

In this book, the reader will learn about the background and shared principles underlying the concept of involvement in mental health research across a number of different countries, including the sometimes major differences both between, but also within, countries regarding a range of issues from basic terminology and traditions to current policies.

Many of the eminent pioneers in the field world wide are authors of chapters of this book. They have included in their rich contributions their substantial experience as well as the work of many others who have significantly shaped the efficient development of this pivotal access to essential evidence.

The World Psychiatric Association and its Institutional Program on Psychiatry for the Person with a participatory agenda and full support for the publication of this book, highlight a focus on person-centredness in all relevant issues ranging from assessment to care and research, as well as policy. This book is intended for a global audience of different players in the field of scientific engagement with mental health.

For researchers seeking to do better involvement work, there are chapters which give practical advice on how to engage with service users/consumers and how to build and maintain research collaboration on a professional level. The book highlights common practical problems in service user/consumer involvement from various countries' research and social policy backgrounds, and gives advice on how to avoid pitfalls and common difficulties.

The book will help researchers decide which level of service user/consumer involvement will be adequate for their research activities and what will be feasible in view of the practicalities involved. It will help researchers and research organizations achieve their respective ambitions and guarantee best practice in successful service user/consumer involvement. It will also help funding bodies decide on adequate levels of requested involvement and evaluate the scale and quality of service user involvement in the projects they are funding.

Jan Wallcraft
Beate Schrank
Michaela Amering

About the Editors

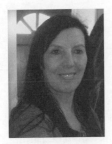

Jan Wallcraft is a consultant at the Centre for Recovery at the University of Hertfordshire. She has previously worked as Manager of the Service User Research Group for England(SURGE), part of the Mental Health Research Network (MHRN). She has written and presented on service-user involvement, recovery and alternatives to the biomedical model, and contributed to many publications. Her PhD was based on narrative accounts of first experiences of psychiatric hospital, which from her own experience she regards as a turning point, not always in the right direction.

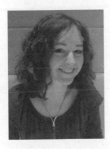

Beate Schrank is a psychiatrist in training at the Medical University of Vienna, Department of Psychiatry and Psychotherapy. While she did a research degree in London (UK) she also had a position as a research worker at SURGE. It was then that she got to know the user movement and service user involvement in mental health research, which fundamentally reshaped her vision of research as well as mental health practice.

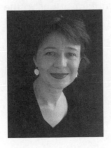

Michaela Amering is a Professor of Psychiatry at the Medical University of Vienna, Department of Psychiatry and Psychotherapy, with a focus of interest on psychosis, and the development of the families' and the users' movements. Her experience also includes work in community psychiatry and research in the UK and USA. She is currently serving as secretary of the AEP Section on Women's Mental Health, and as secretary of the WPA Section on Public Policy and Psychiatry.

About the Authors

Chapter 1

Jan Wallcraft – see 'About the Editors' for author biography.

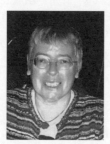

Mary Nettle lives in the UK and is self-employed as a Mental Health User Consultant. She has a particular interest in user-controlled research. She works as a Mental Health Act Commissioner ensuring that the rights of people detained under the Mental Health Act are upheld. She is chair of the European Network of (ex-) Users and Survivors of Psychiatry (ENUSP).

Chapter 2

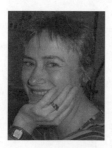

Alison Faulkner is a freelance researcher, trainer and consultant in the mental health field. She has over 20 years' experience of social research, mainly in the mental health field. She has worked for many of the national mental health voluntary-sector organisations in the UK, including the Sainsbury Centre for Mental Health, the Mental Health Foundation, Rethink and Mind. As a user of mental health services, Alison has experience of a range of services including acute inpatient care, crisis services and A&E, psychotherapy and medication. Alison is also a cat lover and one day would like to write a book on the lessons cats have to teach us about mental health.

Chapter 3

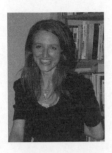

Angela Sweeney is an independent mental health survivor researcher. She has worked for a variety of mental health charities and universities on various research and teaching projects. She is currently completing a PhD at the Service User Research Enterprise (SURE, Institute of Psychiatry, King's College London) in which she has used mixed methods to generate and test a user defined outcome measure of continuity of care.

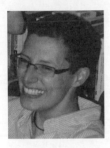

Louise Morgan is a service user researcher based in London. She currently combines freelance work with a service user involvement post at a North London User group called BUG (Brent User Group). Prior to that, she worked for SURGE (Service User Research Group for England), the service user arm of the Mental Health Research Network, before leaving with the rest of her team in a protest resignation. She has also worked at the Service User Research Enterprise (SURE) at the Institute of Psychiatry.

Chapter 4

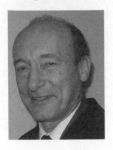

Bill (K.W.M) Fulford is Professor of Philosophy and Mental Health in the University of Warwick Medical School; an Honorary Consultant Psychiatrist and member of the Faculty of Philosophy, University of Oxford; Professor of Philosophy and Psychiatry and Co-Director of the Institute for Philosophy, Diversity and Mental Health at University of Central Lancashire (UCLan, UK). He is also Visiting Professor in Psychology, Institute of Psychiatry and King's College, London University; and Special Adviser for Values-Based Practice in the Department of Health, London. He has published widely on philosophy and psychiatry and is Lead Editor of the journal *Philosophy, Psychiatry, & Psychology* and of a book series from Oxford University Press on International Perspectives in Philosophy and Psychiatry.

Jan Wallcraft – see 'About the Editors'.

Chapter 5

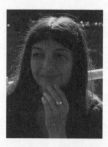

Jasna Russo is a survivor researcher living in Berlin, Germany. She has a degree in clinical psychology and comes from former Yugoslavia where she has experienced forced psychiatric treatment. Jasna has worked on both collaborative research projects (at the Institute of Psychiatry, Kings College London), and on survivor-led and survivor-controlled projects (for the German organisation In Any Case, of which she is a founding member). She is also a Board member of the European Network of (ex-) Users and Survivors of Psychiatry.

Jasna's articles have been published in various different anthologies. Her research reports include *Taking a Stand: Homelessness and Psychiatry from Survivors' Perspective* (together with T. Fink, Berlin 2003); *From One's Own Perspective: Users' Experiences of Person Centred Care* (together with F. Scheibe and A. K. Lorenz, Berlin 2007).

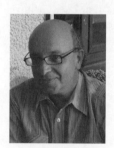

Peter Stastny is Senior Psychiatrist at South Beach Psychiatric Centre. A dissident psychiatrist, he is the author of numerous scholarly papers on psychosocial treatments, advance directives, self-help and empowerment, film history and mental health, and subjective experiences. He has served as expert witness and consultant in legal cases involving standards of care, involuntary treatment, and issues of dangerousness.

Peter has spearheaded innovative programs such as peer specialist services, peer-run businesses, and transitional living groups. He has directed and produced several documentary films addressing mental health subjects. In 2003, Peter was a founder of the International Network of Treatment Alternatives for Recovery (INTAR).

With Darby Penney, he was guest curator of a major exhibit at the New York State Museum in 2004, 'Lost Cases, Recovered Lives: Suitcases from a state hospital attic' and in 2006, Peter and Darby produced a book by the same title (Bellevue Literary Press, New York).

Jasna and Peter met each other in Dresden, Germany at the WPA thematic conference on coercion in 2006. This chapter is their first joint piece of work and they wish to thank the editors for this opportunity.

Chapter 6

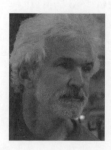

Kim Hopper is Research Scientist at the Nathan Kline Institute for Psychiatric Research, and Professor of Clinical Sociomedical Sciences at Columbia University Mailman School of Public Health. He also co-directs the NIMH-funded Center to Study Recovery in Social Contexts. Kim is most interested in cross-cultural studies of psychosis, alternative perspectives on psychiatry as social practice, and user efforts to enhance participation, and is currently working on adapting Amartya Sen's capabilities approach for use in public mental health.

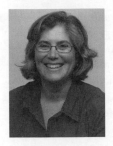

Alisa Lincoln is an Associate Professor of Health Sciences and Sociology and has adjunct appointments at the Boston University School of Public Health and the Division of Psychiatry, Boston University School of Medicine. Her research interests focus on public urban mental health. She was the Principal Investigator of a SAMHSA[2]-funded project which opened and evaluated a Safe Haven Shelter, now known as the Dudley Inn, for people who are chronically homeless, and struggling with both severe mental illness and substance abuse problems. This project included a consumer-driven evaluation. Currently, she is working on two NIMH-funded projects on psychiatric emergency-room care. The first studies staff perspectives of psychiatric emergency-room care and the impact of the culture and climate of a busy, public urban psychiatric emergency room. The second award allowed for the creation of The Boston Community Academic Mental health Partnership (B-CAMHP) a community-based participatory action-research group focused on mental health.

Chapter 7

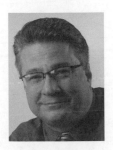

All authors of this chapter work at the Program for Recovery and Community Health at Yale University in New Haven (USA).
Larry Davidson is a Professor of Psychiatry and Director of the Program for Recovery and Community Health of the School of Medicine and Institution for Social and Policy Studies at Yale University. His research and teaching interests focus on processes of recovery, the active role of the person in pursuing recovery, and the active role of people in recovery in transforming mental-health systems to promote recovery-oriented care.

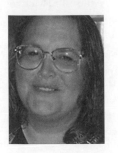

Priscilla Ridgway is an Assistant Professor of Psychiatry at the Yale Program for Recovery and Community Health. Her work experience in the field of mental health ranges from being a psychiatric aide, case manager, and advocate for psychiatric inpatients, program director in an innovative psychosocial rehabilitation agency, and co-ordinator of research and planning for a state mental-health department. For the last 20 years she has worked within organisations committed to innovation and building recovery-paradigm knowledge, including the Center for Psychiatric Rehabilitation at Boston University, the University of Kansas Office of Mental Health Research and Training, and Advocates for Human Potential, Inc. Her work has always concerned human rights, recovery, services that support recovery, and amplifying the voice of mental health consumers. She considers her personal experience of recovery from brain trauma and post traumatic stress disorder as an important background that has taught her a lot in relation to her work.

[2]Substance Abuse and Mental Health Services Administration (SAMHSA).

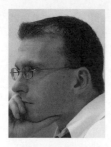

Timothy Schmutte is a clinical psychologist and Associate Research Scientist at the Yale Program for Recovery and Community Health. In his role as the program manager for the evaluation of the federally-funded Connecticut Mental Health Transformation Grant, he works with state departments, advisory councils, and advocacy groups on developing strategies for increasing the level of consumer, youth, and family involvement in system transformation and program evaluation.

Maria O'Connell is an Assistant Professor of Psychiatry and Director of Research and Evaluation at the Yale Program for Recovery and Community Health. She has been involved in local and national recovery-oriented system transformation efforts and is the lead developer of the Recovery Self-Assessment (RSA), a tool designed to assess perceptions of the degree to which a variety of objective recovery-oriented practices are manifest in mental health and addiction service-agencies. Her research interests include recovery and recovery-oriented systems of care, psychiatric advance directives, and self-determination among adults with mental illness.

Chapter 8

Both authors work at the Center for Mental Health Services Substance Abuse and Mental Health Services Administration of the U.S. Department of Health and Human Services (USA).

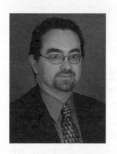

Paulo Del vecchio is currently the Associate Director for Consumer Affairs within the Office of the Director at the Federal Center for Mental Health Services (CMHS) of the Substance Abuse and Mental Health Services Administration in the U.S. Department of Health and Human Services. In this capacity, he manages the Center's precedent-setting activities in addressing consumer participation and education, issues of discrimination and stigma, consumer rights, and others. He was the first Consumer Affairs Specialist hired by this Federal agency. In this capacity, he promoted consumer/survivor participation in all aspects of the Center's policies and operations ranging from public education to efforts at researching effective strategies to address the needs of persons with mental illnesses.

A self-identified mental health consumer/survivor, Paolo del Vecchio has been involved in the consumer/survivor self-help movement for over a decade.

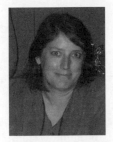

Crystal Blyler is a Social Science Analyst in the Community Support Program Branch, Division of Service and Systems Improvement of the U.S. Substance Abuse and Mental Health Services Administration (SAMHSA) Center for Mental Health Services. She earned her PhD in psychology with a specialization in experimental psychopathology. Prior to joining SAMHSA she conducted schizophrenia research on symptomatology, neurocognition, motor disorders, medication compliance, suicide, and residential alternatives to hospitalization.

As an evaluation specialist at SAMHSA, Dr Blyler has served as a project officer on a diverse range of initiatives, most recently focussing on the design and evaluation of mental-health systems transformation; a variety of evidence-based practice activities, and, most recently, design and evaluation of mental-health systems transformation. Before that, she worked at the Chestnut Lodge Research Institute in Rockville, MD, where she served as a therapist/treatment co-ordinator for people with serious mental illnesses in the hospital's outpatient clinic. The consumer movement has been known to her since graduate school when she served on the Human Rights Committee for the Massachusetts Department of Mental Health in Cambridge, MA.

Chapter 9

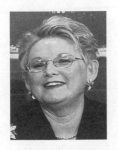

Jean Campbell is a Research Associate Professor in the Department of Psychiatry at the University of Missouri School of Medicine – Columbia, USA, and directs the Program in Consumer Studies and Training at the Missouri Institute of Mental Health. As an internationally-known mental-health consumer researcher, speaker, and consultant, she is a forerunner in the effort to define recovery and well-being of mental health service recipients and to promote multi-stakeholder approaches in evaluation and service delivery. Currently, she is working with the Missouri Department of Mental Health to promote consumer-operated service programs as an evidence-based practice and is part of the national effort to develop the Consumer-Operated Services Program Evidence Based Practices KIT. Dr Campbell was the Principal Investigator of a co-ordinating centre for a large, multi-site federal research initiative to study the cost-effectiveness of consumer-operated programs as an adjunct to traditional mental health services. She was a consultant to the President's New Freedom Commission on Mental Health and a contributor to the Mental Health Report of the Surgeon General.

Dr Campbell is best known for her ground-breaking consumer-directed research study of consumer well-being in California, *The Well-Being Project* (1989 – referred to in Chapter 9) and the supplemental award-winning documentary, 'People Say I'm Crazy'. She has received the NAMI Lionel Aldridge Award (2008), the Silver Key Award from the Mental Health Association of Greater St. Louis, (2004), the New York Association of Psychiatric Rehabilitation Services Executive Directors Award (2003), the International Association of Psychosocial Rehabilitation Services Acknowledgement, (2000), and the Human Rights Diversity Enhancement Award from the University of Missouri-Columbia (1995).

Chapter 10

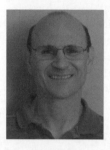

Jonathan Delman is the Executive Director of Consumer Quality Initiatives, Inc., a Massachusetts-based service user directed research and evaluation organization, located in Roxbury, Massachusetts, USA. He is a lead investigator on several research projects, including a recently awarded National Institute of Mental Health (USA) grant to the Boston University School of Public Health (BUSPH) to establish a service user driven community-based participatory action-research partnership, the Boston Community-Academic Mental Health Partnership (B-CAMHP).

Jonathan has written several peer-reviewed articles and book chapters on the significant involvement of consumers in research, and has served on a variety of national and state policy committees, including the President's New Freedom Commission subcommittee on acute care. Mr. Delman has lived with bipolar disorder for many years and is a long-time service user researcher and advocate. He is currently pursuing his doctorate (part-time) in Health Policy and Management at BUSPH.

Alisa Lincoln – see Chapter 6.

Chapter 11

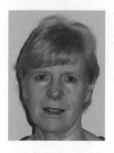

Virginia Minogue works in the NHS as Head of the West Yorkshire Mental Health Research and Development Consortium (UK). Her specific areas of interest are service user and carer involvement in research and service development and planning, partnership working and mentally disordered offenders. She works particularly closely with service users and carers, involving them at all levels of the research agenda, and has published papers in this area and a training package. She was previously a Senior Lecturer in Community Justice in Sheffield. Prior to this she worked for a number of years in the Probation Service as a manager, researcher, Family Court Welfare Officer and probation officer. She is currently Chair of the Editorial Board for the journal *Mental Health and Learning Disabilities Research and Practice*. She is also Chair of a voluntary sector mental-health organisation which offers support, housing and employment services to adults with mental health problems and their carers.

Chapter 12

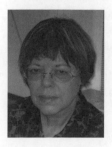

Diana Rose was educated at Aberdeen and London Universities, taking degrees in psychology, and social psychology. Her PhD was about representations of madness in the media. She has also been a mental-health service user all her adult life. After teaching in a university for ten years she was medically retired and spent ten years 'living in the community'. During that time she became active in the user movement. In 1996 she went to work for the Sainsbury Centre for Mental Health (London) and whilst there built on both her research and her consumer experience to develop User-Focused Monitoring (UFM), a model for evaluating mental health services which is wholly user-driven. She has now been co-director of the Service User Research Enterprise (SURE) at the Institute of Psychiatry in London for five years. This is an academic team but nearly all the staff have experience of psychiatric services and treatments and the research done by the team is intended to prioritise the experiences of service users. Leading projects include work on consumers' perspectives on ECT, users' perceptions of detention and compulsion and users' experiences of acute wards.

Chapter 13

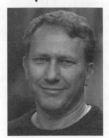

Peter Beresford is Professor of Social Policy and Director of the Centre for Citizen Participation at Brunel University (UK). He is also Chair of Shaping Our Lives, an independent, service user controlled UK organisation and network and a long-term user of mental health services. He has a longstanding interest in issues of participation as a writer, educator, researcher and activist. In England he is a member of the Advisory Board of Involve, which works to support public and user involvement in health, public health and social care research and of the National Institute for Health Research. He is also a member of the Survivor Researchers Network and an active survivor–researcher.

Chapter 14

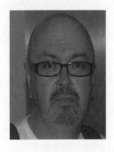

Paddy McGowan, from Omagh in County Tyrone, recovered from schizophrenia with the support of other survivors and professionals. He was involved in organising the first 'Voices' conference in Derry in November 1999. As a member of the Institute for Recovery in Mental Health and a prominent member of the International Network of Treatments Alternatives for Recovery (INTAR) he is respected as a leading and inspirational authority in creating alternatives to the so-called 'medical' or 'maintenance' model. Paddy set up the first user group in Ireland in 1994 and was the founder and first Chief Executive Officer of the Irish Advocacy Network. He has been involved in developing peer-advocacy training alongside staff awareness training in user empowerment and advocacy to an accredited degree level. He served on the National Disability Association's Ad Hoc Focus Group on Mental Health and the Management Committee of the United Kingdom Advocacy Network. Paddy has also been instrumental in designing and implementing user-led research focusing on user-satisfaction with statutory mental health services throughout Ireland, including the Southern Health Board, which led to *Focusing Minds*, the locally-agreed interpretation and implementation of national mental health policy in the Southern Health Board, Ireland. He has been a member of many expert mental health committees and working groups throughout Northern Ireland, gives lectures nationally and internationally, and in 2005 received the prestigious Social Entrepreneurs Ireland Award.

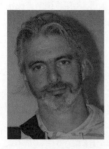

Liam Mac Gabhann qualified as a mental health nurse in 1988 and headed off from Ireland with his new found insights to change the world. Spending most of his early career in England with some brief sojourns in Australia and the Middle East, he consistently worked with people with psychotic illness, and concentrated on acute mental health care. He has been a nurse, researcher/practitioner and worked in practice/service development. In 2001 he returned to Ireland and now works as a lecturer, and in practice. He practises on an acute psychiatric admission ward and co-ordinates the Graduate Diploma/MSc in Health Care Practice/Nursing Practice, and also runs some interesting professional development courses at Dublin City University. His clinical research focus generally centres on the relationships and understandings of mental health professionals and service users in relation to mental health, illness and health care. He is the lead for a research programme 'service user involvement in research' with the aim of creating real partnerships with service users. He has a degree in health studies, a Masters in Sociology of Health and Health Care, and a taught Doctorate in Nursing Science.

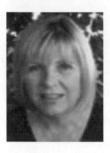

Chris Stevenson trained as a psychiatric nurse in the UK and studied for a degree in psychology and sociology, working on a casual basis in practice. She became a community mental health nurse in a progressive service and learned family therapy 'on the job'. She was challenged in her existing thinking about distress and began to see how patterns of communication, relating and cherished stories could keep the individual and family tied in to a way of living that was not satisfying or fulfilling. She moved from practice to academia, although she maintained her family therapy practice, joining a team with Jim Birch (an alternative psychiatrist) and Alex Reed, now a nurse consultant in family therapy. They immersed themselves in the postmodern/social constructionist therapy literature acknowledging that families are experts on their own lives and she wrote her PhD in the area.

Chris has also worked at University of Newcastle, with Phil Barker, where she led the research underpinning the Tidal Model of psychiatric/mental health nursing as an 'in-system' alternative to existing coercive nursing practices, whilst maintaining her family therapy life. She co-authored a good practice guide on involvement with members of the Irish Institute for Mental Health Recovery (IMHR), Kieran Crowe and Paddy McGowan.

As the first Chair in Mental Health Nursing in Ireland, she established a lectureship open to people with experience of service use.

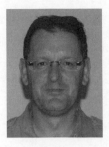

Jim Walsh used mental health services for approximately 14 years. During that time he returned to education completing a degree in psychology at Queens University, Belfast and became actively involved in various mental health initiatives set up with the specific aim of improving the status of people experiencing psychological and emotional distress within mental health care systems. Later he became employed by a health trust in Northern Ireland; first as a Day Care Worker and later coordinating a partnership initiative – the Mental Health Alliance. He is involved in several local, national and international user and carer initiatives – the Irish Advocacy Network, the Institute for Mental Health Recovery, Mental Health Ireland, and the International Network of Treatment Alternatives for Recovery. He now works as a lecturer in mental health at the School of Nursing, Dublin City University.

Chapter 15

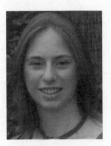

Sarah Hamilton is a senior researcher at Rethink, the leading national mental health membership charity in Great Britain. Sarah's main current research interests are: the role and needs of family members and friends caring for someone with a mental illness; stigma and discrimination against people with a mental illness; and the relationship between debt and mental ill-health.

Chapter 16

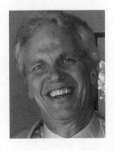

Daniel B. Fisher life's work is to inspire the hope and call forth the voice that helps people recover. This passion comes from his lived experience with mental illness. No-one would have guessed such a calling lay ahead when he obtained a PhD in biochemistry at the University of Wisconsin and carried out neurochemical research at the National Institutes of Mental Health into the possible biochemical basis of schizophrenia. Ironically, however, during the course of that work, he was himself diagnosed with schizophrenia at age 25, and hospitalized several times. In large part, his recovery from schizophrenia was based on the life-changing experiences he witnessed, and he decided he would dedicate the rest of his life to helping others recover from mental illness. To do so, he earned a MD from George Washington University, and was trained as a psychiatrist at Harvard Medical School. He has practised as a Board-certified, community psychiatrist at Riverside Community Care in Wakefield, Massachusetts, USA, for the last 25 years. But he yearned to bring about change at a more extensive level. To do so, in 1992 he co-founded the National Empowerment Center and has served as its Executive Director since then.

Dr Fisher was a Commissioner on the White House New Freedom Commission on Mental Health. He won the Mental Health America's Clifford Beers Award for Mental Health Advocacy in 2002, and he has helped organize the National Coalition of MH Consumer/ Survivor Organizations, which acts as a voice for consumers in the development of national mental health policy.

Chapter 17

Jan Wallcraft and **Beate Schrank** – see 'About the Editors' for author biographies.

History, Context and Language

Jan Wallcraft

Service user Researcher and Consultant, Worcester, UK

Mary Nettle

Mental Health User Consultant, Worcester, UK

This first chapter sets the scene for the chapters to follow. It provides an introduction to the context as well as the history and cornerstones of service user research and service user involvement in research as an evolving discipline. It provides examples which typify the different starting points from which service user involvement in research originated. Examples are given of how and why service users became researchers and the different types of research service users have been, and are being, involved in. There is a brief examination of the politics of research, and how governments are both encouraging involvement and creating further hurdles for service users to overcome. The chapter gives an introduction to the terminology used to describe service users in research, together with the background and history of the respective terms.

INTRODUCTION

Service user involvement in any aspect of mental health must include the possibility that involvement will lead to real change. As the subsequent chapters of this book will demonstrate, service users and survivors of psychiatry have sought to challenge and change the underlying assumptions and world-views on which traditional mental-health research are based, in small, incremental ways and in radical, fundamental ways. This opening chapter sets the scene for the rest of the book by describing the origins of service user involvement in research in the UK, the US and Canada, a few of the countries where involvement in mental health research has taken hold.

Service user involvement in mental health research would not have happened but for the efforts of survivors and users. Power-sharing is rarely initiated from the top, though the contributions in this book also give due credit to the help that political and professional allies have provided.

Service users have, of course, always been involved in research as subjects of tests and as respondents to questionnaires, but it is only in the past 20–25 years that they have been

Handbook of Service User Involvement in Mental Health Research Edited by Jan Wallcraft, Beate Schrank and Michaela Amering
Copyright © 2009 John Wiley & Sons, Ltd

invited in as partners, and have taken part in planning, designing, and carrying out research along with professionals, or as researchers in their own right. This is a new area of development, which has come from a number of different starting points, as this chapter will show.

Although service user groups were active from the late 1970s onwards, for some years they made few inroads into the area of research. Perhaps, in the first ten years, research was not high on the agenda for service user organisations. Primary concerns were providing mutual support and information to their members and campaigning for better services and better public understanding of mental health issues. The world of research was inaccessible to all but clinicians and academics, and the rules of engagement in research were not service user-friendly. Dworkin (1992), in her book *Researching Persons With Mental Illness,* makes no mention of involving the persons being researched in any way, and describes the difficulties of placing reliance on patients' answers to questions, given their illness. In some ways, the 1990s marginalised the nascent service user movement even more firmly than it would have been ten years earlier, as Dworkin shows that in the US at least, mental health was moving away from an earlier public health model and refocusing on the biomedical model. This was reinforced when 'the 1990s were declared the Decade of the Brain. . . with emphasis upon basic neuroscience research' (p7). Though aware that mental illness diagnosis is controversial, Dworkin advises that researchers 'can ill afford to ignore diagnostic issues'.

Though in the late 20th century there was small chance of involving service users in mainstream medical research, there were other forms of research, such as policy-oriented participatory-action research, and service evaluation, concerned with providing high-quality services in the community, where service users/survivors could, and did, get involved and gain experience. Also, as Beresford points out (Chapter 13) user-led research 'has the longest history of any form of user involvement in research' – service users could, and did, begin their own small-scale studies individually and in groups. This type of small-scale study and evaluative, policy-oriented research did not, and still does not, command the status and funding that is given to brain biochemistry, genetics, and drug trials.

Between 'pure' laboratory-based research and 'applied' research such as service evaluation, there has traditionally been a hierarchical division. Some have argued this to be a kind of class distinction, where 'pure' research was carried out by university-educated intellectuals, while messy, real-world, applied research was left to practical-minded working-class engineers.

Rather than a comprehensive history of the origins of involvement in research, we will point out some examples which typify the different routes by which service users and survivors developed skills and confidence and made alliances with professionals which began to create the basis for the establishment of service user involvement.

STARTING POINTS FOR INVOLVEMENT IN RESEARCH

Origins of involvement in research

The origins of involvement in research mirror the origins of the service user/survivor movement generally. They began with efforts by individuals and groups to make sense of their experience, reclaim their identity and have a say in the mental health world. Most of the involvement examples in this book show that it has been the result of people's actions on their personal and collective journeys towards empowerment. For instance, some service users/survivors have found their way into research through their efforts to change things so that others will get a better experience than they did.

Individuals making sense of their own experience

A US example is the work of an individual, Leonard Roy Frank (1978) who researched and compiled an anthology of information about ECT. In testimony, Frank (2001) described his reasons for starting his research on ECT:

> In 1962, three years after moving to San Francisco, I was diagnosed as a 'paranoid schizophrenic' and committed to a psychiatric institution where I was forcibly subjected to 50 insulin-coma and 35 electroconvulsive procedures. This was the most painful and humiliating experience of my life. My memory for the three preceding years was gone. The wipe-out in my mind was like a path cut across a heavily chalked blackboard with a wet eraser. Afterwards I didn't know that John F. Kennedy was president although he had been elected three years earlier. There were also big chunks of memory loss for events and periods spanning my entire life; my high school and college education was effectively destroyed . . ..
> Following years of study re-educating myself, I became active in the psychiatric survivors movement. . . In 1978 I edited and published The History of Shock Treatment. Over the last thirty-five years I have researched the various shock procedures, particularly electroshock or ECT, have spoken with hundreds of ECT survivors, and have corresponded with many others. From all these sources and my own experience, I have concluded that ECT is a brutal, dehumanizing, memory-destroying, intelligence-lowering, brain-damaging, brainwashing, life-threatening technique.

Many other survivors/service users have begun their research similarly, including one of the authors of this chapter, who found Frank's (1978) book in 1985 in a left-wing bookshop. It helped her along her own path to recovery and to use her own experience of ECT as the starting point to a new career as a researcher and writer. Wallcraft carried out a small study of ECT patients' stories as part of her degree (1983–7), and later did a PhD thesis based on narrative first-person accounts of first experiences of breakdown and hospitalisation. Lindow (1990) and O'Hagan (1994) are two other survivors who became academics and researchers as part of their own journeys to mental health activism and recovery.

Service user/survivor groups funded to do consumer studies

While some US survivors began their research, like Frank, as individual pioneers, others chose to work in groups, developing participatory methods. Some of those who developed these methods throughout the 1990s (Van Tosh, Ralph and Campbell, 2000) pay tribute to earlier work, such as the 1984 People First study in California where people with learning disabilities were enabled to talk about the services they needed, and a methodology was developed to use their contributions. The Hill House Project in Ohio was another example, where people labelled 'mentally ill' helped to design the research instruments proved to be reliable and valid, and demonstrated that consumer members had the expertise to identify and classify their feelings (Prager and Tanaka, 1979; Smith and Ford, 1986).

One such was Dr. Jean Campbell (see also Chapter 9) who was principal investigator of the Well-Being Project, which ran from 1986–1989. This was an influential survey programme, based in California, which identified the factors that helped and hindered well-being of those labelled mentally ill. The interviewers were all service users, trained as part of the programme, and carried out over 500 face to face interviews, producing a report (Campbell and Schraiber, 1989) a video documentary, a compendium of statistics, oral history, art and writings.

A Canadian example of local activism as a starting point is the setting up of Second Opinion Society (SOS) in 1990 in Whitehorse, Yukon. As Sartori (2007) recounts, she and two other psychiatric survivors set up SOS in response to their dismay with media portrayals of the 'mentally ill'. The following year, they were funded by the Yukon Ministry of Health to carry out a needs-assessment survey of what psychiatric survivors needed most.

With a good deal of help and support from allies in the Yukon government, SOS completed this study, which was a tremendous learning process for the group, as Sartori (1997) relates in an earlier article:

> The amount of work involved was enormous. For a long time, I felt that it was a mistake to have taken on this project. We'd never done anything like it, so it was this big, big thing that hung over our heads and took our energy away from our other work. I almost wanted to give up. But the wonderful Statistics Department people who were helping us kept telling us this would be important. And, looking back now, they were absolutely right. It took twice as long as we thought it would, but it gave our group a really good foundation. We had the voices of Yukoners and we could say, 'Here, this is what people want'. It gave us a lot of credibility.
>
> (pp 126–7)

SOS's success was not without opposition, according to Sartori (1997):

> There was a huge outcry on the part of people in social services and in the medical profession. For example, the medical council wrote letters to the editor saying things like, 'How dare they let this group interview other people who have experienced the psychiatric system? They'll all jump out of the window!'

Not only did this work give SOS a solid basis of experience and credibility from which they have operated ever since, but their work was recognised by the Federal Health Promotion department as one of the best participatory research projects that had ever been done in Canada.

'Insiders' – professionals with service user experience

Another form of starting point for involvement in research was from the inside of establishments and organisations, from those who were current or former service users/survivors as well as paid workers and professionals. Some were academics, others were mental health professionals, such as nurses, psychologists and doctors, or managers and politicians. They shared a wish to narrow the gap between their personal and working lives and put their experience to good use. Some of these people may have been attracted to their profession because of an earlier mental health problem, others had a breakdown during their working life, sometimes because of the stresses of the job.

Such individuals, such as Dan Fisher, whose chapter is included here (Chapter 16), have contributed tremendously to the establishment of service user involvement in research, as researchers and as allies to service users and user groups.

Reformers in state and non-profit organisations

Service user/survivor involvement in clinical research and large-scale funded community/ social research would not be possible without the work of committed people in government and the large non-profit organisations. They have responded to the rise of organised service user/survivor groups by inviting individuals and groups to join decision-making committees, or have formed partnerships with service users to bid for research grants, or been generous with their knowledge, expertise and contacts. There are many examples of this help offered to service users/survivors throughout this book.

In the UK, we have the example of the setting up of Involve, a state-funded organisation to encourage and support service users to be involved in research. This was originally called Consumers in NHS Research, and was set up in 1996 by the Director of Research and Development in the NHS. It aims to ensure that consumer involvement in research and development improves the way research is prioritised. As stated in the foreword to a progress report of this group (Hanley, 1999).

> *Consumers are the ultimate recipients and beneficiaries of the knowledge derived from research and development. It is therefore not only desirable, but essential that they be involved in developing and implementing strategies for R&D in the NHS.*

Non-profit organisations have enabled innovative work and helped service users/ survivors gain experience as researchers by funding in-house service user/survivor-led programmes such as the Mental Health Foundation, Strategies for Living (Faulkner and Layzell, 2000), Mind's *Coping with Coming off Psychiatric Drugs* (Read, 2005) and Sainsbury Centre for Mental Health's User-Focussed Monitoring work (Rose, 2001).

TYPES OF RESEARCH

An increasingly empowered citizenship, and consumer movements in every type of public service, along with heightened awareness of the costs of public services, have made governments and public bodies more aware of the need for service improvement, cost-benefit analysis and evaluation, and the political benefits of involving the public in making difficult decisions about resources.

This changed climate, along with the growth of the Consumer/survivor/ex-patient (c/s/x) movements, with their emancipatory outlook, has led to service users being involved in different types of research such as participatory-action research, and evaluation, and in the UK, user-led monitoring. Involvement in 'pure' medical research has been a slower process.

US and UK governments, among others, have recently developed policies prioritising evidence-based medicine. As Campbell (Chapter 9) argues, this policy is often worrying to service users, as it can discriminate against the types of service they value, and against the qualitative research, and small-scale studies where service users are more likely to be involved. The writers in this book explore the power-struggles involved in establishing whose evidence is given the highest priority, the need to re-value qualitative research in mental health, and who should determine outcome measures used in studies (see Chapter 8).

Individual research, e.g personal study, literature reviews, academic theses, published collections of narrative accounts

Amongst these would be included many unpublished, self-published and grey-literature studies such as the aforementioned ECT book by Frank (1978), and books such as those by Susko (1991), Shimrat (1997), Pembroke (1994), Leibrich (1999) which are purposeful, edited collections of service user/survivor narrative accounts. There are many, many more such studies which have provided sustenance for other service users/survivors starting out on similar journeys. Given that most of us started out in our journey to becoming researchers without the tools or the encouragement to do research based on our own life experience, the excavation of narrative accounts has been a pioneering enterprise which is only now becoming academically recognised. Webb (2006) has made a strong academic argument for the validity of first-person research using first-person data on experience (which he argues is only directly available to the subject having those experiences), and first-person methods of analysis, based on phenomenology.

Participatory research, or participatory action research

Van Tosh *et al.* (2000) looked back on the process of developing participatory research in the USA.

> *The last decade has witnessed the blossoming of a vibrant consumer research agenda and the growing belief that consumer involvement in research and evaluation holds great promise for system reform, quality improvement, and outcome measurement. The Well-Being Project [1989] made a substantial contribution to understanding the concept of quality of life from the perspective of consumers. Results indicate the validation of personhood, a recognition of common humanity, and a tolerance for individual differences are essential to well-being.*

Since then, consumer/survivor researchers in the USA have been involved in evaluation work and have argued for outcome measures based on the values and desired outcomes of service users. A consumer/survivor mental health research and policy-work group worked in the 1990s to develop tools which incorporated the values of recovery, personhood, well-being and liberty (Ralph and Kidder, 2000).

Demonstration, or pilot projects

The purpose of demonstration projects, or pilot projects, is similar to that of action research, to learn about something by trying to put into practice an idea which already has some evidence base and/or popular force behind it. These are often state-funded 'experiments' with new types of service. Russo and Statsny (Chapter 5) refer to the use of demonstration projects as a tool for change in a resistant system. In England (Haigh, 2007; Haigh *et al.*, 2007) service users were involved (to a greater or lesser extent) at all stages, from policy, to implementation, to evaluation, of a Government funded programme which set up 16 pilot projects for people diagnosed with personality disorders.

Involvement in mainstream biomedical research

In the UK, where the Welfare State is still strong, the impact of efforts to control costs along with a stronger voice of patients and consumers of services, has led to national government policy on involving health service consumers. User involvement is a statutory requirement under the Health and Social Care Act 2001, and has now become a requirement of all government-funded research. As a study by Minogue *et al.* (2003) showed, advocates of involvement believe consumers bring insight and expertise that 'expert' professionals do not have, and legitimise and add value to projects. But on the negative side, others expressed concern that

> ...*current legislation and policy, which makes consumer involvement mandatory, could reduce user involvement to political expediency in order to legitimise a research project and any decisions resulting from it.*

Government directives in England have led to involvement being a high priority in bodies that receive state funding to support mental health research, such as the Mental Health Research Network, and the Institute of Psychiatry. Rose (Chapter 12) describes one such initiative, the SURE project. Such initiatives can be hard to sustain, given the continuing strength of the biomedical model of mental health, especially where studies are funded by the pharmaceutical industry (see also Chapter 16 by Fisher). Increasing closeness between governments and industry do not bode well for the democratic control of research, and service users/survivors and our allies will have to continue to struggle to move our agenda forwards. Service users have argued that qualitative research is often the best way to study issues of meaning and experience, and should be seen as equal in status with quantitative research in mental health.

LANGUAGE AND TERMINOLOGY

It would not make sense to try to provide a glossary of the terms used in different chapters to describe the subject matter of this book. The language we use in this relatively new academic area is evolving, and each country has its own cultural history of terms and meanings. The best we can attempt is to understand each other's language and concepts better. Language, beliefs and philosophies are closely interwoven, so until there is common agreement on what is meant by 'mental illness' there can be no common language for the related concepts of patients/service users/survivors/consumers, etc. We will however discuss some of the language and terminology issues below.

Evolving terms – 'mental patient' to 'survivor' and beyond

In the 1980s people on the receiving end of mental health and psychiatric services began to be seen as 'consumers' with a right to involvement in their services. This was seen as progressive by some, while others rejected the idea of being consumers. In the UK, an early leader of the service user/survivor movement, Eric Irwin, said 'mental patients are consumers in the same way that woodlice are consumers of Rentokil' (personal memory).

The term 'mental patients' itself has been owned by some, especially those who were long-stay patients in the old asylums, but this has become increasingly out-of-date now that these hospitals have closed. In the 1980s some people began to term themselves 'survivors' (of psychiatry, of services, or of the distress or illness itself). This is still a popular term, though some find it too political or controversial.

In the UK, the term 'service user', or 'mental health service user' became widely used, as a compromise, though again, many dissented, saying they had not willingly used services. Some preferred the term 'recipients' of psychiatric services. In the US activists sought to unite their movement by bringing together the terms consumer/survivor, or consumer/survivor/ex-patient, often shortened to c/s/x.

Another widely-used term in the USA is 'persons with psychiatric disabilities'. This term makes a strong link with the disability movement and its rights-based agenda and social model of disability, which places the onus on society to end its disabling exclusions.

Finally, many people argue that we are people first and foremost, and should not accept being labelled at all, simply for the convenience of others.

Ultimately, different people will describe themselves differently, and this is as it should be, since our movement stresses the right to self-define.

Models, discourses and worldviews

Service users working inside or outside the establishment do not all share the same perspectives on psychiatry, mental health and mental illness. As Beresford and Wallcraft (1997) argued, there are some who find the social model of disability helpful because of its stress on social oppression and discrimination, while others do not see themselves in terms of disability. Some reject the medical model, with its pathologising of madness, while others accept the concept of mental illness but seek improved treatment with better outcomes. The rise of 'consumerism' in health provided an opportunity for involvement, though this has been criticised as a 'supermarket' version of choice, not true democratisation based on citizenship and rights.

There are also different views on whether to talk about mainstream psychiatry as a progressive, evolving science, a model, a discourse, or a paradigm. There are similarities between the concepts of models, discourses and worldviews, the main being that one is immediately offered a choice. If current psychiatry can be seen as 'the medical model' or the 'discourse of psychopathology', or as a 'eurocentric worldview' it opens up the possibility of other, very different, ways of seeing and doing things. Many of the chapters in this book refer to these possibilities.

Types of involvement

Several of the chapters look at different types of involvement, such as consultation, collaboration, partnership, and user control of research. These terms may overlap, and in some cases are hotly contentious. For instance, there are different views about whether research carried out within a non-profit organisation by service users can be called 'user-led' when service users do not run the organisation.

Terms for those who get involved

The writers have used a number of terms for service users/survivors who are involved in research, reflecting the different roles and different levels of experience that they may have. These include 'peer specialists', 'experts by experience', 'service user researchers', and 'academic user researchers'. The first two refer to the life experience which is gained by simply being a service user/patient or survivor of mental health services, and the knowledge that has been gained by surviving that experience and from talking to and working with others with similar experiences. Service user researchers are those who bring their personal experience openly to the task of research. Academic user researchers have been defined as those who do the same, but who have research qualifications (see Chapter 15).

The differences in terminology are also a reflection of the emergent nature of these roles. Is there such a creature as a 'service user researcher', or should one have the simple status of 'researcher'? Is a service user researcher of lower status, or does it reflect a new type of research, legitimately and proudly based on personal experience? If so, this new type of research is still nascent. One example might be Webb's (2006) aforementioned PhD thesis, based on his own experiences of suicide attempts and years of contemplating suicide. His thesis is based on the phenomenological method, with the primary aim being to

> ...to give voice to the lived experience of suicidality so that it may contribute to a better understanding of the phenomenon. This voice is my own first-person voice, a narrative voice that gives a detailed description of my suicidality as I have lived it and in my own words.
>
> (p23)

The second aim of Webb's research is to critique of the discipline of suicidology, in which

> the first-person, narrative voice [acts] as a prism through which the discipline is viewed to see what this reveals. That is, the formal, disciplinary knowledge of suicidology effectively becomes the 'data' of this research and my narrative story the analytical tool. This exercise itself can be seen as a phenomenological reduction that deliberately puts to one side the 'natural attitude' of suicidology.
>
> (p23)

The award of PhD for someone arguing a coherent and acceptable academic justification for basing his thesis on his own lived experience, may be an important historic moment for those who have argued that the biomedical discourse of mental illness fails us because it artificially and incorrectly transforms personal experience of distress into categories of 'diseases' which assume the appearance of reality only because of the weight of research behind them.

REFERENCES

Beresford, P. and Wallcraft, J. (1997) 'Psychiatric System Survivors and Emancipatory Research: Issues, overlaps and differences'. In Barnes C. and Mercer G. (1997) (Eds) *Doing Disability Research*, Leeds: Disability Press.

Campbell, J. Ralph, R. and Glover, R. (1993) *From Lab Rat to Researcher: The history, models, and policy implications of consumer/survivor involvement in research*. Fourth Annual Conference Proceedings on State Mental Health Agency Services Research and Program Evaluation. National Association for State Mental Health Program Directors Research Institute.

Campbell, J. and Schraiber, R. (1989) *The Well-Being Project: Mental health clients speak for themselves*, Sacramento, CA: California Department of Mental Health.

Campbell, J. (1997) How consumers/survivors are evaluating the quality of psychiatric care, *Evaluation Review*, **21,** pp. 357–363.

Consumers in NHS Research Support Unit (2001) *Getting Involved in Research: A guide for consumers*, Consumers in NHS Research Support Unit.

Dworkin, R.J. (1992) *Researching Persons With Mental Illness*, London: Sage Publications.

Faulkner, A. and Layzell, S. (2000) *Strategies for Living: A report of user-led research into people's strategies for living with mental distress*, London: Mental Health Foundation.

Frank, L.R. (1978) *The History of Shock Treatment*. San Francisco: Leonard Roy Frank.

Frank, L.R. (2001) Testimony at a Public Hearing on Electroconvulsive 'Treatment' before the Mental Health Committee of the New York State Assembly, Manhattan, 18 May 2001. Available online at: http://www.idiom.com/~drjohn/LFrank.html, accessed 25/10/08.

Haigh, R. (2007) The 16 Personality Disorder pilot projects, *Mental Health Review*, **12**(4) pp. 29–39.

Haigh, R., Lovell, K., Lyon, F. and Duggan, M. (2007) Service user involvement in the National PD Development Programme, *Mental Health Review*, **7,** (12) 4, pp. 13–22.

Hanley, B. (1999) *Involvement Works: The second report of the Standing Group on Consumers in NHS Research*, London: NHS Executive. Available online at: http://www.invo.org.uk/pdfs/involvement_works.pdf, accessed 25/10/08.

Leibrich, J. (Ed) (1999) *A Gift of Stories: Discovering how to deal with mental illness*, Otago University Press, New Zealand.

Lindow, V. (1990) Participation and power, *Openmind*, **44,** April/May, pp. 10–11.

Minogue, V., Boness, J., Brown, A. and Girdlestone, J. (2003) *Making a Difference: The impact of service user and carer involvement in research* (unpublished report), South West Yorkshire Mental Health Trust.

O'Hagan, M. (1994) *Stopovers On My Way Home From Mars*, London: Survivors Speak Out. Prager and Tanaka.

Pembroke, L. (Ed) (1994) *Self-Harm: Perspectives from Personal Experience*, London: Survivors Speak Out.

Prager, E. and Tanaka, H. (1979) A client-developed measure (CDM) fo self-assessment and change for outpatient mental health services. In: *New Research in Mental Health*, Columbus: Ohio Department of Mental Health, pp. 48–51.

Ralph, R.O. and Kidder, K. (2000) *What is Recovery? A compendium of recovery and recovery related instruments*, Cambridge, MA: Human Services Research Institute.

Read, J. (2005) *Coping with Coming Off Psychiatric Drugs*, London: Mind.

Rose, D. (2001) *The Perspectives of Mental Health Service Users on Community and Hospital Care*, London: Sainsbury Centre for Mental Health.

Sartori, G. (2007) 'Second Opinion Society: Without Psychiatry in the Yukon'. In: Stasny P. and Lehmann P. (Eds.), *Alternatives Beyond Psychiatry*, Peter Lehmann Publishing, pp. 199–209.

Sartori, G. (1997) *Call Me Crazy –Stories from the Mad Movement*, I Shimrat Vancouver, Press Gang Publishers, pp. 126–127.

Shimrat, I. (1997) *Call Me Crazy: Stories from the Mad Movement*, Vancouver: Press Gang
    Publishers.
Smith, M.K. and Ford, J. (1986) Client involvement: practical advice for professionals. – *Psychosocial
    Rehabilitation Journal*, **9**(3), pp. 25–34.
Susko, M.A. (Ed) (1991) *Cry of the Invisible*, Baltimore: Harrison Edward Livingstone.
Webb, D. (2006) *A Role for Spiritual Self-Enquiry in Suicidology?* PhD Thesis, Victoria University,
    Australia.
Van Tosh, L. Ralph, R. and Campbell, J. (2000) The rise of consumerism – a contribution to the surgeon
    general's report on mental health, *Psychiatric Rehabilitation Skills*, **4**(3), pp. 383–409.

CHAPTER 2

Principles and Motives

Principles and Motives for Service User Involvement in Mental Health Research

Alison Faulkner

Mental Health Researcher, Trainer and Consultant, London, UK

This chapter considers some of the underlying principles and the motives or incentives for involvement on the part of both researchers and service users. It is easy for researchers to overlook some of these basic principles when driven by deadlines to write a proposal that involves service users. Equally, service users may find themselves in a position where they have not thought through all of the possible implications of becoming involved in a research study. This chapter, then, aims to provide you with some space to think about these things and to encourage you to do so in connection with your own research and involvement activities.

The principles underlying service user involvement, as set out in this chapter, are reflected in certain attitudes and basic pre-requisites necessary for successful and satisfactory involvement. Faulkner's chapter is grounded in experience gained from pioneering work in this field. The chapter also lists some of the tangible reasons for researchers and service users to seek involvement. Awareness of these personal motives is clearly a first and important step to prevent confusion on both sides when establishing and maintaining such involvement. Furthermore, relevant practical benefits that can be expected from service user involvement are summarised, as are challenges that need to be considered. Overall, this chapter gives a comprehensive but concise and practical overview of the basics of service user involvement in mental health research.

INTRODUCTION

The way this chapter is written tends to assume two mutually exclusive categories of service users and researchers. In reality of course researchers can be service users. However, it is

Handbook of Service User Involvement in Mental Health Research Edited by Jan Wallcraft, Beate Schrank and Michaela Amering
Copyright © 2009 John Wiley & Sons, Ltd

assumed here that there is a power differential between the academic researchers who are employed to undertake research and to involve service users in that research, and the service users who are seeking involvement in research from outside the employment world of the researchers. Researchers may choose to recruit service users to positions of employment for the purposes of the research, but this is not the main concern of this chapter. Issues connected to employing service users as paid researchers are discussed in detail in Chapter 10.

UNDERLYING PRINCIPLES

This section is based on two publications which look at the underlying principles for survivor research or service user involvement in research. One is the SURGE[1] *Guidance for Service user Involvement in the Mental Health Research Network* (SURGE, 2005). The other is *The Ethics of Survivor Research* (Faulkner, 2004a), which is based on consultations with survivor/service user researchers and service user groups. These 'underlying principles' are informed both by considerations of ethical research practice and by the wider literature on user involvement. The values and themes to be found in the latter are eminently transferable to user involvement in research, with a few additional issues specific to the academic world. The following shortlist of underlying principles is taken from the SURGE guidance:

- clarity and transparency
- respect
- flexibility
- accessibility
- diversity.

The principle of clarity and transparency reflects the importance of building trust for a collaborative enterprise between researchers and service users. An initial clarity about the extent and nature of involvement on offer from researchers, and any limits on the influence that service users might have on the research, is vital. The practical manifestations of this might include: a written statement of purpose, role descriptions and contracts of involvement. The importance of this honesty cannot be overstated, and is closely connected with the second principle, respect. The establishment of trust between researchers and service users can take time on both sides, and underlines the importance of building relationships over time rather than trying to involve service users at short notice, as so often happens.

The dual principles of flexibility and accessibility reflect the measure of difference or diversity that service users might bring to a research project and a research environment. Some people might not be familiar with the office environment or research context and will need some 'reasonable adjustments', in the language of the Disability Discrimination Act (1995), to begin to establish equitable working relationships. Other people may be perfectly familiar with the office environment but may have other difficulties that make regular work or the demands associated with it difficult to fulfil. All of these can

---

[1] Service User Research Group England (SURGE) is the service user hub of the UK Mental Health Research Network (see www.mhrn.info).

be incorporated with a degree of flexibility and through, for example, checking out any specific access needs in advance of meetings or training. The most important element is probably an *attitude* of flexibility, an openness to difference and an appreciation of people as individuals with something of value to contribute.

Both service users and researchers will have a diversity of views which need to be taken into account when considering involvement in a research project. One of the principles identified in the SURGE guidelines suggested that the diversity of service users to be involved in a research project should reflect the nature of the project itself. It is also important to ensure that, where relevant, involvement includes people on the margins of service use: from homeless people, people of different ages within black and minority ethnic communities, and people with myriad 'overlapping' identities.

Consultations for *The Ethics of Survivor Research* carried out by the author found some additional principles that mental health system survivors and service users held dear to them in the context of research endeavour:

- empowerment
- a commitment to change
- underlying theoretical approach
- accountability.

Empowerment lies at the core of survivor research for many people (Beresford and Evans, 1999; Beresford and Wallcraft, 1997), developing as it has in the wake of feminist, emancipatory and disability research. It is a principle of survivor research to have the empowerment of mental-health service users as a goal.

Clarity about the underlying theoretical approach to the research can help in making explicit some of the values and beliefs held by both researchers and service users and in clarifying any areas of disagreement or incompatibility. Research that takes as read, for example, that a particular diagnosis is incontestable may present difficulties to service users who hold a different set of beliefs regarding either that diagnosis, or diagnoses, in general. Similarly, researchers carrying out research with a black or minority ethnic community who do not recognise the role of racism in mental health and social experience, may not find it easy to involve service users from that community.

A commitment to change leads us into the next section on motives and incentives; it is very often a strong motivation for change that attracts service users to become involved in research. In Faulkner (2004a) a commitment to change is proposed as a principle for undertaking survivor research, on the basis that change and improvement in the lives of people with mental health problems should be at the heart of survivor research. This may be more problematic when it comes to user involvement in research initiated by academic researchers, but it is worth considering as a potential incentive nevertheless.

MOTIVES AND INCENTIVES

No collaboration is without its challenges, and research is no exception to this. One of the key factors that can introduce challenges is a clash or mismatch of motives for embarking upon the research in the first place. It is worthwhile setting these out for discussion at an early meeting in order to 'clear the air' and to ensure that everyone understands each other.

It can help for researchers to write a clear statement of intent outlining why they want to involve service users in their research, and the kind of contribution they hope that the service users will bring.

These potential motives or incentives are separated into two lists for reasons of clarity and to outline where the potential clashes might arise, but there are problems with this approach. Firstly, it assumes that people fall neatly into only one of these categories and secondly, it assumes that we will behave according to the generalisations applied to that category. These lists are not proposed as comprehensive and nor would they apply to every individual; they are simply generalisations based on experience.

What's in it for researchers?

Policy incentives

Policy guidelines have increasingly encouraged the involvement of service users (and carers) as active participants: *Research and Development for a First Class Service* (Department of Health, 1999) requires Trusts holding NHS R&D Support Funding to demonstrate evidence of involving service users in research activity. More recently, the *Research Governance Framework for Health and Social Care* (Department of Health, 2001; revised 2005) called for the active involvement of service users and carers at every stage of research, where appropriate.

Funding requirements

As a result of these policy developments, some research commissioners require research proposals to demonstrate how they are planning to involve service users. The extent to which they impose or monitor this requirement varies and can be no more than a 'tick box' exercise. Nevertheless, researchers will need to be able to refer to some degree of public involvement in their research.

Career progression

It may be that service user involvement in research in some research fields or departments represents the potential for career progression. (This is not often the case, as it is often difficult to achieve publications in peer-reviewed journals where research involves service users or is more qualitative in its approach.)

Quality of research and its outcomes

Some researchers may be motivated by the conviction that involving service users will improve the relevance of research and the likelihood that it will improve services. Similarly, researchers may believe that direct experience of the service, treatment or diagnosis under investigation will add insight and inform the design of research questions.

Social justice

The belief that service users – like all members of the public – have the right to influence publicly funded research.

Increased job satisfaction

Faulkner and Morris (2003) found that researchers reported greater satisfaction and enjoyment from the research they carried out with service users in the forensic mental-health field. This is similarly reported in Telford and Faulkner (2004).

What's in it for service users?

Service improvement

Many service users who become involved in service delivery and planning, training, policy or research are motivated by the desire to improve services. This is an important factor for researchers to take into account in understanding what motivates people. Research is not the quickest way to change things, as many researchers will know. However, projects to monitor or evaluate services may have a more immediate feedback loop to change, and this sort of project is therefore potentially more likely to be of interest to service users.

Giving something back

Similarly, many service users wish to 'put something back' into the system – to give of their time and energy to a system that has benefited them and to help others who are still caught up in it.

Skills development

Involvement in research can act as a springboard for other opportunities through providing people with new skills. Research training might include interviewing skills, literature reviewing, presentation skills, IT skills and/or report writing, all of which are transferable to other arenas of work, education or training.

Employment

Following on from the above, some people may be motivated by the wish to return to work or enter employment or education for the first time. Becoming involved in research on a small scale, with a small and flexible level of commitment, can be a useful introduction to thinking about the future.

Meeting people

Becoming involved in all sorts of things can be valued for the opportunity it gives simply to meet people and to make new friends or colleagues. Research is not different from other involvement opportunities in this, although the focus on a task or goal can be a good way to engage people and to foster collaborative teamwork.

Money

Financial reward is an obvious incentive. However, it is not without its complications. Anyone planning to pay people for their involvement in research needs to be aware of the pitfalls and obstacles presented by the Benefits system. There are a number of useful publications that can provide useful guidance on these matters (McKenna, 2007; Turner and Beresford, 2005).

The real value of understanding each other's motives lies in establishing the foundations of a working collaboration that will satisfy some of everyone's goals or expectations. If researchers and service users share no motives or expectations in common, it will be far harder to achieve a successful project. For example, the researcher who has been driven by funding requirements to involve service users and who is primarily concerned with career progression will be incompatible with the service user who is motivated by the idea of meeting people through involvement and improving services. Barriers may emerge that will remain insuperable if the parties involved are unable to find an area or areas of compromise.

Equally, researchers could benefit from considering some of the factors that might attract service users to becoming involved in their project and building those in to the process: ensuring, for example, that there will be opportunities for people to develop skills or to influence service development.

BENEFITS AND CHALLENGES

Benefits

There is little research 'evidence' available to demonstrate the benefits (or, indeed, the 'disbenefits') of involving service users in research; however a number of researchers have written about the benefits that they have seen or experienced. INVOLVE (see www. invo.org.uk) has established the network INVONET in conjunction with Worthing and Southlands NHS Trust expressly in order to gather this kind of information and evidence together (across the whole health, social care and public health research fields). At the time of writing they are conducting a literature review to establish the evidence base for public involvement in research[2]. In the SURGE (2005) good practice guidance for service user involvement in the UK Mental Health Research Network, the following benefits are explored.

---

[2] By 'members of the public', Involve includes: consumers; patients and potential patients; people who use health and social services; informal (unpaid) carers and parents; members of the public who may be targeted by health promotion programmes; organisations that represent the public's interests; communities that are affected by health, public health or social care issues.

Making research more relevant

Several papers suggest that the user perspective itself brings benefits with it: by offering insight into what it feels like to experience mental health problems, to use mental health services or to receive certain treatments, service users can help ensure that the content of the research is more relevant to clinical practice and the results more relevant to service users (see Hanley *et al.*, 2003; Trivedi and Wykes, 2002; Allam *et al.*, 2004; Goodare and Lockwood, 1999; Rose, 2003).

Contributing to the design and methods

Service users can make positive contributions to the design of research questions and questionnaires and the use of outcome measures. Allam *et al.* (2004) discuss the benefits of involving service users and carers in the design of relevant questions in qualitative research. Such benefits include the fact that questions are more grounded in real experience and in consequence are more meaningful and relevant than those developed by non-service user researchers. Trivedi and Wykes (2002) describe the negotiation needed to determine the outcome measures used in the research since service users and clinicians may regard different outcomes, and hence outcome measures, as important. This also highlights the importance of service users being involved at an early stage of project development in order to allow for enough time to agree on outcome measures relevant to both. Wykes (2003) develops this further, exploring the benefits of service user involvement to the research questions, outcome measures and the overall methods used.

Generating new knowledge and understandings

Ramon (2000) contends that user involvement in the research process leads to the 'generation of new and more in-depth knowledge in the field of mental health'. She also suggests that researchers may gain a better understanding of the lives of service users and of lay perceptions of research as well as those of service users.

Gaining more open and honest responses from participants

Several researchers and service users report that, where service users are engaged as interviewers, they may obtain more open, truthful responses from their interviewees (see Ramon, 2000; Allam *et al.*, 2004; Rose, 2001; Faulkner and Layzell, 2000). Rose reports the findings of two previous authors (Clark *et al.*, 1999; Polowycz *et al.*, 1993) both of whom found a positive difference (or no difference) in the responses made to client as opposed to professional interviewers. A recent project, reported at the UK MHRN scientific conference in March 2008 (Gillard and Turner, 2008) suggests that there are differences in the emphasis placed on issues followed up in interviews between service user and non-service user interviewers. The authors reported that service user interviewers were more likely to follow up issues relating to personal experience and feelings, whereas non-service user interviewers focused more on issues of procedure.

Contributing to the analysis and interpretation of results

Allam *et al.* (2004) suggest that the differences in the interpretation of responses between the service users and carers (and potentially professionals) provide strong justification for involving service users and carers in the research process. They suggest that 'the validity of the findings must be improved by working together and coming to a joint agreement about the meaning of the data.' Faulkner *et al.* (2008) also comment on the value of involving service users throughout the research, including the analysis stage in a complex qualitative research project.

Facilitating access to research participants

Again, several researchers refer to the way in which service users might assist in finding and providing access to potential participants, particularly members of marginalised groups (see Hanley *et al.*, 2003; Fleischmann and Wigmore, 2000). Researchers often find it difficult to access people from marginalised communities. Marginalised communities are often reluctant to have research done 'to' or 'for' them. They are much more likely to work with researchers who want to collaborate with them on research that has been identified by the community as a priority, or researchers who are willing to support them to undertake their own research.

Maximising dissemination

Several researchers and service users report the benefits of service user involvement for the dissemination stage of research (e.g. Telford *et al.*, 2002). Hanley *et al.* (2003) report that voluntary organisations may assist in dissemination by carrying summaries of research in user-friendly language in their newsletters and magazines. This has been demonstrated by research carried out under the umbrella of the Mental Health Foundation's Strategies for Living project and the Sainsbury Centre's User Focused Monitoring projects.

The challenges of involving service users in research

There are a number of challenges involved, some of which are practical, some philosophical and some interpersonal. Some of these issues are not so much challenges as indicators of need; for example, there is a need to provide training and support if the involvement of service users in research is to succeed.

Resources

There is no doubt that involving service users or carers in research brings with it the need for more money and more time, both of which need to be built in to the project from the start.

Training

Some service users may have no research skills and some may have few educational qualifications. They are likely to need training and this will take more resources in terms of both time and money.

Support

People with mental health problems may be vulnerable and need more support than other members of a research team: practical and administrative support, emotional and supervisory support. Mechanisms for support can be built into a project to the benefit of everyone involved. As with training, an assessment of need should take place, rather than a blanket assumption that everyone has the same needs.

Doing things differently

One of the implications of collaborative research is a willingness to compromise and possibly carry out research in a different way. Researchers may need to be more flexible and make procedures explicit and clear. Service users may have good ideas about how to do the research (for example, knowing how or when to access service user participants on an inpatient ward; good practice in interviewing). Researchers need to be open-minded and not assume that they know best; the best research is likely to learn from the expertise of both.

Research quality

Some researchers fear that involving service users will have a negative impact on the quality of research, due to involving people who have no professional research skills and who, they believe, may be biased or lack objectivity; to some extent, this is dealt with above under 'Benefits', p18.

Project management

Many of the above might have an impact on your usual project management responsibilities – taking into account the possibility of people becoming ill or needing more support and supervision may result in the project falling behind schedule and taking more resources than you have predicted.

Power and control

Working with others and sharing your research implies some loss of control over the research. Some researchers may feel reluctant to share control or anxious about doing so for fear of losing power or status. From the service user's point of view, the power issue is central. Service users come to the table with less apparent power over the research process or the way in which the research is conducted. Explicitly sharing power with service users is likely to establish trust and lead to a more productive collaboration.

Interpersonal issues

Stereotypes might lead us to think that researchers may have fears and concerns about working with people who have mental health problems and who are inexperienced in research, and that service users may be intimidated by the idea of 'research' and by the status of research professionals. In some cases, these hold true. Certainly, there is some anecdotal evidence to suggest that the greatest difficulties experienced by service users are attitudinal (see also Faulkner, 2004b). At the basis of this are issues of power and control, but an open and flexible approach to working with each other can overcome these difficulties.

NEGOTIATING DIFFERENCE

One of the aims of this chapter has been to minimise the possibility of difficulties further on down the line by encouraging collaborating researchers and service users to consider some of the important principles, values and goals that (should) underlie this work from the start. Giving space for this kind of open discussion early on and approaching a project with openness and a willingness to learn from each other should prevent difficulties and the need for major negotiations later on.

It is often the interpersonal issues that create the greatest barriers. Attitudes on both sides can be difficult to negotiate. Several years ago, when I approached someone in the Department of Health to advocate for user involvement in some policy initiative, I received the response 'but they're always so angry!'. My response was something along the lines of 'Yes, they may be angry and have good reasons to be angry. You need to listen to that properly and respond to it before you can move on to work together.' I have also had the experience of helping service users and researchers find a satisfactory ending to a project, after intense interpersonal difficulties that never found a resolution during the course of the project (Faulkner, 2004b). If researchers commence this kind of enterprise with the view that they alone are the experts, then the prospect of collaboration is considerably weakened.

In the process of interviewing researchers about projects involving service users for the National Programme for Forensic Mental Health R&D, Faulkner and Morris (2003) found examples of useful strategies for negotiating differences of opinion concerning the research. In one project, the researcher reported having a voting strategy for points of difference; he said he was voted down on occasions despite believing he was right. In another project, the researchers thought it important that the service users were not outnumbered in the research advisory group and consequently able to override the opinion of the researchers on occasions.

LAYING THE FOUNDATIONS

The following suggestions for laying the foundations for a good collaborative enterprise are adapted from the SURGE Guidance and are directed primarily at researchers considering involving service users in their research:

- Involve service users from the start of a project in order that they can have the maximum influence and involvement.
- Resources should be planned in advance to take into account the time and money required to involve people fully.
- Communicate clearly and regularly with service users, particularly if they are not attending the work place on a regular basis.
- Plan for flexibility and periods of absence.
- Adequate support for service users is vital: practical, emotional and research related support.
- Training in relevant knowledge and skills is vital for both service users and researchers.
- Be prepared to be flexible and to negotiate about the research process in an atmosphere of collaboration and respect.
- It is advisable for researchers (particularly in large institutions) to communicate well in advance with their Finance department and Human Resources department about their intention to involve or employ mental health service users in research – in order to facilitate the process and pre-empt any difficulties that may arise.

REFERENCES

Allam, S., Blyth, S., Fraser, A. *et al.* (2004) Our experience of collaborative research: service users, carers and researchers work together to evaluate an assertive outreach service, 'Commentary', *Journal of Psychiatric and Mental Health Nursing*, **11**, 365–373.

Beresford, P. and Evans, C. (1999) Research Note: Research and empowerment. *British Journal of Social Work*, **29**, 671–677.

Beresford, P. and Wallcraft, J. (1997) Psychiatric System Survivors and Emancipatory Research: Issues, overlaps and differences. In C. Barnes and G. Mercer (Eds) *Doing Disability Research*, Leeds: Disability Press.

Clark, C.C., Scott, E.A., Boydell, K.M. and Goering, P. (1999) Effects of client interviewers on client-reported satisfaction with mental health services. *Psychiatric Services*, **50**(7), 961–963.

Department of Health (1999) *Research and Development for a First Class Service*, London: DH. Department of Health (2001; revised 2005) *Research Governance Framework for Health and Social Care*, London: DH, pp. 24–26.

Faulkner, A., Gillespie, S. and Imlack, S. *et al.* (2008) Learning the lessons together. *Mental Health Today*, **8**(1).

Faulkner, A. (2004a) *The Ethics of Survivor Research: Guidelines for the ethical conduct of research carried out by mental health service users and survivors*, Bristol: Policy Press on behalf of the Joseph Rowntree Foundation.

Faulkner, A. (2004b) *Capturing the Experiences of Those Involved in the TRUE Project: A story of colliding worlds*, London: INVOLVE, www.invo.org.uk

Faulkner, A. and Morris, B. (2003) *Expert Paper on User Involvement in Forensic Mental Health Research and Development*, National Programme on Forensic Mental Health Research and Development.

Faulkner, A. and Layzell, S. (2000) *Strategies for Living: A Report of user-led research into people's strategies for living with mental distress*, London: Mental Health Foundation.

Fleischmann, P. and Wigmore, J. (2000) *Nowhere Else to Go: Increasing choice and control within supported housing for homeless people with mental health problems*, London: Single Homeless Project.

Gillard, S. and Turner, K. (2008) *'Does who we are make a difference to the research that we do?'* presentation to UK Mental Health Research Network National Scientific Conference, March 2008.

Goodare, H. and Lockwood, S. (1999) Involving patients in clinical research. *British Medical Journal*, **319**, 724–725.

Hanley, B. *et al.* (2003) *Involving the public in NHS, public health and social care research: Briefing notes for researchers*, (second edition), London: INVOLVE.

McKenna, R. (Ed.) *Valuing Involvement: Payment and reimbursement policy guidance*, Making a Real Difference Project, London: National Institute for Mental Health in England, 2007. Available online at: http://www.nimhe.csip.org.uk/silo/files/payment–reimbursement-policy-guidance–mar-08.pdf, accessed 1/11/08.

Polowycz, D., Brutus, M., Orvietto, B.S., Vidal, J. and Cipriana, D. (1993) Comparison of patient and staff surveys of consumer satisfaction. *Hospital and Community Psychiatry*, **44**(6), 589–691.

Ramon, S. (2000) Participative mental health research: users and professional researchers working together. *Mental Health Care*, **3**(7), 224–228.

Rose, D. (2001) *Users' Voices: The perspectives of mental health service users on community and hospital care*, London: The Sainsbury Centre for Mental Health.

Rose, D. (2003) Collaborative research between users and professionals: peaks and pitfalls. *Psychiatric Bulletin*.

SURGE (2005) *Guidance for Service user Involvement in the Mental Health Research Network*, London: SURGE (part of the UK Mental Health Research Network, see, www.mhrn.info).

Telford, R. and Faulkner, A. (2004) Learning about user involvement in mental health research. *Journal of Mental Health*, **13**(6), 549–559.

Telford, R., Beverley, C.A., Cooper, C.L. and Boote, J.D. (2002) Consumer involvement in health research: fact or fiction? *British Journal of Clinical Governance*, **7**(2), 92–103.

Trivedi, P. and Wykes, T. (2002) From passive subjects to equal partners. *British Journal of Psychiatry*, **181**, 468–472.

Turner, M. and Beresford, P. (2005) *Contributing on Equal Terms: Service user involvement and the benefits system*, London: Social Care Institute for Excellence.

Wykes, T. (2003) Blue skies in the *Journal of Mental Health*: Consumers in research. *Journal of Mental Health*, **12**(1), 1–6.

CHAPTER 3

Levels and Stages

The Levels and Stages of Service User/Survivor Involvement in Research

Angela Sweeney
Survivor Researcher, London, UK
Louise Morgan
Survivor Researcher, Brent User Group, London, UK

Service user involvement is an evolving and multi-faceted area in mental health research that can occur at various stages in the research process and carry varying levels of influence. For researchers who are required to describe service user involvement in funding applications as well as for funding bodies and for users who seek involvement, it is important to draw on a common language and understanding of what involvement actually means in each particular instance.

Drawing on the literature, as well as on the authors' practical experience, this chapter clarifies the terminology to describe service user involvement in mental health research. The authors offer a revised version of a classification system currently used in the UK of the potential levels of involvement at all stages of a research project. Descriptions of the possible levels and stages are provided and a contingency table is offered to help researchers identify a realistic level of involvement to aim for in their project, setting out the respective tasks for both researchers and involved service users in order to establish successful involvement at each level and stage.

Many thanks are due to James Mitchell and Jo Maltby for their invaluable contributions to an earlier version of this chapter.

INTRODUCTION

Recent years have seen a growing tendency to involve service users/survivors in mental health research. At its simplest, service user/survivor involvement can be defined as people with experience of using or surviving mental health services being involved as 'active partners in the research process rather than "subjects" of research' (Hanley *et al.*, 2000, 2004). This means that service users/survivors involved in research will actively participate in the *research process*, rather than simply being research participants or sources of data. A service user/survivor involved in research would not just fill in a questionnaire or answer questions in an interview, but instead could be involved in designing the questions or in interviewing others. In essence, they would have some influence on how the research is conducted, whether through steering group membership, employment as an interviewer or researcher or even through having control of the research from conception to dissemination.

However, there is currently some confusion surrounding the terminology to describe service user/survivor involvement in research, largely because of the complexity and diversity of involvement. The most commonly used existing terms – *consultation, collaboration and control* – lack firmly agreed definitions and do not always reflect what is happening on the research scene. This can make it difficult to clearly distinguish which of the terms should be applied.

By drawing on the existing literature, this chapter will offer a basic overview of the levels of service user/survivor involvement in research and the use of the terms consultation, collaboration and control. This will highlight some of the confusion in their application. A further aim of this chapter is to attempt to resolve some of these problems. As a result we will propose an additional level of service user/survivor involvement, *contribution*.

The second section of this chapter will explore how different levels of service user/survivor involvement in research can occur at different stages of the research process. This will provide readers with concrete examples of how terminology should be applied throughout the cycle of a research study. Through discussing the levels and stages of service user/survivor involvement in research we hope to enable a more nuanced understanding of involvement, and thereby clarify the meaning and application of existing terminology.

WHAT'S IN A NAME?

The need to define language is not just a matter of semantics. It is vitally important that all those connected to mental health research (researchers, participants, service users/survivors, funders, commissioners and so on) understand the meaning of the terms used to describe service user/survivor involvement and apply language in a standardised way. Without a shared, common language, researchers can claim to be involving service users/survivors in research, or to be conducting user-focussed research, when this is not the case. In the UK, for example, Telford and colleagues (2002) surveyed researchers and NHS Research and Development (R&D) managers across a number of NHS Trusts and found that most claimed to be involving service users/survivors in research. However, on further examination, it became clear that service users/survivors were typically 'involved' as traditional subjects (participants) of research with no involvement in or influence on the research process (Telford *et al.*, 2002). Furthermore, Beresford and Evans (1999) reported techniques for respondent validation (checking the results of data analysis with participants) being used inappropriately as measures of service user/survivor involvement. These findings echo the experiences of one of the authors (AS) who has reviewed research grant applications where applicants have claimed to be conducting 'user-focused research' when *no* service user/survivor involvement was evident.

As researchers are increasingly required to describe service user/survivor involvement in research funding applications, there is a strong motivation to inflate the level of involvement, increasing confusion around terminology. It is therefore more important than ever that the terms available for use clearly describe and communicate involvement activity and accurately reflect the work taking place. Having a shared language would mean that we understand what others have done and are able to accurately express what we have done ourselves. Through honesty, clarity and the use of shared language we may better judge where service user/survivor involvement is simply a 'tick box exercise', and where there is a genuine commitment to changing the way research is carried out so that service users/survivors have a real impact on research[1].

THE LEVELS OF SERVICE USER/SURVIVOR INVOLVEMENT IN RESEARCH

Service user/survivor involvement in research is widely understood as being on a continuum, from low to high involvement. This extends from Arnstein's initial, and frequently cited, ladder of citizen participation, first described in the 1960s (Arnstein, 1969). Within UK-based mental health research, the most frequently employed continuum is that of INVOLVE (Hanley *et al.*, 2000, 2004). In it, Hanley and colleagues identified three levels of service user/ survivor involvement in research, *consultation*, *collaboration* and *control*. These were defined in the following ways (pp 8–10):

- **Consultation:** 'When you consult people who use services about research, you ask them for their views and use these views to inform your decision-making'. In consultations, power is firmly held by traditional researchers.
- **Collaboration:** defined as 'active, on-going partnership with members of the public in the R&D process'. Although collaborative research takes many forms, the defining feature is that power is *shared* between traditional researchers and service users/ survivors.
- **Control:** 'User-controlled research might be broadly interpreted as research where the locus of power, initiative and subsequent decision making is with service users rather than with the professional researchers'. Crucially then, in user-controlled research power is held by service users/survivors.

As these levels are on a continuum they do not have sharply defined boundaries. This has meant that it can be difficult to apply these definitions in the real world; a single project may contain more than one level of service user/survivor involvement at different stages or may not conform to any of these levels as they are widely understood. For example, Telford *et al.* (2002) attempted to classify service user/survivor involvement in research in a number of NHS Trusts in the UK in order to capture the range and diversity of involvement activity. However, they encountered difficulties in classifying involvement, and in particular in

---

[1] We acknowledge that there is much debate around the terms used within research to describe the people who take part. We have decided to use the term 'traditional researchers' to describe researchers, typically academics with a clinical background, who do not declare any experience of using mental health services. We have selected the term 'user researchers' to describe those researchers who have a declared experience of using or surviving mental health services and who actively draw on those experiences to inform their research.

determining a boundary between consultation and collaboration. This was largely because service users/survivors could be engaged using the same methods of involvement but for different purposes and therefore with very different impacts on the research process. For this reason Telford and colleagues concluded that more work is needed to define the levels of involvement.

We agree with Dixon *et al.* (1999) that further classification and refinement of models of consumer involvement is needed. Improved clarity of the definitions of levels and stages of involvement and some consistency in the use of terms is likely to help researchers, clinicians and consumers to identify appropriate methods of involvement.

Whilst the INVOLVE model has been found to be highly valuable in defining the levels of involvement in research, there is a growing tendency for traditional researchers to involve service users/survivors in more in-depth and profound ways than simply consultation, without necessarily sharing power through collaboration. An obvious example is where a research study employs a user researcher, or user interviewers, without giving them access to decision-making processes.

Because of these difficulties in accurately classifying real-world research and the subsequent need to define the levels of service user/survivor involvement in more depth, we would like to propose a fourth level to sit between consultation and collaboration: *contribution*. This would describe research where the team has moved beyond simply consulting with service users/survivors, asking their opinion and then choosing what they do with that information (if anything), to involving service users/survivors more actively *without* sharing decision-making power. This idea is, however, very much in its infancy and we hope that in the future, researchers will further develop and test its utility.

Consultation

During consultations service users/survivors are invited to comment on the research, but crucially, the power to act, or not, on those comments resides with traditional researchers. In practice this usually means that the research team invites comments through informal discussion groups, workshops, panels, interviews, visits to user groups or written feedback. This can be on any aspect of the research, but most commonly focuses on the research topic or data collection tools (such as questionnaires or outcome measures).

Because service users/survivors' comments are not necessarily acted upon, this has been seen as the lowest level of involvement. However, this does not mean that it has no value, or should be seen as the poor relation to user-controlled research. For example, Boote *et al.* (2002) describe organisations (citing the NHS Health Technology Assessment Programme) consulting service users/survivors about their priorities for research, thus giving them a genuine opportunity to influence the research agenda. Furthermore, INVOLVE describe consultations as an easy way for traditional researchers to begin to acclimatise themselves to new ways of working. However, Jordan *et al.* (1998, quoted in Telford *et al.*, 2002) have warned of one-off consultations. For consultations to be meaningful and of high quality, service users/survivors should be adequately informed, prepared and provided with opportunities for deliberation and discussion.

For an in-depth consideration of service user consultation in research and its practical implications see also Chapter 11.

Contribution

We propose 'contribution' as a useful concept for the level of service user/survivor involvement that sits between consultation and collaboration. We define this as research where service users/survivors make a significant and meaningful contribution to research but with power and decision-making still residing with traditional researchers. The most obvious example of contribution is where a service user/survivor is employed as part of a larger research team. This could be as a user researcher, user interviewer or data analyst. The key is that the employed service user/survivor is able to draw on their experiences of using/ surviving mental health services to inform the work. However, as for most research assistants, interviewers or analysts, access to and influence over wider decision-making is limited.

Central to the concept of contribution then, is the fact that service users/survivors do not have opportunities to influence the broader research study that they are involved in. Through openly acknowledging this lack of power our aim is not to devalue the contribution that service users/survivors make. Instead the value of user researchers on wider teams is beginning to be recognised and the employment of service users/survivors in research roles represents an important step forward for service user/survivor involvement in research. A significant advantage of contribution is that there is a commitment to involvement, even though it is contained. This contrasts with consultations where there is a choice whether to accept or reject the advice of service users/survivors. Furthermore, we argue that the introduction of the concept 'contribution' is necessary to accurately describe an existing level of involvement which is currently subsumed under collaboration.

Further details and examples for contribution as a form of service user involvement can be found in Chapter 10.

Collaboration

The crucial, defining feature of collaborative research is that power is genuinely shared between service users/survivors and traditional researchers, with decisions taken jointly. However, the specific ways in which power is shared vary widely and this means that there is no single model of collaborative research. Even within a single project, power may be shared collaboratively at some stages but not others (see next section p31). For these reasons it is important to be clear about where power has been shared, where it has been held by service users/survivors and where it has been retained by traditional researchers. The key is transparency in order that the research is not making claims that do not hold.

Rose has begun to classify the types of collaborative research that she has experienced whilst at the Service User Research Enterprise at the Institute of Psychiatry, England (Rose, 2003). To date she has identified the following models: where user researchers influence or generate outcome measures in trials; where service user/survivor research teams conduct a user-led component of a larger project; and finally, where the empirical part of a project is conducted by service users/survivors. However, as data collection and analysis does not necessarily imply shared decision-making, this latter model may at times be classified as 'contribution'. Undoubtedly other models of collaborative research will be identified, and the boundaries between the levels of involvement will be further explored as service user/survivor involvement in research evolves.

As the ultimate aim of collaborative research is to share decision-making power, it is perhaps the hardest form of service user/survivor involvement to successfully achieve. Turner and Beresford (2005) have found that service users/survivors are wary of collaborative research, feeling that it is difficult to move from an inherent power imbalance to genuine partnership working and shared decision-making. This is echoed in the writings of Trivedi and Wykes (2002) who state that little has been written on:

> *[the] philosophical, conceptual and practical challenges which may arise for clinical researchers when they seek to involve users in research, especially in the field of mental health where the massive imbalance of power that exists in services between professionals and users may make working together in research particularly challenging.*
>
> (p468)

Clearly, sharing power is not easy. However, as it is the defining feature of collaboration, it is vital that collaborators honestly appraise the extent to which joint decision-making was achieved at each stage of the research.

A detailed description and practical examples for collaborative research are also provided in Chapter 12.

Control

User-controlled research, also referred to as user research, survivor research or user-led research, refers to research where service users/survivors have absolute control over the process. This means:

> *service users controlling all stages of the research process; design, recruitment, ethics, data collection, data analysis, writing up and dissemination*
>
> (Rose, 2003, p404)

Although user-controlled research can be seen as being at the furthest end of the involvement continuum, it is in fact a unique form of research with its own distinct traditions and history. In the UK, Beresford (2002) has described how different approaches to providing welfare have generated different approaches to research. He describes user-controlled research as being rooted in a democratic model that values citizenship, inclusion, autonomy and collective agendas. This has led to research that values experiences and aims to empower service users/survivors at individual and collective levels (Wallcraft, 2003). By contrast the 'consumerist model', more strongly allied with consultation, collaboration and contribution, emphasises notions of choice, information and accessibility. Research within this model tends to be conducted by traditional researchers who may involve service users/survivors as a way of increasing the relevance of research to consumers.

In practice, this means that a single research project will not contain consultation at one stage and control at another. Instead, service user/survivor control will occur from the planning of the research project to the dissemination of findings. This differs from consultation, contribution and collaboration which may occur at different stages of a single research study.

User controlled research and its practical implications are also discussed in-depth in Chapter 13.

THE STAGES OF SERVICE USER/SURVIVOR INVOLVEMENT IN RESEARCH

Different levels of service user/survivor involvement in research may be achieved at different stages of the research process. Even within a single project, consultation may occur in the early stages, for example, with collaboration occurring later. The following table (Table 3.1) explores some of the more common ways that service user/survivor involvement in research occurs at each stage of the research process. Note that this table is not exhaustive and service user/survivor involvement in research will vary greatly. Instead, the aim of the table is to illustrate the main stages of the research process and how the levels are more commonly applied. It is hoped that this will help researchers move beyond, for example, a single line on a research funding application form claiming 'collaborative research', to achieving a more sophisticated and honest reporting of how service user/survivor involvement has been or will be achieved at various stages.

To this end, the table contains a column describing the absence of service user/survivor involvement in the research process. This column clarifies some of the more common misunderstandings regarding involvement by demonstrating what service user/survivor involvement is *not*. So, for example, a clinical academic initiating research in an area that patients have raised in clinical practice is not involving service users/survivors in research. Likewise, including a user component in a broader research project that focuses on users' experiences is not involvement, unless service users/survivors are actively involved in the research process. By including these examples we hope to add to the body of work that breaks down the misunderstandings around involvement in research.

It is common for service users/survivors to be more heavily involved in a specific arm of a research project. For example, one component may explore service users/survivors' experiences, nested within a larger, traditional research project. How is this best classified? There is no single answer and the classification of a user component will be largely dependent on the nature of the studies and how they inter-relate. The following questions (in line with the table below) may help in assessing the level of involvement:

- Was the research topic/question identified by service users/survivors?
- Was the design of the user component generated by service users/survivors?
- Were outcome measures generated or modified by service users/survivors?
- Who collected, analysed and interpreted the data?
- Was the write-up separate, marginalised or embedded in the main findings?
- Who had editorial control?
- How was the research disseminated, and was a service user/survivor audience considered?

Depending on the answers to these questions, the component may be considered user-controlled (where service users/survivors hold power from design and identification through to dissemination) or may variously achieve the levels of consultation, contribution and collaboration at different stages. The fact that there is no catch-all classification for all studies with a user component demonstrates the need for a clear and shared language enabling transparent and honest reporting.

Table 3.1 Examples of levels and stages of service user/survivor involvement in research

Stages of research process	No involvement	Consultation	Contribution	Collaboration	Control
Identifying research topics	Research topic identified by traditional researchers/research funders. This may reflect issues that users have raised with clinicians in practice.	Users asked their views of (typically pre-identified) research topics. Traditional researchers decide whether to adopt ideas.	An employed user may work with other users to identify research topics. Traditional researchers take final decisions.	Users and traditional researchers jointly identify a topic for research.	Ideally the research topic is generated entirely by users. Alternatively, users may tender for research that reflects users' priorities.
Designing research	Study designed by traditional researchers. This may include a focus on users' experiences.	Users asked for their views on existing or proposed study design. Traditional researchers have the final say.	Users may contribute to a specific part of the study design. Traditional researchers take the final decisions.	Users and traditional researchers jointly design the study.	Users design the entire research study. Traditional researchers might be consulted for technical advice.
Outcome measures	Traditional researchers select outcomes they believe it is important to measure. These might not reflect the outcomes users' prioritise.	Users' views of outcome measures sought e.g. their importance. Traditional researchers take final decisions.	A user may be tasked with generating an outcome measure that reflects users' concerns.	Users and traditional researchers jointly identify, select and modify outcome measures.	Users select all outcome measures, potentially generating user focussed outcome measures where needed.
Data collection	Users are research participants with no influence over how data is collected.	Users' views of data collection plans sought. Traditional researchers take final decisions.	A user may be employed to collect data. This is a common form of 'contribution'.	Users and traditional researchers jointly decide data collection strategy/ collect data.	Users develop data collection strategy and collect all data. Occasionally users may commission others to collect data.

Data analysis and interpretation	Traditional researchers analyse and interpret data. Interpretations may be checked with research participants (validation).	Users asked their opinion of analysis and interpretation strategies. Traditional researchers have the final say.	Users may be employed to analyse and interpret data.	Users and traditional researchers jointly engage in data analysis and interpretation, each bringing their unique perspectives.	Users analyse and interpret data. They may consult traditional researchers for technical advice.
Write-up	Traditional researchers write up the research results and retain editorial control (although constraints may be set by funders/ commissioners).	Users consulted on (near) final draft e.g. its accessibility. Traditional researchers decide whether to make changes.	Users may contribute to write-up but traditional researchers retain editorial control.	Users and traditional researchers jointly undertake writing and share editorial control.	Users undertake write-up and ideally have full editorial control. However, constraints may be set by funders/ commissioners.
Dissemination	Traditional researchers plan dissemination strategy. This may include dissemination to user audiences.	Users consulted on dissemination strategy, often how to reach a user audience. Traditional researchers make final decisions.	Users may have a key role in disseminating research findings to other users.	Users and traditional researchers jointly plan dissemination strategy.	Users plan dissemination strategy, typically seeking to reach a wide user audience in a variety of innovative ways.

Whilst the table provides a useful overview of what service user/survivor involvement can look like throughout the research process, it also raises some important points. The first is that there is a clear difference between a research area and the specific research question that determines a study. This means that research may occur in an area that ostensibly reflects service users/survivors' priorities (such as self-help) whilst the specific research question remains rooted in mainstream perspectives (such as defining self-help as computer-aided therapist interventions rather than empowerment and recovery). Once again, to ensure clarity and consistency it is important that this distinction is noted when researchers describe the involvement within a study.

Secondly, whilst it is possible for service users/survivors to make a contribution to the design of a project, with ultimate decision-making laying with traditional researchers, it is more common in practice for a user researcher to be recruited once major design decisions have been made.

Thirdly, we have classified a service user/survivor employed to collect data as making a contribution. This is because in this scenario, the employee is recruited to perform a specific task and decisions regarding who will participate and how data are collected are likely to remain with employers.

Finally, even within user-controlled research there may be some limitations placed on the amount of control that service users/survivors have. Whilst this is the same as for all researchers (for example, receiving funding on a pre-determined topic or having final editorial control rest with host organisation or research funder), this is of greater concern for user-controlled research because external bodies are likely to represent traditional and mainstream approaches, excluding a service user/survivor perspective. However, it is our belief that this does not mean that the user-controlled research that operates within these constraints needs to be reclassified, simply that these constraints should be acknowledged.

CONCLUSION

In this chapter we have provided a basic description of the levels and stages of service user/survivor involvement in research. We described how confusion surrounding the terminology used to describe involvement has led to difficulties in applying the most commonly used terms, *consultation*, *collaboration* and *control*. The boundary between consultation and collaboration is particularly hazy. Furthermore, these three categories of involvement do not reflect all that is now happening in research, in particular the growing tendency to employ service users/survivors as researchers or interviewers. In practice, this means that 'collaboration' is used as an umbrella term for all the involvement falling between consultation and control. We therefore proposed a fourth level of involvement to sit between consultation and collaboration, that of *contribution*.

Contribution describes research where service users/survivors have significant and concrete input, for example as user interviewers or researchers, but have no access to major decisions about the research. We hope that through identifying a fourth level of involvement, researchers will be able to use the term collaboration more accurately by applying it only to research where power has genuinely been shared between service users/survivors and traditional researchers.

In the second section of this chapter we described how different levels of involvement can occur at different stages of a research project. We also described some common areas of controversy, disagreement and confusion surrounding the levels of involvement at different stages of a research project, including some of the more widespread misunderstandings about what is and is not service user/survivor involvement. In doing so we hope to have contributed to the literature that encourages and defines a shared language amongst all those connected with research. This is important because, as Townend and Braithwaite (2002) have commented

> *we must move away from the tendency to consider we have 'done' user involvement in research when users have solely been used as interviewees or participants in controlled trials.*
>
> (p118)

There is also an ethical motivation to be clear about the level of involvement. Working with integrity with service users/survivors means a commitment to honesty about the extent of power sharing. This honesty would enable service users/survivors to choose whether to get involved in research, and would also enable funders to know exactly what they are funding. Of course, there will be times when involvement is limited including through funding, capacity or time restrictions. The key is that researchers are clear and honest about what could and could not be achieved. Only then will we be in a position to understand and evaluate the impact of service user/survivor involvement on research.

REFERENCES

Arnstein, S.R. (1969) A ladder of citizen participation, *Journal of the American Institute of Planners*, **35**(4), 216–224.

Beresford, P. and Evans, C. (1999) Research Note: Research and empowerment, *British Journal of Social Work*, **29**(5), 671–677.

Beresford, P. (2002) User involvement in research and evaluation: liberation or regulation? *Social Policy and Society*, **1**(2), 95–105.

Boote, J., Telford, R. and Cooper, C. (2002) Consumer involvement in health research: a review and research agenda, *Health Policy*, **61**, 213–236.

Dixon, P., Peart, E. and Carr-Hill, R. (1999) A database of examples of consumer involvement in research, Centre for Health Economics, York.

Hanley, B. *et al.* (2000, 2004) *Involving the Public in NHS Public Health and Social Care Research: Briefing Notes for Researchers*, London: INVOLVE Support Unit, First and Second Editions.

Jordan, J., Dowswell, T., Harrison, S., Lilford, R. and Mort, M. (1998) Whose priorities? Listening to users and the public, *British Medical Journal*, **316**, 1668–1670.

Rose, D. (2003) Collaborative research between users and professionals: peaks and pitfalls. *Psychiatric Bulletin*, **27**, 404–406.

Telford, R., Beverley, C.A., Cooper, C.L. and Boote, J.D. (2002) Consumer involvement in health research: fact or fiction? *British Journal of Clinical Governance*, **7**(2), 92–103.

Townend, M. and Braithwaite, T. (2002) Mental health research – the value of user involvement, *Journal of Mental Health*, **11**(2), 117–119.

Trivedi, P. and Wykes, T. (2002) From Passive Subjects to Equal Partners: qualitative review of user involvement in research, *British Journal of Psychiatry*, **181**, 468–472.

Turner, M. and Beresford, P. (2005) *User Controlled Research: Its meaning and potential*, London: INVOLVE.

Wallcraft, J. (2003) Service User Led Research: Towards a model of empowerment, Mental Health Foundation on-line conference.

CHAPTER 4

Values

Values-Based Practice and Service User Involvement in Mental Health Research

Bill (KWM) Fulford
St Cross College, Oxford, and University of Warwick Medical School, Coventry, UK
Jan Wallcraft
Service user Researcher and Consultant, London, UK

This chapter introduces a new skills-based approach to working with complex and conflicting values, called values-based practice, and outlines its potential contribution to supporting service user involvement in research. The chapter is in three parts: Part I introduces values and values-based practice; Part II gives a more detailed account of values-based practice and illustrates each of its ten main elements (partly by reference to other chapters of this Handbook); and Part III shows how values-based practice fits together respectively with ethics and with evidence-based practice, drawing on practical examples from current developments in the field. In a brief concluding section the chapter indicates, from the perspective of values-based practice, the importance of service user involvement in research in mental health for the future development of research in healthcare as a whole.

INTRODUCTION

It is widely assumed that research, whether in healthcare or in any other area, should be or should aim to be value-free. The American philosopher of science, Carl Hempel, for example, gave a lecture in the late 1950s that was to prove highly influential on the development of modern classifications of mental disorder (Fulford and Sartorius, forthcoming), in which he equated values with bias in research. He argued that many psychiatric diagnostic terms such as '. . .inadequacy of response, inadaptability, ineptness, and poor judgment clearly have *valuational* aspects. . .' and hence that '. . .their use in concrete cases will be influenced by the idiosyncrasies of the investigator' (Hempel, 1961, p322 in 1994 reprint, emphasis added).

Handbook of Service User Involvement in Mental Health Research Edited by Jan Wallcraft, Beate Schrank and Michaela Amering
Copyright © 2009 John Wiley & Sons, Ltd

Hempel's words will ring true to many, particularly those in medical research. Yet Hempel was perhaps the last great philosopher to advocate a positivist model of science of this value-excluding kind[1]. The positivists emphasised the importance of science being based on observation – and careful observation is indeed fundamental to science. But much work in the philosophy and sociology of science in the second half of the 20th Century has shown the extent to which, as an essentially *human* activity, scientific research, as well as being based on observation, is embedded in human wishes, needs, drives, motivations, in a word, 'values'. A glance through this Handbook will show directly the extent to which research, in all its many aspects, is indeed a deeply value-laden human activity. The chapter titles themselves speak to the importance of values – 'principles and motives', 'roles', 'purpose and goals', 'consultation' and 'collaboration', 'control', 'power' and 'politics'.

PART I: VALUES AND VALUES-BASED PRACTICE

The term 'values' is used in many different ways and 'values-based practice', correspondingly, could mean different things to different people. In this first Part, therefore, we introduce both concepts before looking at values-based practice in more detail in Part II.

What are values?

The first point to make is that values are wider than ethics. Ethical values are nowadays the most widely discussed values in healthcare. But there are values of many other kinds, such as aesthetic and prudential, for example; and values extend to needs, wishes, preferences, indeed to any and all of the many different ways in which we express negative or positive evaluations and value judgments. There is also a considerable diversity in the values held by different individuals, by different cultures, and at different historical periods. As Sackett *et al.* (2000), put it, in their training manual on evidence-based medicine,

> By patient values we mean the unique *preferences, concerns and expectations each patient brings to a clinical encounter and which must be integrated into clinical decisions if they are to serve the patient.*

(p1, emphasis added).

The way in which the term 'values' means different things to different people, is illustrated by Table 4.1. This shows the responses of a small training group when asked to write down three words or short phrases that they associated with 'values'. As Table 4.1 shows, every member of the group came up with a different set of associations. Some values are shared, however: the values of autonomy (freedom of choice) and of acting in a person's best interests, for example, are widely shared values, as Table 4.1 also illustrates. We return to the importance of these shared values in Part III. For the moment, though, it is the diversity of individual values that is the starting point for values-based practice.

An outline of values-based practice

Values-based practice is a new approach to balanced decision-making where complex and conflicting values are involved (Fulford, 2004). It is based on work in analytic philosophy

---

[1] Hempel's variant of positivism was called Logical Empiricism.

Table 4.1   What are values?

Faith	How we treat people
Internalisation	Attitudes
Acting in best interests	Principles
	Autonomy
Integrity	Love
Conscience	Relationships
Best interests	
Autonomy	
Respect	Non-violence
Personal to me	Compassion
Difference … diversity	Dialogue
Beliefs	Responsibility
Right/wrong to me	Accountability
What I am	Best interests
Belief	What I *believe*
Principles	What makes me tick
Things held dear	What I won't compromise
Subjective merits	'Objective' core
Meanings	Confidentiality
Person-centred care	Autonomy
A *standard* for the way I conduct *myself*	Significant
Belief about how things *should* be	Standards
Things you would not want to change	Truth

(Hare, 1952) as applied to concepts of disorder (Fulford, 1989), and combines analytic with empirical social science research (Colombo *et al.*, 2003). Values-based practice thus represents a strong 'philosophy into practice' development within the wider field of the philosophy of psychiatry (Fulford *et al.*, 2003). As described further below, there have also been important developments internationally (Mezzich, 2007; Van Staden and Fulford, 2007), particularly through the World Psychiatric Association's Institutional Program on Psychiatry for the Person (IPPP) (Mezzich and Salloum, 2007).

Values-based practice is of course only one among a number of new resources from different disciplines that can support more effective ways of working with values in medicine: these include, for example, decision theory (Hunink *et al.*, 2001) and health economics (Brown *et al.*, 2005). The distinctive contribution of values-based practice, however, is that rather than seeking to prescribe 'right values', it starts from *respect for differences of values* and relies on 'good process' for balanced decision-making where values conflict. To put it another way, values-based practice, focuses not on *what* is done but on *how* it is done. Values-based practice is in this respect similar to evidence-based practice: where evidence-based practice offers a *process* for working more effectively with complex and conflicting *evidence*, values-based practice offers a (different although complementary) *process* for working more effectively with complex and conflicting *values*.

The ten key elements that make up the 'good process' of values-based practice are summarised as ten pointers in the arrow diagram in Table 4.2. We will be referring to this diagram, which is taken from the first training manual in values-based practice,

Table 4.2 Ten key pointers to values-based practice

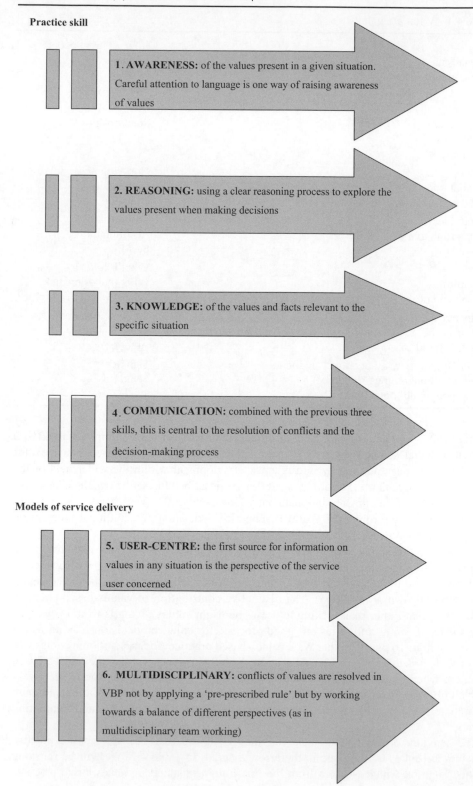

Practice skill

1. AWARENESS: of the values present in a given situation. Careful attention to language is one way of raising awareness of values

2. REASONING: using a clear reasoning process to explore the values present when making decisions

3. KNOWLEDGE: of the values and facts relevant to the specific situation

4. COMMUNICATION: combined with the previous three skills, this is central to the resolution of conflicts and the decision-making process

Models of service delivery

5. USER-CENTRE: the first source for information on values in any situation is the perspective of the service user concerned

6. MULTIDISCIPLINARY: conflicts of values are resolved in VBP not by applying a 'pre-prescribed rule' but by working towards a balance of different perspectives (as in multidisciplinary team working)

Table 4.2   (*Continued*)

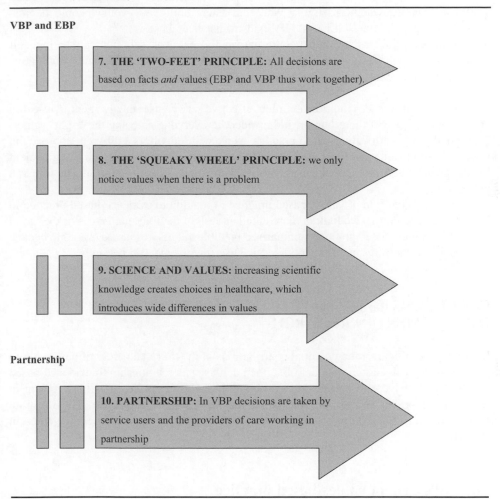

VBP and EBP

7. **THE 'TWO-FEET' PRINCIPLE:** All decisions are based on facts *and* values (EBP and VBP thus work together).

8. **THE 'SQUEAKY WHEEL' PRINCIPLE:** we only notice values when there is a problem

9. **SCIENCE AND VALUES:** increasing scientific knowledge creates choices in healthcare, which introduces wide differences in values

Partnership

10. **PARTNERSHIP:** In VBP decisions are taken by service users and the providers of care working in partnership

Whose Values? (see below, Woodbridge and Fulford, 2004), throughout the chapter. As the diagram shows, at the heart of values-based practice are four key areas of clinical skills (pointers 1–4). Also important, however, are two aspects of service delivery, that services should be user-centred and multidisciplinary (pointers 5 and 6), close links between values-based practice and evidence-based practice (pointers 7–9), and, perhaps most important of all, partnership in decision-making between service users and service providers (pointer 10).

The importance of a values-based approach for effective involvement of service users in research is clear throughout this book. Values, as noted in the last section, are everywhere! But what is also evident is that it is *differences* of values that are crucial to many of the themes raised by the Handbook. To take just one example, on the topics chosen for research, Del Vecchio and Blyler (Chapter 8) note the wide differences between the topics that researchers tend to prioritise and those that are prioritised by service users:

- Researchers' priorities across the world include: epidemiology, cost effectiveness and efficaciousness, awareness, stigma. War + disasters, children + young people, depression, epilepsy, suicide/self harm, HIV/Aids, substance abuse.
- Consumers' priorities are: holistic alternatives to treatment, safe houses, healing, self help, damaging effects of treatment, involuntary treatment, cultural issues, qualitative methods, community surveys, consumer needs/preferences.

Given such differences in priorities, then, effective service user involvement in research could not even get off the ground if it depended on everyone agreeing the 'right' values. The 'good process' of values-based practice, as we will see, offers a different approach in which different value priorities are converted from a source of conflict and disagreement into a positive resource for balanced decision-making at every stage in the research process.

We return to the role of values-based practice in relation to evidence-based practice in Part III. First, in Part II, we look in more detail at each of the four main areas of the 'good process' of values-based practice summarised in Table 4.2, the resources available in each area, and how these resources support service user involvement in research.

PART II: VALUES-BASED PRACTICE AND SERVICE USER INVOLVEMENT IN RESEARCH

In this Part we illustrate the potential contributions of the four main areas of values-based practice – its skills base, its model of service delivery, its relationship to evidence-based practice, and its basis in partnership – to building effective service user involvement in research. In practice, all four areas have to work together. But we will illustrate them separately and return to examples of how they have been brought together in Part III.

The skills base of values-based practice

Table 4.3, which is based on the first training manual for values-based practice, '*Whose Values?*' (Woodbridge and Fulford, 2004; see below), gives further details of the four skills areas that are at the heart of this approach (pointers 1–4 in Table 4.2, above).

As Table 4.3 shows, raising awareness of values and of the often surprising extent to which our values differ, is the first and perhaps the most important training step in value-based practice. A word association exercise, like the one from which Table 4.1 is derived, is one way of doing this. Other exercises described in '*Whose Values?*' (Woodbridge and Fulford, 2004) include thinking through real decisions we have taken, or looking at the words used in actual documents, such as ward policies or referral letters.

Given the extent of the values issues raised by this Handbook, it may seem that raising awareness is unnecessary. However, as Alison Faulkner (Chapter 2) points out, it is easy for researchers to overlook what may be important from a service user's perspective when they are driven by deadlines, and, conversely, service users may not always have 'space' to think through the implications of becoming involved in research.

Table 4.3   The four skills areas for values-based practice

Skills area	Applications in values-based practice
1. Raising awareness of values	Values, our own and those of others, are often implicit. The first step in values-based practice is thus to raise awareness: 1) of values 2) of differences of values.
2. Reasoning about values	In ethics and law, different methods of reasoning are used to try to decide what ought to be done. These include principles, casuistry (case-based reasoning), utilitarianism (balancing utilities, used especially in health economics), deontology (rule-based reasoning, used especially in law). In values-based practice, the same range of methods is used but primarily to *explore and open up the range of values* bearing on a given situation.
3. Knowledge of values	Values-based practice draws on evidence about values using: 1) empirical methods (including service user narratives) 2) philosophical methods 3) combined methods.
4. Communication skills	Communication skills are central to: 1) understanding individual values 2) resolving conflicts of values, for example by negotiation and conflict resolution.

Experience in other areas of values-based practice suggests that raising awareness of values is always important even where it may seem unnecessary. This is illustrated by Figure 4.1 which is taken from an exercise that one of the authors of '*Whose Values*?', Kim Woodbridge, did with an assertive outreach multidisciplinary team. The team already had a strong ethos of service user-centred care and they had asked for training in values-based practice to support their approach. As a first step, they agreed to the perspectives expressed in one of their Care Programme Review meetings being recorded. Figure 4.1 shows the

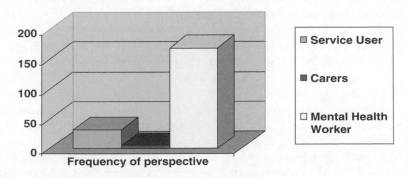

Figure 4.1   Perspectives referred to in a Care Programme Review meeting.

results. As you will see, despite the strong service user-centred ethos of the team, their perspectives as mental health workers dominated the meeting, there being only occasional references to the perspectives of the service users concerned and almost no references to the perspectives of carers. The team were understandably very surprised by this result. But it raised their awareness of how strongly their own values were influencing their work despite their commitment to a service user-centred approach, and this formed the basis for the rest of their training in values-based practice.

Raising awareness, however, although important, is only the first step in training in values-based practice. As Table 4.3 indicates, reasoning about values, knowledge of values, and particular aspects of communication skills, also have key roles to play.

- *Reasoning* – the reasoning skills for values-based practice draw on all those used in ethics (such as principles reasoning, casuistry, utilitarianism and deontology) but with a distinctive twist – values-based reasoning is employed not to support a particular ethical position but *to explore the range* of often very different values that may be present in a given situation (Fulford *et al.*, 2002). We return to the relationship between ethics and values-based practice in Part III.
- *Knowledge* – evidence-based approaches, 'listening to the evidence' rather than relying on intuition alone, are just as important to finding out about values as in more obvious areas of evidence-based practice such as the effectiveness of different treatment options. We return to the links between values-based and evidence-based practice in Part III. For now, it is important to be aware of the wide range of well-developed methods available: in addition to empirical approaches, such as surveys (Rogers *et al.*, 1993), these include personal narratives of patients and family carers, a number of powerful philosophical methods – phenomenology (Stanghellini, 2004), hermeneutics (Widdershoven and Widdershoven-Heerding, 2003) and discursive philosophy (Sabat, 2001) – and combined philosophical and empirical methods (Colombo *et al.*, 2003).
- *Communication skills* – communication skills are central to values-based practice, in particular as applied to individual cases (Hope *et al.*, 1996), and are clearly central to effective service user involvement in research at all levels, from consultation (as Virginia Minogue shows, Chapter 11), through collaboration (Diane Rose, Chapter 12), to effective resolution of such contentious issues as payment (Sarah Hamilton, Chapter 15). In these and other areas, methods and resources from management theory may be particularly helpful both for exploring differences of values and for resolving conflicts between values (Fulford and Benington, 2004).

Resources for training in values-based practice include the first training manual, 'Whose Values?' (Woodbridge and Fulford, 2004), developed and piloted with front-line mental health and social care staff, and launched by the Minister of State in the Department of Health, Rosie Winterton, at a conference in London in 2005. 'Whose Values?' has subsequently been used successfully in a wide variety of clinical contexts and particular sections of it have also been published as a CD-Rom (Woodbridge and Fulford, 2005).

'Whose Values?' has subsequently become the basis for the 10 Essential Shared Capabilities (the 10 ESCs), a national training programme in England in the generic skills for mental health and social care, which brings together evidence-based with values-based resources (Department of Health, 2004). The 10 ESCs support a number of other key policies, in particular as these involve multidisciplinary and user-centred care (Department of Health, 2005). Internationally, there have been key developments in a number of countries, including Sweden, France, Belgium, Spain, Brazil and South Africa, and through the World Psychiatric Association (Fulford *et al.*, 2004).

The policy framework for values-based practice

However well developed the skills of service users and service providers in working with values, they will have little effect unless they are able to work within an appropriate service delivery model supported by a strong policy framework.

Recognising this, a National Framework (see Table 4.4) setting out a number of key principles of values-based practice has been developed by the National Institute for Mental Health in England (NIMHE, 2004). NIMHE is responsible to the UK government's Department of Health for implementing policy in mental health. As such, the NIMHE Values Framework has in turn supported a number of policy and service development initiatives in such areas as recovery practice, black and minority ethnic services, audit, commissioning, and the development of mental health law in relation to involuntary treatment and capacity (Fulford *et al.*, 2004). As Table 4.4 indicates, person-centred and multidisciplinary working are both essential to values-based practice (Pointers 5 and 6, in Table 4.2). Correspondingly, the NIMHE Framework has also been the basis for a series of specific policy and service development initiatives concerned with improving multidisciplinary and multi-agency teamwork as the basis of more effective patient-centred care (see e.g. Department of Health, 2004a, and 2004b; and NIMHE, 2008).

The NIMHE Values Framework (which explicitly acknowledges the importance of research), and related policy initiatives, thus provide a strong basis for balancing up the power inequalities that, as several contributors to this Handbook make clear, are among the most important barriers to effective partnership between service users and service providers. Specifically in relation to research, such inequalities crucially distort the processes by which the very topics of research are decided (Chapter 8, Paolo del Vecchio and Crystal Blyler); and they are also important at every other stage in the research process, including the development of research instruments (such as questionnaires), the way in which findings are interpreted, and, not least, the effectiveness with which the results of research are applied in practice. At every stage of the research process, then, the NIMHE Framework, by empowering service users, offers a basis for a more equal relationship with researchers, one result of which, as Davidson (Chapter 7) so clearly argues, will be better quality research.

Values-based practice and evidence-based practice

Pointers 7–9 in Table 4.2 spell out the importance of the relationship between values-based and evidence-based approaches. As Pointer 7 indicates, everything we do is based on values as well as evidence, and as several contributions to this Handbook show, this is true not least in research: Paolo del Vecchio and Crystal Blyler (Chapter 8), in particular, illustrate the extent to which differences of values between traditional researchers and researchers with service user experience, ultimately impact on practice in such areas as recovery. Similarly, in her chapter on methods, Jean Campbell (Chapter 9) gives a detailed account of the significance of the service user 'voice'. Yet, despite the best efforts of many of those leading the movement in evidence-based care (see the quote from David Sackett *et al.*, 2000), evidence-based practice, from the framing of research through to the development of guidelines, is carried out to all intents and purposes in a values vacuum.

Table 4.4   The NIMHE National Framework for values-based practice

The NIMHE Values Framework

The National Framework of Values for Mental Health
The work of the National Institute for Mental Health in England (NIMHE) on values in mental health care is guided by three principles of values-based practice:

1) Recognition – NIMHE recognises the role of values alongside evidence in all areas of mental health policy and practice.
2) Raising awareness – NIMHE is committed to raising awareness of the values involved in different contexts, the role/s they play and their impact on practice in mental health.
3) Respect – NIMHE respects diversity of values and will support ways of working with such diversity that makes the principle of service user centrality a unifying focus for practice. This means that the values of each individual service user/client and their communities must be the starting point and key determinant for all actions by professionals.

Respect for diversity of values encompasses a number of specific policies and principles concerned with equality of citizenship. In particular, it is anti-discriminatory because discrimination in all its forms is intolerant of diversity. Thus respect for diversity of values has the consequence that it is unacceptable (and unlawful in some instances) to discriminate on grounds such as gender, sexual orientation, class, age, abilities, religion, race, culture or language. Respect for diversity within mental health is also:

- user-centred – it puts respect for the values of individual users at the centre of policy and practice;
- recovery oriented – it recognises that building on the personal strengths and resiliencies of individual users, and on their cultural and racial characteristics, there are many diverse routes to recovery;
- multidisciplinary – it requires that respect be reciprocal, at a personal level (between service users, their family members, friends, communities and providers), between different provider disciplines (such as nursing, psychology, psychiatry, medicine, social work), and between different organisations (including health, social care, local authority housing, voluntary organisations, community groups, faith communities and other social support services);
- dynamic – it is open and responsive to change;
- reflective – it combines self monitoring and self management with positive self regard;
- balanced – it emphasises positive as well as negative values;
- relational – it puts positive working relationships supported by good communication skills at the heart of practice.

NIMHE will encourage educational and research initiatives aimed at developing the capabilities (the awareness, attitudes, knowledge and skills) needed to deliver mental health services that will give effect to the principles of values-based practice.

One reason for the 'values vacuum' of research is that the paradigms available for doing research on values are relatively undeveloped (even literature search methods are at only an early stage of development, see Petrova *et al.*, 2006). Yet there are a number of powerful methodologies available. Values-based practice itself is underpinned by a branch of analytic philosophy, called philosophical value theory (see for example, Hare, 1952; and Fulford, 1989) that, as an analytic discipline, is a natural partner both of empirical research, as in the example described immediately below, and of other philosophical disciplines such as phenomenology (Stanghellini, 2004) and of the philosophies of science and of mind (Thornton 2006; 2007). As the American psychiatrist and neuroscientist, Nancy Andreasen (2001) has argued, these and other philosophical disciplines, have a growing practical importance not only in mental health and social care, but in the new neurosciences.

An example of a combined philosophical and empirical approach to eliciting implicit values (i.e. the values actually driving actions, as opposed to the values people claim), is a study by the social scientist, Anthony Colombo, of the models of mental disorder of different team members and of service users and carers, involved in the community care of people with a diagnosis of long-term schizophrenia (Colombo *et al.*, 2003). It will be worth looking at this study in some detail because it shows the importance of service user involvement in the design of research as well as in its implementation. Thus, Peter Campbell, a prominent service user and survivor in the UK, made key contributions to the details of the questionnaire used in the research as well as to other aspects of the methodology. In addition, service users and carers were included throughout on an equal basis with service providers, for example being recruited through their representative organisations rather than through healthcare services (Fulford and Colombo, 2004).

This 'level playing field' approach, consistently with Davidson's claim in this Handbook (Chapter 7) that full service user involvement leads to better quality research, led to some unexpected but important results. These are illustrated by the two part Figure 4.2. This Figure looks complicated but it is just the overall similarities between the two tables in the two parts of the Figures that we want to concentrate on. What these show is that the pattern of responses in this study from service providers (Part 1 of the figure) is very similar to the pattern for service users (Part 2 of the figure). Based on their respective *explicit* values, we had expected that the values of the two groups elicited in the study (i.e. their respective *implicit* values) would be very different. Yet as Figure 4.2 shows, the service users in the study formed two (overlapping) groups whose responses were broadly similar to the two (overlapping) groups of psychiatrists and social workers.

The methods developed in this study have subsequently been incorporated into the skills training resources of values-based practice (in '*Whose Values?*'; Woodbridge and Fulford, 2004). The study has also given a completely new significance to the importance of a broadly based multidisciplinary approach, representing different perspectives, in providing care that is genuinely person-centred. What it showed is that, in addition to a range of different *skills*, the different *perspectives* on a mental health problem of different team members are also important in matching the different perspectives of individual service users. This work has continued through a pilot study supported by the Mental Health Foundation in London (King *et al.*, forthcoming) that has been led by a researcher and ex-service user, Colin King, with extensive personal experience of the abusive consequences of a 'values blind' approach (King, 2007).

Values-based practice and partnership

Pointer 10 to good process in values-based practice (Table 4.2 above) reminds us of the importance of partnership. This goes to the heart of what values-based practice is all about – building alliances, not (solely) through shared values, important as these may be (see Part III), but (also) through an overarching principle of mutual respect that allows groups and individuals with *different* values to work together in an effective way.

The development of values-based practice is itself an example of the power of partnership in that it has been developed throughout by a University-based organisation (the Philosophy and Ethics of Mental Health programme at Warwick University) working in partnership with national and international organisations representing the three key stakeholder

	MODELS: Psychiatrists (P) and Social workers (S)					
ELEMENTS OF MODELS	A Medical (Organic)	B Social (Stress)	C Cognitive behavioural	D Psycho-therapeutic	E Family (Interaction)	F Conspiratorial
1 Diagnosis/description	P			S		
2 Interpretation of behaviour	P			S		
3 Labels	P			S		
4 Aetiology	P			S		
5 Treatment	P	S			S	
6 Function of the hospital	P S	P S				P
7 Hospital and community	P	S		S		
8 Prognosis	P			S		
9 Rights of the patient	P S	S				S
10 Rights of society	P S					
11 Duties of the patient	P		P S			
12 Duties of society	P	S				

Figure 4.2 (Part 1)   Models of disorder comparing psychiatrists (P) with social workers (S).

| ELEMENTS OF MODELS | MODELS: Two groups of service users – similar to Psychiatrists (UP) and similar to Social workers (US) | | | | | |
	A Medical (Organic)	B Social (Stress)	C Cognitive behavioural	D Psycho-therapeutic	E Family (Interaction)	F Conspiratorial
1 Diagnosis/description	UP			US		
2 Interpretation of behaviour			UP	UP US		
3 Labels	UP		US	US		
4 Aetiology	UP			US		
5 Treatment	UP	US		US		
6 Function of the hospital	UP US	UP				UP US
7 Hospital and community		UP US		UP US		
8 Prognosis	UP			US		
9 Rights of the patient	UP US	US				UP US
10 Rights of society		UP US				
11 Duties of the patient		UP US	UP US			
12 Duties of society	UP		UP US			UP US

Note: The two parts of this figure compare the models of disorder of two groups of service users (second Part, respectively 'UP' and 'US') with those of psychiatrists and social workers (first Part, respectively 'P' and 'S'). Comparing the two parts of the figure shows that the models of disorder of the two groups of service users ('UP' and 'US') are overall very similar to those respectively of psychiatrists ('P') and social workers ('S').

Figure 4.2 (Part 2)   Models of disorder comparing two groups of service users (UP and US).

groups of patients, professionals and policy makers. Partner organisations have included, in particular, major mental health NGOs such as The Sainsbury Centre for Mental Health and the Mental Health Foundation, the UK government's Department of Health, the World Psychiatric Association, and the Mental Health and Substance Abuse Section of the World Health Organization. In addition to the research described above, service users and carers have continued to make full contributions, as equal partners with clinicians and researchers, in the development of the new training and policy initiatives to be described in Part III.

Partnership, however, is not always easy, particularly where the issues of unequal power noted above are in play. It is for this reason, as Peter Beresford (Chapter 13) notes in this

Handbook, that there may be a need for research that not only involves service users and carers, even on an equal basis, but is actually led by them. Others (for example, Diana Rose, Chapter 12) suggest more collaborative models of service user involvement. In this respect, as Kim Hopper (Chapter 6) shows, there are well established methods for increasing the capacity of service users to play a full and equal role in research.

A values-based approach here would be that as far as possible, research should be based on collaboration. Given current power differentials, as graphically outlined by both Paddy McGowan (Chapter 14) and Dan Fisher (Chapter 16), however, there is a case for more user-controlled research, to balance up the extent to which research is currently dominated by other interests. As part of an overall research field, that is to say, having some projects user-controlled, may help to balance up power differentials and hence to provide better quality research overall.

Ultimately, partnership working in research should be the normal practice. The history of mental health, as the German historian and philosopher, Paul Hoff has pointed out, is of repeated collapses into single model mythologies (Hoff, 2005). The significance of this danger, moreover, is evident in the fact that the worst abuses of psychiatry have arisen, not through ill intent but through one set of values coming to dominate all others (Fulford *et al.*, 2003). It is to practical examples of partnership in the development of values-based approaches, therefore, that we turn in Part III.

PART III: VALUES-BASED PRACTICE IN ACTION

In this final part of the chapter we give two examples of values-based practice in action. In Part II we looked at a number of examples of the practical applications of some of the key elements of values-based practice used separately, respectively in regard to training, to policy and service development, to research, and to the overall theme of partnership. Here we describe how these elements have been brought together in two recent programmes of work for the UK government's Department of Health, one concerned with ethics, the other with evidence-based practice.

To anticipate a little, we should point out that neither of the programmes to be described is, as such, a research programme. Indeed, Anthony Colombo's work (2003, 2004, 2005, described above) aside, we believe the development of research paradigms that are fully values-based as well as evidence-based, is a task waiting to be done, and one in which, as we will indicate in our Conclusions, service user involvement in research has a key role to play. Whatever form such paradigms take, however, the relationships between values-based practice and both ethics and evidence-based practice will be crucial. Hence, the particular relevance of the examples to be described here.

Values-based practice and ethics

As noted earlier, where ethics is mainly outcome focused, values-based practice is process-focused. The approaches are complementary, however, both offering practical tools to support decision-making, and in this Part we look at how they fit together. The relationship between them can be summarised briefly as follows: the tools of ethics, being outcome-focused, are based on rules and regulations prescribing 'right outcomes' for different situations; the tools of values-based practice, on the other hand, being process-focused, support training and other resources described in Part II. In a word, ethics tells us 'what to do', values-based practice tells us 'how to do it'.

The need for both approaches, i.e. rather than relying on ethics alone, arises from the growing complexity of values and hence the tensions that arise between them. 'Autonomy' and 'best interests', for example, although both shared ethical values, are often in tension. In the past, people were often content to allow doctors to decide what is in their best interests and this is still the case in many so-called developing countries (Okasha, 2000). Increasingly, though, a growing emphasis on autonomy has led to complex interactions between autonomy and best interests. This is notably the case, for example, in relation to issues of compulsory treatment, as we describe further below. Then again, 'best interests' has highly complex applications, what is 'best' for one person often being very different from what is 'best' for another, according to differences in their personal values and the values of others concerned.

One response to such difficulties is to write ever more detailed rules and regulations and indeed the size and variety of ethical codes and guidelines has increased enormously in recent years. Relying solely on such codes and guidelines, however, may be counter-productive: it leads to defensive practice, for example, that may be a major barrier to full service user partnership in decision-making in clinical care (Fulford *et al.*, 2006) and, through similar processes in Research Ethics Committees, in research (Osborn, 1999).

This is where values-based practice may be helpful. The approach is based on the idea that, while codes provide a vital framework of *shared values* to guide practice, coming to balanced judgments where values *conflict*, and interpreting the applications of *complex* values, are matters, primarily, not for reference to a rule book but for good clinical skills operating within an appropriate service framework (Fulford, 2004). The theory underpinning this is derived from work in jurisprudence by a former professor of philosophy in Oxford, H. L. A. Hart (Hart, 1968). The approach has also been applied to Human Rights legislation by Lord Woolf, at the time Lord Chief Justice in the UK. As Lord Woolf put it, the Human Rights Act is not about rights as conventionally understood by lawyers (and by implication by ethicists); it is rather a framework of values within which balanced judgments have to be made according to the particular circumstances of each individual situation (Lord Woolf, 2002).

This 'framework of values' approach has been adopted in relation to recent legislation covering the use of compulsory treatment in the UK. There is of course a large literature on the ethical and legal issues around the use of compulsory treatment (see several chapters in Bloch *et al.*'s seminal *Psychiatric Ethics*, 1999), and it might be thought something of a paradox that compulsory treatment could be 'values-based'. However, as Roberts *et al.* (2008) have recently argued, compulsory treatment in psychiatry requires no less than any other area of mental health, a positive and recovery-oriented approach as the basis of good practice. Values-based practice, moreover, goes to the heart of what is so contentious about the use of compulsory treatment, namely that it involves a direct *conflict of values*: by definition, the person concerned wants one thing (not to be treated) while everyone else wants something else (i.e. that the person concerned accepts treatment).

The key to using values-based practice in this case, was a set of Guiding Principles that was developed to support the application of the new legislation in practice. The Guiding

Principles, which are given in full in Table 4.5, are set out in the Code of Practice to the legislation and hence have a strong degree of legal force. In terms of values-based practice, then, the Guiding Principles represent a framework of shared values which fit together with the Code of Practice and the legislation itself as follows:

1. The law tells us *what to do*
2. The Code of Practice tells us *how to do it*
3. The Guiding Principles provide a framework of shared values as the basis for applying the law guided by the Code of Practice *in a balanced way to individual cases*.

As a framework of shared values, the Guiding Principles have not been produced 'out of the blue'. Rather, they draw together the many expectations, concerns and other values that were expressed from a wide variety of different stakeholder perspectives during the extensive consultation that preceded the introduction of the new legislation. Following the 'framework of values' approach, we can thus understand the Guiding Principles as shown diagrammatically in Figure 4.3, i.e. as providing a framework of shared values that have to be balanced in applying the new legislation in individual cases; and the skills-base and other elements of values-based practice, as summarised in Table 4.2, provide the key to carrying out this process in a balanced way.

Table 4.5   The Guiding Principles in the Code of Practice for the new Mental Health Act

Purpose	Decisions under the Act must be taken with a view to minimising the undesirable effects of mental disorder, by maximising the safety and wellbeing (mental and physical) of patients, promoting their recovery and protecting other people from harm.
Least restrictive alternative	People taking action without a patient's consent must attempt to keep to a minimum the restrictions they impose on the patient's liberty, having regard to the purpose for which the restrictions are imposed.
Respect	People taking decisions under the Act must recognise and respect the diverse needs, values and circumstances of each patient, including their race, religion, culture, gender, age, sexual orientation and any disability. They must consider the patient's views, wishes and feelings (whether expressed at the time or in advance), so far as they are reasonably ascertainable, and follow those wishes wherever practicable and consistent with the purpose of the decision. There must be no unlawful discrimination.
Participation	Patients must be given the opportunity to be involved, as far as is practicable in the circumstances, in planning, developing and reviewing their own treatment and care to help ensure that it is delivered in a way that is as appropriate and effective for them as possible. The involvement of carers, family members and other people who have an interest in the patient's welfare should be encouraged (unless there are particular reasons to the contrary) and their views taken seriously.
Resources (effectiveness, efficiency and equity)	People taking decisions under the Act must seek to use the resources available to them and to patients in the most effective, efficient and equitable way, to meet the needs of patients and achieve the purpose for which the decision was taken.

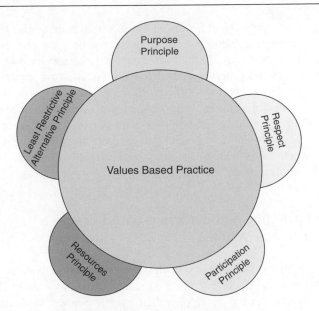

Figure 4.3   Guiding Principles and values-based practice.

We do not have space here to look in detail at how each of the ten elements of values-based practice summarised in Table 4.2 contribute to making balanced decisions about compulsory treatment within the framework of values represented by the Guiding Principles. This is set out fully, with worked examples, in a module of the training materials produced to support the new legislation (CSIP and NIMHE, 2008a) and in a supporting article (Fulford, King and Dewey, forthcoming).

That such an approach is needed, however, will be clear from the evident conflicts between the Guiding Principles: for example, the Purpose Principle, which includes 'protecting other people from harm', may conflict with the Principle of Least Restriction. In applying the law to individual cases, therefore, the different Principles, each of which is important in its own right, have to be applied in a balanced way according to the circumstances of the individual case. Similarly, it will be clear that in this process of balancing, again to take just one example from Table 4.2, *raising awareness* of the different values bearing on a particular case (Pointer 1 in Table 4.2) will be the key to understanding what the Respect Principle will mean from the often very different perspectives represented by different cultural groups. The service delivery context (Pointers 5 and 6) will also be crucial, as will partnership (Point 10), directly reflected in the Principle of Participation.

We believe that a similar approach may be helpful in relation to resolving some of the values issues raised by service user involvement in research. Alison Faulkner (Chapter 2), for example, is among those in this Handbook who set out what are in effect Guiding Principles for such involvement: she includes clarity and transparency; respect, flexibility, accessibility, diversity, empowerment; commitment to change, clarity about theoretical approach and accountability. As a mere 'checklist' such a list would have little effect. As a framework of values to guide decision-making at each stage of the research process, it could prove powerful indeed.

A further important values-based feature of the approach is that, reflecting Pointers 7–9 (Table 4.2), it is strongly evidence-based, drawing not only on conventional research sources (e.g. Sheehan and Burns, 2005), but also directly on service user narratives from people with direct personal experience of different aspects of the impact of compulsory treatment in practice. These narratives, reflecting a wide range of both positive and negative experiences of compulsory treatment were drawn together by a member of the team that produced the training materials, Sarah Dewey, with personal experience of compulsory treatment, and thus represented a crucial service user derived evidence-base for the programme as a whole[2]. It is to the relationship between values-based and evidence-based practice that we turn in the next section.

Values-based practice and evidence-based practice in mental health assessment

As noted earlier, the process-based approach of values-based practice is complementary not only to ethics but also to evidence-based practice. This has been well recognised by many of those involved in the development of evidence-based medicine. Thus, David Sackett and his colleagues in their book (2000, p1) on *Evidence-Based Medicine: How to Practice and Teach EBM* emphasise that evidence-based practice combines three distinct elements. The first element, as you would expect, is best research evidence. But best research evidence, Sackett *et al.* say, has to be combined with the experience and skills of practitioners and, crucially, with *patients' values*. The importance of values in evidence-based practice noted by Sackett *et al.* correspond directly with Pointers 7–9 of values-based practice (Table 4.2, above). The NIMHE Values Framework (Table 4.4, above) also emphasises this, both in the first principle, of 'Recognition' and in its explicit endorsement of the need for research.

The importance of evidence, however, raises the question of 'whose evidence?'. In traditional research, personal narrative has often been neglected. But in research on values, it is through personal narrative that the 'unique perspectives', referred to by Sackett *et al.* (see quote in Part I, above), are identified. In this Handbook, for example, Jasna Russo (Chapter 5) and Larry Davidson (Chapter 7) both emphasise the importance of drawing on individual real world experiences in coming to understand the variety of different roles and perspectives of researchers as well as of service users, and thus to identify the motives, values, aims and issues of power, that make up the very different perspectives from which they engage in research.

The importance of personal narratives as part of the evidence base for values-based practice is illustrated by recent work in the UK on assessment in mental health. Assessment (which includes but is wider than medical diagnosis) is an area that is often taken to be somehow 'purely' scientific and hence value-free, (i.e., like taking a blood test or doing an x-ray). The theory of values-based practice, however, shows that assessment, how we *understand* a problem, is matter as much of values as of evidence (Fulford, 1989; Fulford *et al.*, 2005); and the American psychiatrist and philosopher, John Sadler, has shown that the American Psychiatric Association's own diagnostic manual, the Diagnostic and Statistical

---

[2] In addition to the training materials, these narratives have been published in the form of a CD-rom (available from NIMHE).

Manual (American Psychiatric Association, 1994), is deeply value-laden as well as being explicitly evidence-based (Sadler, 2005). The value-ladenness of assessment, correspondingly, is noted both in the NIMHE Values Framework (Table 4.4); and in Sackett et al.'s definition of evidence-based practice (as above), they write of the need for a '*diagnostic* and therapeutic alliance' between clinicians and patients (Sackett *et al.*, 2000, p1, emphasis added).

In light of all this, NIMHE, working in partnership with a number of international organisations, including both the World Psychiatric Association and the Mental Health and Substance Abuse Section of the WHO, have supported a series of international research seminars that brought together clinicians, service users and policy makers to explore the role of values in mental health assessment. These conferences culminated in a national programme set up by the UK's Department of Health exploring best practice in assessment in mental health and social care, the aim of which was to provide evidence of the aspects of assessment that all stakeholders – service users, carers, different service providers within the multidisciplinary team, and managers – all agreed were important. The processes, as well as aims, of the programme were values-based in a number of key respects:

1. The programme was co-led by one of us (KWMF) as Department of Health Lead for Values-Based Practice, with the NIMHE Service User and Carer Leads, respectively Laurie Bryant and Lu Duhig.
2. It was supported by a steering group co-chaired by Professor Sheila Hollins, at the time President of the Royal College of Psychiatrists, for mental health, and Lord Adebowale, Chief Executive of a major social care NGO in London (Turning Point); and by an extensive Development Group representing all stakeholders.
3. The examples of positive practice collected came from service user and carer-led organisations as well as from mental health and social care services (there was also an extensive consultation exercise including minority groups (www.3keys.org.uk/downloads/3keys.pdf).

The findings from this programme, summarised as '3 Keys' in Table 4.6 and published in full as '3 Keys to a Shared Approach in Mental Health Assessment' (Care Services Improvement Partnership (CSIP) and NIMHE, 2008b), may not seem very startling! It is well recognised, as the 3 Keys indicate, that 1) active participation of service users and carers in a shared approach (Key 1), 2) inputs from different specialist perspectives (Key 2; also reflected in the work of Colombo *et al.*, noted in Part II), and, above all, 3) a strengths-based approach that emphasises strengths, resiliencies and aspirations as well as needs and difficulties (Key 3), are all essential to recovery and developing self-management skills.

Table 4.6   The 3 keys to a shared approach to assessment in mental health and social care

The 3 keys to the Shared Approach are:

1) **Active participation** of the service user concerned in a shared understanding with service providers and where appropriate with their carers
2) Input from **different provider perspectives** within a multidisciplinary approach, and
3) A person-centred focus that builds on the **strengths, resiliencies and aspirations** of the individual service user as well as identifying his or her needs and challenges.

All stakeholders recognised these as, literally, three key aspects (i.e. values) guiding how assessments are carried out. Yet – and this is a further example of the importance of the awareness raising principle of values-based practice (Pointer 1, Table 4.2) – we found *few if any examples of all three in action together*. The '3 Keys' document includes many wonderful examples of innovative approaches to all three 'keys' but the consistent finding from service users and carers was that all three keys needed to be brought together in a fully shared approach.

The next stage in the programme will be to respond to this finding by extending the partnership approach to the development and sharing of positive practice. This work will be coordinated by NIMHE and involve partners in all stakeholders groups. Importantly, we are looking for funding to support a programme of research and development in a partnership between a service user organisation, Commensus, and the Institute for Philosophy, Diversity and Mental Health, at the University of Central Lancashire (www.uclan.ac.uk/ipdmh). There will also be continued collaboration with international organisations, in particular the World Psychiatric Association through its Institutional Program on Psychiatry for the Person (IPPP) (Mezzich and Salloum, 2007). The IPPP is particularly active in this area with a number of key initiatives, including important innovations in person-centred diagnosis (Mezzich, 2007); and there have also been significant developments in various European countries and in South Africa (Van Staden and Fulford, 2007).

Values-based approaches to assessment, it is important to emphasise finally, are fully complementary to more traditional objective diagnostic criteria (Fulford *et al.*, 2005). Objective criteria provide the basis for general categorisations related to evidence of effectiveness of treatment, epidemiological data and so forth. But these objective categories need to be related to *individuals* and the particular circumstances in which they find themselves, and it is here that as the evidence of 'The 3 Keys' shows, a values-based approach, working alongside and in partnership with evidence-based approaches, is vital.

CONCLUSIONS

This chapter has introduced the concepts of values and values-based practice and shown how these are woven through the issues and concerns raised by other chapters in this Handbook around the involvement of service users in mental health research. As noted at the start of the chapter, there has been and remains a widespread assumption that scientific research is, or should be, somehow 'value free'. This is very far from the case, however. As we have seen, values come into all stages of the research process, from commissioning, through design and implementation, to the interpretation of results and their applications in practice. Rather than seeking artificially to exclude values from research, therefore, our aim should be to develop processes for working with them more effectively, and this is where values-based practice comes in. Values-based practice, as we have described, offers a process for working more effectively with complex and conflicting values that complement the processes for working with complex and conflicting evidence provided by evidence-based practice. Key points about values-based practice are summarised in Table 4.7.

We would like to add a final point in conclusion about the wider significance of service user involvement in research. As noted several times, the traditional stereotype has been that scientific research is value-free. According to this stereotype, therefore, service user 'involvement' is at best irrelevant, at worst prejudicial to the objectivity of research. Yet,

Table 4.7   Key points from the chapter

1. Values are wider than ethics and include all the many ways in which we express positive and negative evaluations, i.e. preferences, needs, wishes, etc as well as ethical values
2. Values-based practice is a new approach to working with complex and conflicting values that focuses on "good process", including skills training in: 1) awareness of values and of diversity of values, 2) reasoning about values, 3) knowledge of values, and 4) communication skills (including skills in such areas as negotiation and conflict resolution)
3. Values-based practice is one of a number of potential practical resources to support service-user involvement in research arising from the new philosophy of psychiatry
4. In mental health, values-based practice is supported by 1) a wide range of training materials, 2) a strong policy framework, 3) developing links between values-based and evidence-based approaches, and 4) an overall model of partnership (as in the work described in the chapter on a shared approach to assessment)
5. Values-based practice is also the basis of a number of both national and international developments aimed at building a strong diagnostic and therapeutic alliance between service users and service providers in mental health and social care
6. Ethical principles provide a framework of shared values – such as 'best interests' and 'autonomy of patient choice' - that guide the *outcomes* of clinical decision-making supported by codes of practice and regulatory bodies
7. Values-based practice is complementary to ethics in focusing on the *process* of clinical decision-making: ethics focuses on 'right outcomes' (reflecting shared values); values-based practice focuses on 'good process' (for balancing complex/conflicting values)
   Example in text: the framework of values provided by the Guiding Principles supporting new mental health legislation on compulsory treatment in the UK
8. In focusing on process rather than outcomes, values-based practice (concerned with complex and conflicting values) is fully complementary to evidence-based practice (concerned with complex and conflicting evidence) in clinical decision-making
   Example in text: the NIMHE programme in the UK leading to the '3 Keys' to a shared approach to assessment in mental health and social care
9. Values-based practice is only one resource for working with complex and conflicting values in healthcare: other important disciplines include ethics, health economics and decision theory
10. In meeting the challenges of effective service user involvement in research in mental health, we are leading the way for the rest of healthcare.

as Davidson (Chapter 7) so clearly argues, the whole point of service user involvement in research is to *improve the quality of research itself*. The vital importance of this is not confined to mental health, however. Indeed, as Pointer 9 of values-based practice itself reminds us (Table 4.2), future advances in science and technology, by increasing the range of choices available, will bring ever more complex values issues into play not just in mental health but in all areas of healthcare. In being 'first in the field' with tackling the challenges of service user involvement in research in mental health, therefore, we are leading the field for research in twenty-first century healthcare as a whole.

ACKNOWLEDGEMENTS

Table 4.1 was first published in Fulford, forthcoming. Table 4.2 is based on material first published in Woodbridge and Fulford, 2004. Table 4.4, the NIMHE Values Framework, is published in various places including Department of Health, 2004 and 2005, and in Fulford and Woodbridge, 2004. Table 4.5 and Figure 4.3 were first published in CSIP and NIMHE, 2008a. Table 4.6 is based on material in CSIP and NIMHE, 2008b. Figure 4.1 was published in Fulford and Woodbridge, 2008. The information on which Figure 4.2 is based is derived from the study of models of disorder described in the text and first published in Colombo *et al.*, 2003.

REFERENCES

American Psychiatric Association (1994) *Diagnostic and Statistical Manual of Mental Disorders*, (fourth edition, DSM-IV), Washington, DC: American Psychiatric Association.

Andreasen, N.C. (2001) *Brave New Brain: Conquering Mental Illness in the Era of the Genome*, Oxford: Oxford University Press.

Bloch, S., Chodoff, P. and Green, S.A. (1999) *Psychiatric Ethics* (Third edition), Oxford: Oxford University Press.

Brown, M.M., Brown, G.C. and Sharma, S. (2005) *Evidence-Based to Value-Based Medicine*, Chicago: American Medical Association Press.

Care Services Improvement Partnership (CSIP) and the National Institute for Mental Health in England (NIMHE) (2008a) *Workbook to Support Implementation of the Mental Health Act 1983 as Amended by the Mental Health Act 2007*.

Care Services Improvement Partnership (CSIP) and the National Institute for Mental Health in England (NIMHE) (2008b) *3 Keys to a Shared Approach in Mental Health Assessment*, London: Department of Health.

Colombo, A., Bendelow, G., Fulford, K.W.M. and Williams, S. (2003) Evaluating the influence of implicit models of mental disorder on processes of shared decision making within community-based multi-disciplinary teams. *Social Science & Medicine*, **56**, 1557–1570.

Department of Health (2004) (40339) *The Ten Essential Shared Capabilities: A Framework for the Whole of the Mental Health Workforce*, London: The Sainsbury Centre for Mental Health, the NHSU (National Health Service University), and the NIMHE (National Institute for Mental Health England).

Department of Health (2005) *New Ways of Working for Psychiatrists: Enhancing effective, person-centred services through new ways of working in multidisciplinary and multi-agency contexts, (Final report 'but not the end of the story')*, London: Department of Health.

Fulford, K.W.M. (1989, reprinted 1995 and 1999) *Moral Theory and Medical Practice*, Cambridge: Cambridge University Press.

Fulford, K.W.M. (forthcoming) In: M.G. Gelder, N. Andreasen and J. Geddes (Eds.) *Values and Values-Based Practice in Clinical Psychiatry*, Chapter for Oxford Textbook of Psychiatry (Second edition), Oxford: Oxford University Press.

Fulford, K.W.M. and Benington, J. (2004) VBM²: A Collaborative Values-Based Model of Healthcare Decision-Making Combining Medical and Management Perspectives. In: R. Williams and M. Kerfoot (Eds) *Child and Adolescent Mental Health Services: Strategy, planning, delivery, and evaluation*, Oxford: Oxford University Press, pp. 89–102.

Fulford, K.W.M. and Colombo, A. (2004) Six models of mental disorder: a study combining linguistic-analytic and empirical methods, *Philosophy, Psychiatry & Psychology*, **11**(2), 129–144.

Fulford, K.W.M. and Sartorius, N. (forthcoming) 'A Secret History of ICD and the Hidden Future of DSM'. In: M. Broome and L. Bortolotti (Eds.) *Psychiatry as Cognitive Neuroscience: Philosophical Perspectives*, Oxford: Oxford University Press.

Fulford, K.W.M. and Woodbridge, K. (2008) Practising Ethically: Values-Based Practice and Ethics: Working together to support person-centred and multidisciplinary mental health care. In:

T. Stickley and T. Basset (Eds) *Learning About Mental Health Practice*, Chichester: John Wiley & Sons Ltd., pp. 145–160.

Fulford, K.W.M., Dickenson, D. and Murray, T.H. (2002) Introduction: Many Voices: Human Values in Healthcare Ethics. In: K.W.M. Fulford, D. Dickenson and T.H. Murray (Eds) *Healthcare Ethics and Human Values: An Introductory Text with Readings and Case Studies*, Malden, USA, and Oxford, UK: Blackwell, pp. 1–19.

Fulford, K.W.M., King, M. and Dewey, S. (forthcoming) Values Based Practice and Involuntary Treatment: A new training programme in the UK. *Advances in Psychiatric Treatment*.

Fulford, K.W.M., Stanghellini, G. and Broome, M. (2004) What can philosophy do for psychiatry? Special Article for *World Psychiatry (WPA)*, **3**(3), October, pp. 130–135.

Fulford, K.W.M., Thornton, T., and Graham, G. (2006) Natural Classifications, Realism and Psychiatric Science. In: Fulford, K.W.M., Thornton, T., Graham, G. (Eds) *The Oxford Textbook of Philosophy and Psychiatry*, Oxford: Oxford University Press, pp 316–383.

Fulford, K.W.M., Broome, M., Stanghellini, G. and Thornton, T. (2005) Looking with both eyes open: fact *and* value in psychiatric diagnosis? *World Psychiatry*, **4**(2), 78–86.

Fulford, K. W. M., Morris, K. J., Sadler, J. Z. and Stanghellini, G. (2003) Past Improbable, Future Possible: the renaissance in philosophy and psychiatry. In: K.W.M. Fulford, K.J. Morris, J.Z. Sadler, and G. Stanghellini (Eds.) *Nature and Narrative: an Introduction to the New Philosophy of Psychiatry*, Oxford: Oxford University Press, pp. 1–41.

Hare, R.M. (1952) *The Language of Morals*, Oxford: Oxford University Press.

Hempel, C.G. (1961) Introduction to Problems of Taxonomy. In: J. Zubin (Ed) *Field Studies in the Mental Disorders*, pp. 3–22, New York: Grune and Stratton. Reproduced in J.Z. Sadler, O.P. Wiggins and M.A. Schwartz (1994) *Philosophical Perspectives on Psychiatric Diagnostic Classification*, Baltimore, The Johns Hopkins University Press, pp. 315–331.

Hoff, P. (2005) Die psychopathologische Perspektive. In: M. Bormuth, U. Wiesing (Eds) *Ethische Aspekte der Forschung in Psychiatrie und Psychotherapie*, Deutscher Aerzte-Verlag, Cologne, pp. 71–79.

Hope, T., Fulford, K.W.M. and Yates, A. (1996) *The Oxford Practice Skills Course: Ethics, Law and Communication Skills in Health Care Education*, Oxford: The Oxford University Press.

Hunink, M., Glasziou, P. and Siegel, J. *et al.* (2001) *Decision Making in Health and Medicine: Integrating Evidence and Values*, Cambridge: Cambridge University Press.

King, C. (2007) They Diagnosed Me a Schizophrenic When I Was Just a Gemini: The Other Side of Madness, Chapter 2. In: M. Chung, K.W.M. Fulford and G. Graham (Eds) *Reconceiving Schizophrenia*, Oxford: Oxford University Press, pp. 11–28.

King, C., Bhui, K. and Fulford, K.W.M. and Williamson, T. (forthcoming) *Model Values? Race, Values and models in mental health (provisional title)* London: The Mental Health Foundation.

Mezzich, J.E. (2007) Psychiatry for the person: articulating medicine's science and humanism. 'Editorial'. *World Psychiatry*, **6**(2), 1–3.

Mezzich, J.E. and Salloum, I.M. (2007) Towards innovative international classification and diagnostic systems: ICD-11 and person-centered integrative diagnosis, 'Guest Editorial'. *Acta Psychiatrica Scandinavica*, **116**, 1–5.

Okasha, A. (2000) Ethics of psychiatric practice: consent, compulsion and confidentiality. *Current Opinion in Psychiatry*, **13**, 693–698.

Osborn, D. (1999) Research and ethics: leaving exclusion behind. *Current Opinion in Psychiatry*, **12**(5), 601–604.

Petrova, M., Dale, J. and Fulford, K.W.M. (2006) Values-Based Practice in primary care: easing the tensions between individual values, ethical principles and best evidence. *British Journal of General Practice*, **56**, 703–709.

Roberts, G., Dorkins, E., Wooldridge, J., and Hewis, E. (2008) Detained – what's my choice? Part 1: Discussion, *Advances in Psychiatric Treatment*, **14**, 172–180.

Rogers, A., Pilgrim, D. and Lacey, R. (1993) *Experiencing Psychiatry: Users' Views of Services*, London: The Macmillan Press.

Sabat, S.R. (2001) *The Experience of Alzheimer's Disease: Life Through a Tangled Veil*, Oxford: Blackwell Publishers.

Sackett, D.L., Straus, S.E. and Scott Richardson, W. *et al.* (2000) *Evidence-Based Medicine: How to Practice and Teach EBM* (*2nd Edition*). Edinburgh and London: Churchill Livingstone.

Sadler, J.Z. (2005) *Values and Psychiatric Diagnosis*, Oxford: Oxford University Press.

Sheehan, K.A. and Burns, T. (2005) *Patient and Clinician Perceptions During Psychiatric Hospital Admissions* (Poster presentation). Cairo, Egypt: World Psychiatric Association Conference.

Stanghellini, G. (2004) *Deanimated Bodies and Disembodied Spirits: Essays on the psychopathology of common sense*, Oxford: Oxford University Press.

Thornton, T. (2006) Tacit Knowledge as the unifying factor in EBM and clinical judgement. *Philosophy Ethics and Humanities of Medicine*, **1**(2), Online journal.

Thornton, T. (2007) *Essential Philosophy of Psychiatry*, Oxford: Oxford University Press.

Van Staden, C.W. and Fulford, K.W.M. (2007) Lead Guest Editorial. Hypotheses, neuroscience and real persons: The theme of the 10th International Conference on Philosophy, Psychiatry and Psychology. *South African Journal of Psychiatry* **13**(3), 68–71.

Widdershoven, G. and Widdershoven-Heerding, I. (2003) Understanding Dementia: A Hermeneutic Perspective. In: K.W.M. Fulford, K.J. Morris, J.Z. Sadler and G. Stanghellini (Eds) *Nature and Narrative: An Introduction to the New Philosophy of Psychiatry*, Oxford: Oxford University Press, pp. 103–112.

Woodbridge, K. and Fulford, K.W.M. (2004) *'Whose Values?' A workbook for values-based practice in mental health care*, London: The Sainsbury Centre for Mental Health.

Woodbridge, K. and Fulford, K.W.M. (2005) Values-Based Practice. Module 4. In: T. Basset and L. Lindley (Eds) *The Ten Essential Shared Capabilities Learning Pack for Mental Health Practice*. For The National Health Service University (NHSU) and the National Institute for Mental Health in England (NIMHE).

CHAPTER 5

Roles

Beyond Involvement: Looking for a Common Perspective on Roles in Research

Jasna Russo
European Network of (ex) Users and Survivors of Psychiatry, Berlin, Germany
Peter Stastny
South Beach Psychiatric Centre, New York, NY, USA

This chapter considers, from both perspectives, different roles and positions service users and traditional academics can hold in joint research endeavours. The authors enter into a dialogue, drawing on their respective real world experiences as a service user researcher and an academic researcher/clinician in order to explore critical issues relating to their roles and find some common ground. Openly critical and self-critical they touch on important topics related to the realities of service user involvement in mental health research, referring to motives, values, aims and (im)possibilities, risks, and crucial issues of institutional and societal power as they have experienced them in their different roles throughout their careers. This allows the reader to gain insight into how it can feel for people from differing perspectives seeking to work together and make a real difference.

INTRODUCTION

Points of departure

We approached working on this chapter as an exchange of our experiences between someone who was subjected to psychiatric treatment and someone who works in the psychiatric system, along with offering our different experiences of collaborative research. Without

Handbook of Service User Involvement in Mental Health Research   Edited by Jan Wallcraft, Beate Schrank and Michaela Amering
Copyright © 2009 John Wiley & Sons, Ltd

ambition to represent all users/survivors[1] and all academic researchers we decided to pay attention to our two different personal perspectives. This honest but not too comfortable approach of letting our differences talk to each other enabled us to seek a common base for collaborative research instead of simply presuming that there was such a thing.

> *Being honest and open about the motives and incentives for involvement is an important starting point for collaboration. If there is no meeting point between the respective parties, then perhaps it will not and should not happen, but at least both parties will have shared where they are coming from and raised the possibility of starting in an atmosphere of trust.*
>
> (Faulkner, 2003)

Our thinking about roles in the research process started with briefly asking ourselves about the reasons for collaborating; this is when we noticed how disparate our perspectives actually are.

Peter: the academic perspective

Never meaning to be a purely academic researcher, I always saw research as a tool to foster change in a system that was highly resistant to progress and transformation. Research demonstration projects that provided federal dollars to evaluate innovative interventions were a way to prod mental health services in the direction of enhancing the status of service users, while at the same time improving outcomes. Setting out from the anti-institutional politics of the 1970s, it took me a few years to realize the potential of service users as partners and innovators in a professionally dominated system. This newly found collaboration between the most and the least powerful players in the mental health system generated excitement, insights, new alliances, but little change in actual power structures. One of the first major studies that involved user/survivors as collaborators, provided evidence for a positive contribution of peer specialists (current or former service users with expertise based on their experiences) to clients' recovery and quality of life, and we were able to create a new entry-level position for former psychiatric patients (Felton *et al.*, 1995).

Nevertheless, hampered by administrative and labour politics that would not go beyond minimal adjustments in the redistribution of power, the path of transformation through collaboration seemed insurmountably blocked. As a result of this experience I have come to believe that new structures for research and practice need to be created collaboratively, where partnerships and newly formulated power relationships between survivors/service users and those who are lacking such experiences could be carried out to its fullest extent.

Jasna: the survivor perspective

Collaborative research is, in most cases, the only way for survivor researchers to contribute to the production of knowledge. It is very difficult for user/survivor-controlled research to get funding and recognition, so collaboration often remains the only way for us to take part in research. My personal experiences of collaborative research projects have always given

---

[1] Having noticed that 'user involvement in research' excludes the notion of 'survivor', we decided to keep including the latter throughout this article.

me fewer and fewer reasons to want to collaborate, and more and more reasons to initiate user/survivor-controlled projects.

Parallel paths

After clarifying our different motives for collaborating, we continued exchanging ideas and expectations from research, our experiences of collaborative projects and articles that we liked. We decided to split the process into two in order to deepen our different experiences of collaboration and be able to reflect on them first for ourselves. We wanted to see what we have learned individually, and whether or not we could come up with a platform that we both agreed upon. Here is what we came up with on our independent journeys.

Jasna: four roles of experts by experience in research

The following distinction between the first, the ideal, the common and the final role for users/survivors in research is my attempt to frame the way I perceive and reflect our collaborations with academics. They are based both on my own research experiences as well on my knowledge about other researchers with whom I share the 'expert by experience' identity.

The first role: making sure that there is one!

Collaboration usually starts by academics inviting user researchers to contribute to their projects and not the other way around. The way someone joins the project – on whose initiative and for what reasons – defines their role, at least at the beginning. Users are invited at various stages of someone else's project. They are rarely invited to plan and seek funding for the research and to define the roles and responsibilities.

   Whoever has the power and the resources to issue such invitations always feels more at home than the one who joins in. The fact that we are invited, or that posts for user researchers are advertised, makes us expect that there will be room for us. But this is not always the case.

> . . . when I join an advisory group or steering group it is in the hope of being recognised as an *'expert by experience'*, as having my own expertise to contribute to the group, not in order to *be further pathologised in the process. Put quite simply, there is no pleasure in attempting to be 'involved' where you are not wanted.*
>
> (Faulkner, 2003)

   The invitation to collaborate can happen for various reasons or for no real reasons at all, and the one who joins has a sense of that very quickly. The amount of 'room' for user researchers in the project varies, but there is often no clarity about why we are there and what exactly is expected from us.

> *The power is usually held by the academic researchers who give away as much or as little of it as they wish, and the service users can feel exploited in the process.*
>
> (Faulkner, 2003)

We are often expected to demonstrate why it makes sense that we are there. The expectations of user researchers are often far smaller than what they could and would like to contribute. We experience collaboration as an effort and a process of enlarging our role rather than being equal partners from the beginning. Collaboration is often not the starting point but something to be developed in the course of the research project – or sometimes not. So the first role for survivor researchers is to make sure that they will *have* a role. This means investing additional work which is often not even recognised as such.

The ideal role: making substantial change

When talking about roles in collaborative research it is important not to concentrate exclusively on the role of user/survivor researchers. This is usually the only topic of interest, while at the same time there is no discussion of what is considered to be 'self-evident' and 'natural', such as the role of academics in the research process.

> *Those who hold power can ensure that their values are seen as self-evident, as unquestionable common sense. To a large extent and for long periods they can be successful in resisting challenges to their knowledge and authority.*
>
> (Wallcraft, 2003)

True collaboration questions and changes everybody's role and also requires that such change is wanted. There is a lot of collaboration taking place within the traditional mental health research frame where service users/survivors are somehow inserted without really being let in. This 'letting–in' cannot take place without 'letting go' of some of the traditions on which mental health research is based. The roles in research are based on perceptions and expectations of each other, as well as of the research which should be explored.

> *I think the idea of user involvement in research raises fundamental issues for research; for our understandings of the nature, principles and purpose of research, which need to be worked through, not sidestepped.*
>
> (Beresford, 2003)

If there is openness to substantial changes, what starts as 'involvement' can grow into a working partnership between user/survivor and other researchers, But 'user involvement' can also remain stuck within a more traditional research and 'scientific' discourse.

What are the fundamental issues in research? If the research starts with a hypothesis, it will make a big difference whether this hypothesis addresses the social reality of participants or the researcher's definition of it, however 'scientifically proven' the latter might be. If the purpose of mental health research is to increase the understanding of different phenomena, it makes a major difference whether the understanding comes from an insider or an outsider perspective. If the basis of psychiatric research is the need for more knowledge, the question is – whose need is it? Is it the need of those treating or selling treatment? Or is it the need of those who are subjected to treatment? If the research is about the comparison between what works and what doesn't, the question is – for whom does something work? Whose definition of 'positive' and 'negative symptoms' is applied? Usually, these and other fundamental issues are never revealed.

User involvement in research can have both liberatory and regressive potential and there is a distinction between a consumerist and a democratic approach:

> While service user researchers, organisations, and movements have tended to see user involve-ment in research and user-controlled research as part of a process of developing their own knowledge and discourses (as a basis for change), for service providers, the focus is essentially service-led, and for mainstream researchers tied in to developing new domains for professional and academic activity.
>
> (Beresford, 2002)

Thinking exclusively in terms of user involvement in mental health research implies recognition of a territory where users should be let in, in a controlled way, through *user involvement*. User involvement is an *a priori* reduction of all the roles that users/survivors can take.

> For as long as service users continue to be involved (in the historical sense of involvement), they reinforce the power of the dominant discourse.
>
> (Stickley, 2006)

Mental health research, like the mental health system, is a territory which has been occupied for a very long time. User involvement might be a way of reclaiming this territory, but this will not happen as long as service users are given only a limited 'involvement role'. If mental health research is to be reclaimed, this will not take place through allowing users to have some roles in it. If the process aims for fundamental changes, user/survivors cannot be offered less than access to all the possible roles, including decision-making on what research will be funded or ethically approved.

Some of us feel that by agreeing to the existing role division we help psychiatric research open new markets. We are extending topics and methodologies but we are not turning the research culture into something we can stand behind and identify with. Influencing the research projects that we are working on to the point that we can call them 'ours' is often not possible. Instead of feeling free to make contributions we believe in, we are busy compromising with someone else's conceptions in a careful and constructive way, in order to get some share in power. That share is rarely fair.

> [...] there are salary and status differentials so that even experienced user researchers in a collaborative project will be perceived as 'junior'. Some user-researchers acting as con-sultants to research projects do not get a salary at all, they receive therapeutic earnings despite substantial input.
>
> (Rose, 2003)

The common role: being useful

The 'usefulness' of user researchers for academics seems to be the most attractive aspect of user involvement. Apart from increasing the funding chances, the perceived 'usefulness' usually relates to peer-to-peer interviewing. The psychiatric thinking remains not only unquestioned, it becomes even more sustained through turning the diagnoses of user researchers into a central criterion for their involvement and pairing them up with the diagnoses of the research subjects.

> *The project has demonstrated the ability of service users with a PD[2] diagnosis to learn to conduct good quality, ethical interviews in a relatively short time, adding another confirming case study to the existing evidence of the usefulness of user-researchers (Oliver, 1992; Rose,). Interviewees were offered a unique opportunity to share their experiences with the person they could more easily trust than a professional researcher.*
>
> (Ramon, Castillo and Morant, 2001)

Service user researchers are also more trusted when it comes to conducting surveys among users' organisations and obtaining permission to do so. The fact that user researchers turn out to be better than academics in making and maintaining contact with 'subjects' can easily become functionalised into 'improving recruitment' and 'reducing the drop-out rate'.

The bewailed 'permitted work' rules in the social welfare system can become useful for the researchers by saving considerable money through user involvement, which is generally cheaper than hiring non-user staff. And finally, it is often stressed that users can acquire new knowledge and abilities, increase their self-confidence and – in distinction to academics – might also experience 'empowerment' through having a role in research. There are several ways to involve users in research without really letting them in – either 'for their own good' or in order to improve some of the research technicalities.

> *If we continue to work within existing models of service user involvement, then the change that is wrought within mental health services will only ever be mediated by those in control of services, to comply with their agenda.*
>
> (Stickley, 2006)

Solely allowing users to collect data or even to carry out the research will not turn the subjects into research participants or shift the ethics of research. But enabling participants to become more than 'information givers' or 'treatment responders' could change the existing research culture.

> *Research is seen as an essentially political activity, rather than a 'neutral fact-finding mission'. The disabled people's movement has highlighted the importance of changing (and equalising) the social relations of research production [...]*
>
> (Beresford, 2002)

We will have to stop being 'useful' to the psychiatric and mental health research as it is now, if we want it to become different.

> *We are being sold short if we accept a tame, sanitised, toothless form of government-controlled patient and public involvement.*
>
> (Wallcraft, 2008)

---

[2] Personality disorder.

The final role: growing out of collaboration

The users' role of assisting in ongoing research by refreshing and extending it, also has its other side. Paid work contracts have their seductive power for everybody and we are far more likely to get them in collaborative than in user/survivor-controlled projects. It is hard to leave after you have just entered and if we are determined to do research; leaving to go nowhere is a crazy decision to make. On the other hand, acting as expert-by-experience can turn into a chronic identity that precludes actually becoming an expert.

> *The institution of psychiatry however is very powerful and the notion of service users ascending the power hierarchy is illusory and does not pay adequate regard to the institutional powers that exist within a wider society.*
>
> (Stickley, 2006)

From the point of view of those who have not ascended the hierarchy it is hard to say how the top feels and whether or not the whole process is illusory or real. It is also hard to decide in which direction one is going – up or down. Most of us are not familiar with academia's rules such as career-building, competition and the notion of 'intellectual property'. It takes time to learn that our ideas have market value and that the innovation we bring to a project can also bring money and fame, but for someone other than us. It is important to be aware of the context but we might find ourselves refusing to learn the rules.

> *Service users call for openness and democratic decision-making, while the academics and commercial sectors are used to top-down, professionally-controlled decision-making behind closed doors.*
>
> (Wallcraft, 2008)

There are many parallels between psychiatric research and psychiatry, between mental health research and the mental health system. The division of roles in research can repeat the clinical division of roles. We often arrive at similar questions – who has the power to name? Who writes the (case) history? Who owns the research? In the same way that there came a time when we had to leave the mental health system behind, in order to survive, our final role in collaborative research might as well be to grow out of it.

Peter: lessons of a pioneer manqué

In my section I will focus exclusively on the experience and resulting perspectives of an academic/clinician/researcher who has attempted, on a number of occasions, to create partnership scenarios in research and program development.

Motivating forces and the counterpunch

In the past three decades, science involving human subjects, and especially mental health research, has become significantly more diverse with respect to its methods, moving from simple experimental designs, to complicated, triangulated studies with multiple vantage points and data sets. In addition, opportunities for service-demonstration projects, such as existed in the USA during the 1970s and 80s, allowed researchers, to ride the wave's crest between scientific ambition and institutional change. This was an opportunity for a practitioner such as myself who did not want to be bound by traditional specialisation/ stratification guidelines. Thus I was able to grow into a considerably more elastic role, encompassing scientific, transformative, and 'fraternizing' elements.

At the onset of my career as a psychiatrist, consumer/survivors were never seen outside the box of their assigned patient roles. Even the advent of social and community psychiatry did not change this equation, it simply considered the relationship between the institution and its patients as problematic, and advocated for a disbanding of the former and a relocation of the latter. For me, the rupture of my image of patients in their embalmed roles ('loques autistizées' – 'wrecks turned autistic' – Deleuze and Guattari, 1983) began when a patient on the ward (an open ward, where no one was held against their will, but in truth, the residents did not have anywhere else to go) proposed that patients start saving surplus food for the benefit of others who were still homeless in the streets of New York. The staff on this ward had begun to espouse the idea of mutual support by adapting a social engineering project called Fairweather Lodge (Fairweather et al., 1969). We believed that people consigned to institutional life could progress further, if they were invited to form peer groups with the dual goal of encouraging and supporting each other. Social control was being transferred from the institutional pyramid to the artifice of a peer-group hierarchy. Our peer approach was less structured than Fairweather's, encouraging patients to become friends to each other and live together, if they so desired. In this environment the idea of collecting surplus food and distributing it to those in greater need, fell on fertile ground in a situation where mutual trust was emphasized over traditional clinical approaches.

Among the first dialogues that broke the mould was a conversation I had with William Brown, the budding leader of Share Your Bounty around 1987, who helped me understand where he was coming from: having been helped, he now wanted to help others. Such dialogues began to replace the doctor–patient relationship and enabled me to envision endless opportunities of engagement and collaboration. Share Your Bounty became a federally funded demonstration project (Van Tosh and Del Vecchio, 2000); it spawned several user-run projects in the areas of housing and business development, and led to a major research project testing the impact of peer workers with personal experience on the lives and well-being of intensive case-management clients. This million-dollar project was developed by a group of people that included several survivor-advocates who already had established a formidable track record. We believed that the personal experiences of peer specialists would have a positive impact on a variety of factors, such as the nature of the service relationship and clients' quality of life. We hired people to collect data who clearly had distressing personal experiences of their own. They needed much reasonable (and a certain degree of unreasonable) accommodation, which nearly resulted in a hostile take-over of the project by state bureaucrats. We barely succeeded in obtaining the findings that we expected, but ultimately were able to show that peers could make positive contributions on many levels – as supporters to their peers, data collectors, supervisors and co-investigators. Even though the project was highly successful by laying the groundwork for creating a new civil service title in New York State for 'peer specialists', soon thereafter the state turned into a hotbed of cooptation. Certain user-survivor activists were appointed to coveted government positions, and a small number of user-run organizations were handpicked to receive the lion's share of government funding, while other grassroots efforts were sidelined, especially if they were vocal about their critical views. Research fell into increasingly tighter control of government officials, who were especially keen on suppressing any voices that were critical of their programs. The last peer-run research project (Crisis Hostel in Ithaca – Dumont and Jones, 2002), folded in 1997 despite finding that the availability of a user-run crisis respite house ('hostel') significantly reduced the number of hospitalizations for a population at risk. There have been no collaborative or user-run research projects since. Clearly, the political environment had crushed any hopes for greater inclusion and partnerships, especially in the research arena. No one knew, or cared to figure out, how the forces unleashed by the user-survivor movement in the late 1980s and early '90s could be engaged in an equitable and productive fashion.

Pitfalls and pratfalls

While the experience in New York State may be quite different from recent developments in the UK, where user involvement in research and services on all levels has become de rigueur, it highlights many of the risks of partnerships and user engagement under 'unsafe' political and institutional conditions. The fickleness of powerful government officials, who purportedly were pursuing an agenda that favoured 'self-help and empowerment' and user involvement, made it clear that liberation and autonomous agendas would be subject to selective endorsement, rejection, or worse.

My own pursuit of an agenda that was openly critical of institutional psychiatry, especially with regard to its coercive practices which became a huge part of the State's agenda in the 1990s (for example, outpatient commitment), led to my stigmatization and banishment. The invitation from an earlier government to use our critical energies as a way to transform the system, had turned into its opposite – a methodical exploitation of user-input for the sake of a threadbare public image that endorsed 'consumer involvement' and 'recovery'.

Naivety of blending a transformative and a scientific agenda

Saddling research projects with political reform agendas generates problems on several levels. Action-oriented research that proposes to insert 'change agents' into a system that is not prepared to change, ends up burdening those very individuals with the impossible mission that has been foisted upon them. Creating larger organizational structures that rely less on the impact of individuals could be a way out of this dilemma, but leads to the problem of sustainability. Quite often we have been able to secure start-up grants for research demonstrations and after three (or rarely five) years, we were faced with the dilemma of securing permanent local funding, which usually was not forthcoming. The system and its officials are eager to accept 'outside' moneys that are meant to stimulate change, but are not likely to follow up with the money from their own pockets that would be required to sustain and broaden such change. In the end, the influx of 'foreign' money for such projects results merely in demonstrating 'good will' but not fundamental transformation.

In terms of persons such as myself who are in the position of developing such research, we must decide whether it would not be more honest to propose research that simply relies on its findings, rather than weigh it down with an overt or covert political agenda. In my case, this has led me to suspend the role of researcher and focus on activities that are more directly transformative. The bold-faced lie that the public mental health system is building its services on a so-called evidence-base, has led me to focus on other, alternative sources of evidence that have been sidelined or marginalized by the powers that be. User/survivors, who are clued into those alternative sources of evidence, and who may want to promote a research agenda that broadens this non-traditional evidence-base, will have an important role in moving this process forward.

Dependence on whims of the political/institutional system
In the US, any type of system-transforming research must be administered by the very system it is designed to change. This immediately creates a conflict of interest for researchers who are at once beholden to their administrators and to the transformative research agenda. Truly independent research outfits with an ability to garner serious financial support are essentially non-existent. Academic institutions are often forced to enter partnerships with government outfits for the purpose of conducting research, which puts them into a similar dilemma. User-run organizations have rarely, if ever, been able to establish a sufficiently autonomous base along with adequate funding for serious research projects. It has long been argued that advocacy and system transformation has to be supported by funding streams that are independent of traditional mental health agencies, governmental or otherwise. However, such a separation of purposes is still awaiting a more widespread reform.

Lack of an autonomous base for transformative research
Extending the previous point into the personal situation of researchers who are often wearing several hats and working for several masters, leads to a rather pessimistic outlook. The neutrality expected of researchers who must be open to any outcomes of the hypotheses they are testing, is in itself a harrowing proving ground for their ethics and political perspectives. Several of my colleagues who were in their hearts dedicated advocates, have become embroiled in a series of experimental studies that left little room for political agitation. I consider them a loss to the movement for change, even though their contributions may become important foundations for system change at some point in the future. My own choices of forgoing power and abandoning traditional research have allowed me to establish a fairly independent foothold, which, however, is still too narrow for any fanciful moves.

Slowness of science and urgency of need
Finally, one of the most fundamental problems I choose to mention at this point is my impatience with the slow and unpredictable progression of scientific inquiry while facing evermore pressing needs, embodied by an endless succession of people coming through the clinic doors. The gaping chasm between the evidence that is being created for interventions (and perspectives) that might improve the lot of user/survivors and their broad availability is revealed to me every day by the wounds, disparities, stigmatization and lack of opportunities faced by users/survivors of the system. I know that responding to those daily needs is merely a stopgap measure, and might indeed take important energy away from tasks likely to benefit a much wider swath of people.

TOWARDS TRUE RESEARCH PARTNERSHIPS

Our independent contemplations and lessons learned about roles in research made us realize that behind our different experiences there is a ground on which we share similar visions of research. It is because of this common ground that we also share an urgent need to communicate on a different level and to find a different language, which could bring us far beyond 'user involvement in research'.

The following points are our attempt to summarize some of the necessary conditions and our suggestions for roles that we could all take in moving towards true research partnerships:

- **Start from scratch** instead of pretending equality exists – begin by talking about fundamental issues in research. Don't be scared of differences and dare to display them openly. Partnership between us is something to be created in every single project, not just proclaimed.
- **Create standards of collaboration** which are to be fulfilled when advertising posts for user/survivor researchers and employing them. These should be protective of their rights in a similar way as 'equal opportunity policies' or 'Americans with Disabilities Act'.
- **Position users/survivors strategically** in funding agencies, institutional review/ethics boards, and grant review committees, rather than merely engaging them as consultants, data collectors or co-investigators.
- **Establish networks of user/survivor researchers** in order to combat isolation within single collaborative projects and create possibilities of exchange, support, joint reflections of work and undertaking joint research.
- **Develop and broaden user/survivor-run and partnership NGOs** to redefine the nature of evidence and conduct international studies.

REFERENCES

Beresford, P. (2002) User involvement in research and evaluation: liberation or regulation, *Social Policy and Society*, **1**(2), 95–105.

Beresford, P. (2003) *User Involvement in Research: Connecting lives, experience and theory*, from, www.2warwick.ac.uk.

Deleuze, G. and Guattari, F. (1983) *Anti-Oedipus: Capitalism and schizophrenia*, Minneapolis: University of Minnesota Press.

Dumont, J. and Jones, K. (2002) Findings from a consumer/survivor defined alternative to psychiatric hospitalisation. *Outlook*, **4–6**.

Fairweather, G.W., Sanders, D.H., Maynard, H. and Cressler, D.L. (1969) *Community Life for the Mentally Ill*, Chicago: Aldine, Chicago.

Faulkner, A. (2003) The emperor's new clothes. *Mental Health Today*, **3**(8), 23–25.

Felton, C.J. *et al.* (1995) Consumers as peer specialists on intensive case management teams: impact on client outcomes. *Psychiatric Services*, **46**(10), 1037–1044.

Oliver, M. (1992) Changing the social relations of research production, *Disability, Handicap & Society*, **7**(2),101–113.

Ramon, S., Castillo, H. and Morant, N. (2001) Experiencing personality disorder: a participative research, *International Journal of Social Psychiatry*, **47**, 1–15.

Rose, D. (1999) Do it yourself, *Mental Health Care*, **2**(5), 174–177.

Rose, D. (2003) Collaborative research between users and professionals: peaks and pitfalls. *Psychiatric Bulletin*, **27,** 404–406.

Stickley T. (2006) Should service user involvement be consigned to history? A critical realist perspective. *Journal of Psychiatric and Mental Health Nursing*, **13**, 570–577.

Van Tosh, L. and Del Vecchio, P. (2000) *Consumer-Operated Self-help Programs: A Technical Report*, Rockville, MD: U.S. Center for Mental Health Services.

Wallcraft, J. (2003) *The Role of Experts by Experience*, full paper for the Mental Health Foundation's online conference on 4th December 2003: *Different Truths: User Control and Involvement in Mental Health Research and Evaluation*, www.mentalhealth.org.uk.

Wallcraft, J. (2008) View point. *Mental Health Today*, **8**(1), 41.

CHAPTER 6

Capacity-building

Participation in Public Mental Health Research: A Conceptual Framework and Report from Practice

Kim Hopper
Center to Study Recovery in Social Contexts,
The Nathan S. Kline Institute for Psychiatric Research, NY, USA
Alisa Lincoln
Northeastern University, Bouvé College of Health Science, Boston, MA, USA

The first part of this chapter explores in detail the philosophical, historical and sociological background of participation in the context of mental illness. The second part then looks at the issue from a practical point of view. An example is given of the establishment of a mechanism to promote the participation of consumers in mental health services research in Boston (US). On the basis of this example, the processes and practical challenges connected with the establishment of truly inclusive participation are discussed. Special attention is paid to practical issues arising in relation to diversity, flexibility and power as well as to the relationship between research and advocacy.

INTRODUCTION

When, mid-20th century, Erving Goffman decided to examine the nature of 'personal proprieties' (and so to update 'Durkheim's chapter on the soul'), he figured 'a logical place' to study them would be 'among persons who have been locked up for spectacularly failing to maintain them' – on a psychiatric ward (Goffman, 1956, p475). The ward was a convenient and, as it happened, a moribund venue. *Asylums* (Goffman, 1961) was essentially the final dispatch from the front of mass psychiatric confinement, a practice already in decline out

---

when the book appeared. But the infractions that brought people there – serious, sometimes flamboyant rule-breaking (and real need) – and the toll paid for breaking them, are still much in evidence. By most measures, even the crude tallies of comparative bills of mortality (Colton and Manderscheid, 2006), de-institutionalization has not been a success. It failed as reform, not only because adequate material provision for an unconfined life worth living was never made, but also because it never seriously engaged issues of social identity. Fighting stigma (Goffman, 1963; U.S. Department of Health and Human Services, 1999) is only partly a matter of educating a misinformed anxious public, and of reassuring the acutely distressed that competent help is available. It is also one of reckoning with the symbolic costs of seeking help. Outside the oasis of the clinic, it is still the case that 'stigma defines the limits of treatment' (Rosenfield, 1997, p670; cf. Link *et al.,*1997).

For their part, research endeavours, even when progressive in intent, can unthinkingly reinforce and extend 'what goes without saying' (Bourdieu, 1977) with respect to 'the mentally ill'. The starting point of this chapter is thus twofold: first, diluting stigma is less a matter of fixing attitudes than it is one of re-engaging the excluded. Beliefs do a job, Luhrmann reminds us (1989, p351), and stigma's job is to *justify* behaviour and policy that would never be applied to 'one of us'. Until persons grappling with a diagnosis of mental illness are regarded as fully fledged citizens – until they enjoy 'participatory parity' (Fraser, 1998; Olson, 2001) – the ideological corrective will be at odds with pragmatic and political realities. Second, as it seeks to understand (and even to rectify) those realities, research must also actively embody the inclusionary principle. This is more than a nod to consistency; it speaks to how we know what we report. When social scientists (anthropologists especially) talk about participation (e.g. Favret-Saada, 1990), it's usually their own participation they're worried about – the terms and conditions of justifiable engagement that can be put forward to establish their fieldwork's *bona fides* and ratify the quality of their reportage without impugning its 'objectivity'. Such a methodological confession is meant to show the reader how the author secured access to the social reality described there, how s/he came to grasp what life is like 'from the native's point of view' – and thus what makes this ethnographic account trustworthy. The participation at issue here also goes to 'how we know what we report,' but it does so by convincing some of the 'natives' to be part of that inquisitive 'we' from the start.

FRAMING PARTICIPATION

The approach developed here rests critically upon a robust sense of agency, or capacity for intentional action. Following Sen, we're particularly concerned with 'people's ability to act on behalf of goals that matter to them' (1999, p53). So it may be useful to revisit why that construct is so central to any serious discussion of participation on the part of persons carrying diagnoses of severe psychiatric disorder.

Reclaiming agency in public mental health

So categorical and consequential was mental illness thought to be that until recently, it was uncontested common sense that a diagnosis of severe psychiatric disorder sufficed to eclipse and displace agency. For official intents and purposes, a patient's agency was reduced to the docile acts of compliance with prescribed regimens of treatment and the repetitive routines of batch-processed life. Departures from this 'legitimizing identity' (Castells, 2004, p8) were seen less as gestures of thought-through insubordination than as reflex-like resistance. For the most part, being a patient meant subordinating personal initiative to institutional inertia. Admittance to the hospital was not only a 'degradation ceremony' (Goffman, 1961, p139), stripping away residual markers of a former life; it was also the installation of – or a crossing over into – a surrogate status. Most traces of individual identity disappeared in the acid rinse of ward inmate.

De-institutionalization did more than empty gaslight-era institutions. Unlike shop-floors, which (though designed for efficiency) inadvertently brought workers together in ways that facilitated collective organizing during off-work hours, the temporal rhythms and spatial confines of the asylums were all inclusive. There was no down time or off-premise place for assembly, and what overt resistance could be mounted was likely to be short-lived and costly. De-institutionalization changed that and, in the process, re-drew the staging areas of agency. Though in practice much of the early policy was 'trans-institutionalization' (with nursing homes and proprietary 'adult homes' shouldering the shifted burden), this was also a period in which 'the movements of patients. . . . [became] the stuff of which markets are made' (Lewis *et al.*, 1989, p178). Housing options – whether rented hovels, family homes or shared makeshifts – expanded. A fledgling freedom found tenuous footholds in the humdrum routines of everyday life. So, eventually, did venues for assembly and social interaction. These are crucial to bringing together people who are effectively barred from many common 'third places' (between work and home), let alone competitive employment. Even so, formation of what Castells calls 'resistance identities' – identities that openly confronted those legitimized as 'appropriate' for subjects whose very capacity for self-determination was in question – had to await the arduous work and slow coming-together of former patient collectives. But by the late 1970s, they are documented fact (e.g. Chamberlin, 1979) and near textbook in quality. Produced by actors in 'positions/conditions devalued and/or stigmatized by the logic of domination' and committed to 'building trenches of resistance and survival on the basis of [alternative] principles' (Castells, 2004, p8), these early efforts were local and fragile; but they were also vital to producing the first cohorts of opposition spokespersons. Without them, a later 'recovery' movement (Jacobson, 2004) would have looked very different.

Agency in the sense of *intentional action in pursuit of self-determined ends* first comes to prominence in public mental health during the present-day recovery era. It had survived as resistance to stigmatized social identity, flourished *samizdat*-style in user-produced memoirs and howls of protest, and informed a still-influential archipelago of alternative treatment and re-integration programs (e.g., Stastny and Lehmann, 2007). A few progressive rehabilitation programs were quick to integrate what they could get away with billing for; others set themselves up as protective sanctuaries at odds with mass-[pharma-] production as therapeutic rule, and proceeded to chart the possibilities of peer-run alternatives (Clay, 2005). With official embrace of recovery, these once-sectarian experiments were belatedly hailed as pioneering works whose lessons need to be re-examined and re-appraised. In the process, agency itself comes in for closer scrutiny even if, at the time, it was only the exceptional practice of a few that attracted attention.

Consider how thoroughly the institutional fortunes of psychiatric disorder have been transformed over the last half-century. As an abeyance mechanism (Mizruchi, 1987), asylums served to warehouse people who were economically redundant, a burden to their families, and sometimes troublesome in civic life. Come de-institutionalization, and a de facto mental health system – sprawling, unplanned, ill co-ordinated, with no governing institutional authority – lurched into being. And with it, a stigmatized, outcast and forgotten population became a visible, ambiguous and (at times) freshly politicized social presence. Contained and closeted so long, a newly independent agency might have invited direct social attention, as, say, the reintegration prospects of demobilized soldiers (once) did. It didn't happen: institutional locus may have changed but social identity had not. Persons with psychiatric disabilities remained patients – if, at times, neglected or abandoned patients (Scull, 1977). Socially, their exile hadn't ended; living outside did not mean 'living outside mental illness' (Davidson, 2003). In the eyes of most others, when seen at all, their exercise of agency (homeless on the pavement, in the news for some extravagant crime) defaulted to pathology. As a factor in social reproduction, the de-institutionalized patient (no less than hospitalized forebears) figured primarily by providing means of livelihood for others.

Lest we be misunderstood: we're not arguing (anymore than Goffman did) that hospitalization robs people of any trace of agency. Nor, more to the point here, are we suggesting that being (and even benefiting from being) a patient necessarily negates all agency. But in the strong sense of pursuing self-defined ends – of constructing and working to realize 'life projects'– reclaiming agency is a more ambitious, risk-friendly, and singular undertaking. It's what Sen refers to as 'commitment' – and not in the sense of involuntary hospitalization.

Capabilities and participation

Developed over the course of several decades, Amartya Sen's 'capabilities' framework provides one way of recapturing agency in the strong sense (1992; 1993; 1999; Nussbaum, 2000; Alkire 2002; Hopper, 2007). Sen's approach revolutionizes the way we think of 'well-being' – especially as that goal takes shape in 'assisted development' schemes – and his founding premise provides the direct tie-in to participation that we mean to exploit here. Sen argues that development programs should explicitly make provision for 'persons [being] actively involved – given the opportunity – in shaping their own destiny and not just passive recipients of the fruits of cunning development [or treatment] programs' (1999, p53). 'Capabilities' is Sen's term for such practical opportunities. Income or goods alone do not suffice to capture the full complexities of well-being. Instead of resources alone, he argues that we need to appreciate the value of what people can be or do. In this sense, capabilities refer to substantive freedoms: these are the actionable options that open to someone as the combined result of resources, capacities and an enabling socio-cultural environment. How difficult it is to 'convert' such combinations into real opportunities is one measure of social distinctions such as gender, race, class or disability. Inequalities, from this perspective can be understood as constraints on substantive freedoms. Functionings, in turn, refer to concrete choices made or practices undertaken in a given context (including more complex 'social functionings' like the activities it takes to exercise citizenship).

The basic deprivations of poverty (ill health, premature mortality, inadequate shelter and nutrition, limited literacy, etc.) can be tallied in the ledger of functionings. But Sen refers to poverty as 'capability deprivation' to underscore the deeper forms of disadvantage and damage he means to take stock of. To be able to appear in public (or send one's children to school) without shame is one such capability that seems universally applicable. (Adam Smith's example (1776) of the 'linen shirt' that every 18th working man required for reputable public appearances is Sen's favorite illustration.) His basic point is the one we've already encountered with respect to stigma: poverty, like the long shadow of psychiatric diagnosis, not only erodes purchasing power but also poisons social regard and cramps participation in civic life (see also Sayer, 2005). Truly corrective interventions, then, will need to deal not only with material resources but also with symbolic representations, social practice and everyday engagements.

How well anti-poverty measures *actually enlarge the local field of genuinely available and valued life options* becomes Sen's preferred metric of development of any social group. Quality of life, in turn, becomes a richly textured matter of both basic securities and more complex capabilities, especially those that have to do with 'practical reason' and social 'affiliation' (Nussbaum, 2000). The first refers to the tricky business of reflective assessment, good judgment, wide-ranging imagination and courage that goes into planning a life of one's own authorship. The second takes in both opportunities for social interaction and what Rawls (2001, p59) calls 'the social bases of self-respect:' those elemental institutional provisions that must be in place 'if citizens are to have [or develop] a lively sense of their own worth as persons and to be able to advance their ends with self-confidence'. Sen has one last trick up his sleeve: the capabilities framework explicitly allows for – it actually *builds in* – a tension between being well provided for ('well-being') and pursuing one's own life projects/sense of dignity ('agency').

As participants in public mental-health systems understand only too well, that tension can become a problem in the most fundamental acts of care and custody. Agency is not only the wounded faculty ostensibly being treated; it also conditions – it enables, constrains and shapes – how effective care and basic securities are to be provided. Even when delivered with the best of intentions, 'cunning development [or treatment] programs' (Sen, 1999, p59) may come to grief if they ignore this fact. Put differently, the provision of needs-meeting goods may be stymied, and their intended purposes negated, if the terms of receiving them violate locally/culturally prized aspects of persons. When the costs of being a 'beneficiary' are reckoned in terms of damage to one's sense of oneself as an active agent of one's own destiny, for example, offers of assistance may be refused even if one suffers as a result (Hopper, 2006). People accused of 'spectacular violations' of social proprieties in the past, to take a ready instance, may place great stock in such conventions being scrupulously honored in the present.

Our contention here is that what is true of development in general should hold for knowledge development in particular – that is, should also pertain to research. After sketching how Sen's framework translates into participation as principle, the remainder of the chapter culls from our experience to show how this principle might practically be implemented in public mental health research.

Participation in public mental health

If capabilities supply a framework, participation is its working principle. And here we draw on the strong meaning it has acquired in the new development literature. Participation refers to a method of decision-making in which those who are directly affected by the action make the choice. In development work, it refers to a procedural rule for recognizing and negotiating those inescapable '"value judgments" that poverty-reducing (or, we might suggest, illness-managing) activities embody' (Alkire, 2002, p127; cf. Sen, 1992, p64). As bitter experience in both development and rehabilitation shows (Alkire, 2002, 2004; Abraham and Platteau, 2004; Wade and de Jong 2000), formal embrace of this principle still leaves plenty of room for inefficiency, misunderstanding, unintended consequences, and perceived injustice in practice. Participation takes time, demands commitment to process, and can be messy; it requires up-front investment of resources, committed stakeholders, clear rules (appeal, adjustment, etc.), a process for modifying rules as they become obstacles or obsolete, accommodating schedules and a tolerance for sub-optimal efficiencies. Of particular relevance here, effective participation may hinge on the cultivation of domain-specific competencies (Ibrahim and Alkire, 2007). More broadly, the resource demands of effective participation would inevitably force us to confront issues of equity (Anand *et al.*, 2006), the larger social debate that was effectively tabled while de-institutionalization got quietly under way. Our concern here is narrower and more manageable: what might 'maximizing participation' in public mental health research mean and how it might work – not, for our purposes, as an ICIDH-approved goal of rehabilitation (WHO, 2001), but as the presumptive *rule for research design and conduct*.

Like the diagnostic entities that define membership in the class 'mentally ill,' participation as used here is local, consequential and contested. Ideally, too, it is *informed* and the process in which it is engaged will be *transparent*, but invariably those aspects are matters of degree. Technical knowledge, the state of the relevant rehabilitative art, pertinent resources, individual effort and collective commitment will all affect how well participation is translated in practice. Consider basic treatment decisions, and let's assume for argument that access to evidence-based knowledge (where available) and practice- and/or experience-based information is assured. For a given diagnosis, then, various drug regimens can be described, the ranges of anticipated effects and 'side-effects' specified, and their respective likely impacts and probabilities of effect indicated to the extent possible. Assume, too, that competent counsel (an engaged provider, an informed user group) is available. Collect all these information resources and add an interested agent/patient – and the stage has still only been set for informed participation.[1]

To reiterate: Sen posits an 'irreducible' difference between two perspectives on quality of life: *well-being* views people as beneficiaries, whose needs and interests are addressed by others;[2] the second, or *agency* perspective, considers people in their capacity as 'doers and judges' – as discriminating actors accountable for their actions. The first considers people's interests from the standpoint of 'basic securities' – the elemental guarantees that must be in place for citizenship to be exercised; the second considers people as 'moral agents'. For Sen, this latter concern includes not only those zealously guarded remnants of self-respect that can get in the way of (much-needed but badly offered) help, but also 'commitments' (1977) – valued 'objectives, allegiances, obligations' the pursuit of which derives from an individual's conception of the good (Sen, 1985; p203f). Such projects extend the exercise of freedom in ways that move well beyond basic securities, and may even compromise or put them at risk. (Again, Sen explicitly recognizes and allows for such eventualities.) Research

---

[1] To anticipate a bit: The same considerations apply in research, but with a significant difference: in research, the participant's own welfare is rarely directly at issue.

[2] Tellingly, he sometimes refers to this as the 'patient' perspective.

falls clearly into the latter camp. If any direct value is to be realized, it will come from the exercise of agency itself and the deliberation that is ingredient to collective undertakings.

The challenge for mental health researchers is to make that possible. The remainder of this chapter considers how we might do that.

Putting participation into practice in research: five questions

What determines the limits of participation in research in actual practice?

This ultimately relates to issues of power and authority. Many of us have been involved with projects that make diligent provision for 'consumer advisory boards' or appoint consumer members to steering committees. Symbolic (and possibly token) inclusion aside, the real question is what role do these members play? Who has the authority and power to make decisions? Community participation in research means that community members, however defined (more below), are *involved in every stage of the research*, from developing the questions of interest, choosing methods of research, conducting research activities, analyzing data, developing findings and conclusions, and disseminating results. And by 'involved' we mean that community members (see below for defining 'community') identify the area of focus for the research. They review the existing literature, conduct key informant interviews with 'experts in the field' and speak with their colleagues and friends to gain an understanding of what is known on the selected topic. Community members then identify the research question to be examined. Then, with an understanding of the limitations and strengths of various research methodologies garnered through cross-trainings, the community members decide how the study should be conducted. They gather data and conduct analyses. All of this occurs in a context in which often the academics hold more power and authority, for despite efforts to level the playing field one must acknowledge the imbalance in training and knowledge concerning research. Finally, we would suggest that they also play substantive roles in thinking about how best to link the research to social change and activism. Here there may be more balance as often community members have greater experience than their academic partners.

What specific lessons can we draw from our experiences with collaborative research?

In Boston, several non-profit mental-health advocacy groups, the Department of Mental Health, and Consumer Quality Initiatives (a consumer-run research organization – see also Chapter 13 for issues on user-controlled research) came together with an academic partner (AL, co-author of this chapter) to create a mechanism to promote the participation of consumers of mental health services in research in Boston. While Boston is a community rich with academic research in mental health, few mechanisms for participation existed. This group initially received pilot funding from the Massachusetts Department of Mental Health and later federal funding. Representatives from each of the partner agencies began meeting monthly (as the Boston Community Academic Mental Health Partnership B-CAMHP Steering Committee) and with a clear and shared commitment to increasing participation. The first step was to define the community. This proved to be surprisingly difficult. Our initial working definition was 'consumers of mental health services in Boston'. But the well-known (if too little regarded) issue of *language* quickly rose to the fore. Several group members were offended by the use of the term 'consumer'; others at the table were strongly attached to the term. So before we could even structure an exploratory discussion we had to find a way to talk about our community that each partner could sit with. Ultimately, we grappled with these questions: are people with addiction issues part of the community? Do we use illness, disorder or disability language? How do we demonstrate a recovery perspective?

Ultimately, we arrived at the cumbersome but acceptable phrasing: 'people with mental health and addiction-recovery needs in Boston (MHARN)'. This first step, while time-consuming, involved critical discussions of difficult topics, and a consensus-building process. While in some ways this was 'merely' symbolic it was critical in order for each partner to feel included in the community and comfortable with our process.

Next we struggled with who should be at the table to develop an infrastructure that would enable us to conduct community-based participatory research within our newly defined community. At that point, this included representatives from each of the local advocacy groups engaged with the people with MHARN in Boston as well as academic partners and the state Mental Health Department. There is ongoing discussion about the expansion of the group and whether providers of services should be included. Certainly the academic partners and the state DMH are involved as stakeholders, and services providers might be defined similarly. Currently the group partners with service providers on specific research projects, when they are relevant or necessary for the conduct of the research; however, the core group has not been expanded to include service providers in the decision-making bodies of the partnership.

Full participation meant very different things to different partners. The development, design, conduct and activation of research is a complex process with many stages. With the traditional conduct of research, without participation of the community, full participation most often means role differentiation among the research team. For instance, the biostatistician might consider herself a full participant, but only actually be involved in certainly analytic aspects of the research. However, as we struggled with participation it was clear that for some participation meant being fully involved in all key decision-making; others preferred to be informed of key decisions but were not invested in making the decisions themselves. Participation for us thus came to mean that each partner determined the level of participation that worked for her. This of course, created a situation with unequal participation of partners so we created minimum guidelines for participation of partner agencies.

Full participation of people with MHARN in Boston – how did we capture this?

Developing a strategy to garner participation from the diverse community of people in Boston with mental health and addiction recovery needs has been perhaps our biggest challenge. There are a lot of ways to parse/describe diversity in the this community of 'consumers' and advocates: racial/ethnic, gender, age, diagnoses, severity of illness, role of substance abuse, stage of recovery, positive and negative experiences with services/treatment providers, etc. Our Steering Committee was initially composed of representatives from our collaborative partner agencies; this created several immediate and important challenges. First, our representation was solely limited to people who had chosen to affiliate with formal advocacy groups. These agencies in Boston are over-represented by whites, people with more stable life circumstances and people who are commonly considered to be at later stages in their recovery. As we looked around the table at the Steering Committee meetings it was evident that we did not reflect the diversity of people with MHARN in Boston.

As we began to develop our pilot study we explored multiple methods for recruiting research associates. The group was committed to hiring 6–8 people with MHARN to serve as the RAs for the project. The easy option would have been to recruit 6 research assistants from within these partner agencies. But we were acutely aware of the types of people who would be excluded by this all too handy process. For this reason, we chose to post flyers at treatment sites, resource centres and universities, take out ads in local newspapers and online,[3] and make use of the networks of each partner to distribute the job description. We indicated in that description that preference would be given to people who had used psychiatric emergency room services (PER) themselves, as our pilot study was of PER services. This would ensure that our researchers would have in common the lived experiences of our research participants. This recruitment strategy proved surprisingly effective. In two weeks we received more than 100 applicants for the 5–10 hours/week research assistant positions.

The letters and emails only reinforced our suspicion that we had not even begun to understand the extent of our community's diversity. There was tremendous variation in education level and work history. We had inquiries from professionals, who were working full-time and who often had lived quietly with their depression, anxiety or other symptoms for many years. These full-time workers were interested to see if they could participate, in addition to maintaining their regular employment. A few noted that this was the first time they had seen a job posting where their life experience of having used psychiatric emergency services was considered an asset. Other applicants had been out of the workforce for many years; some sought us out independently, others in partnership with job coaches, treatment providers or family members. The pool kept growing: people were referred from our partner agencies, students from local colleges applied, and clients from psychiatric rehabilitation work programs. A small committee was formed to cull through the applications; 18 were selected to be interviewed and rated by multiple reviewers. Our interview protocol was developed in Steering Committee and included questions about work history, work ethic, schedule flexibility, problem-solving, any research experience, and the interviewee's experience with our partner agencies and formal mental health advocacy. This last question was included in order to ensure that we did not inadvertently hire a pool of RAs all of whom were connected with advocacy agencies.

Finally, while our interviewers were non-clinicians the group quickly realized that we could not avoid a discussion of people's level of functioning in the assessment process, especially since a large part of their role would be to conduct interviews. Discussions of diversity of level of functioning were difficult, and it was often the community members who were foremost proponents of hiring people at 'higher levels of functioning' or 'later

---

[3] **Craigslist** is a central network of online communities, featuring free online classified advertisements – with jobs, internships, housing, personals, for sale/barter/wanted, services, community, gigs, resume, and pets categories – and forums on various topics (Wikipedia, accessed fall 2008).

stages of recovery'. We resolved this issue by agreeing that while all the RAs would receive training in all aspects of the research project, we would allow for flexibility in the actual job tasks. For example, if an RA was not able to conduct interviews, she could become more active transcribing their colleagues interviews.

This related closely to another important aspect of participation for people with MHARN in research. The uncertain course of most severe psychiatric conditions, even when well managed, is such that most people have periods of time when their symptoms and/or their functioning changes. Actually, this is true for all of us: whether it be our health, flagging commitment, or pressing demands from other aspects of our lives, our work takes on fluctuating patterns of functioning and productivity. For partners in a research team, periods of lower functioning necessitate substitutions or adjustments in work assignments. For example, we have had several periods of a week or more when a community member RA was out for health-related reasons. We have been able to accommodate these patterns by minimizing the number of project related tasks that must be done by one specific person. In order to sustain that degree of flexibility, we have trained multiple people in each aspect of the conduct and management of the project.

The larger challenge has been in creating a process of 're-entry' back in to the team following an extended absence. As our research is a developmental process it is often hard to return to where someone left off. In our experience, it was the high level of motivation among our community RAs that facilitated this process. RAs are sent minutes of meetings, all documents, and even audiotapes of events that have been missed during their time away from the project. These protocols set high expectations on all involved and helped equip us to address the issue of power differentials discussed below.

As academics engaged in community-based participatory-action research, we look to our partners to inform us as to the extent to which we have promoted full participation and included the diversity of the community in the work. Typically, these partners hail from non-profit or advocacy leadership. Thus, the greatest difficulty in achieving diversity in community involvement in research may be in discussing with advocacy groups the ways in which their good efforts do not, and really could never, capture the true diversity of people with MHARN in the community. Clearly, the easier path is to work with existing advocates and groups and declare that the community has been represented. The tougher challenge lies in determining who is not represented and developing strategies to reach out to those excluded voices. Expanding the reach of participation in this way ultimately benefits both the research and advocacy communities: it compels each group to examine and justify the de facto criteria of membership.

How can we acknowledge and deal with power differences among the participants?

There are some concrete factors that determine power differences in these types of partnerships. The first is resources. Our partnership was ultimately funded by a federal grant to the University. Thus, no matter how great the effort to balance power across the participants, the academic partners ultimately controlled the resources. This formality also meant that the academic partners bore the ultimate responsibility of reporting to the funders and ensuring the integrity of the project. And so the academic partners were the formal interface with institutional review boards and NIMH. This included attendance at IRB meetings to discuss the project, the institutional management of budgets and sub-contracts, and both financial and research activity annual reporting.

The literature on CBPR typically describes a clean power differential (favouring the academics) and identifies the focus of capacity-building on the community side. In our case, this oversimplified matters greatly. In the first place, some of our researchers are part of the 'community' of MHARN in Boston; overlap, not distinction, was built in from the start. Second, for purposes of the research at hand, 'expertise' was clearly a distributed good and in some instances favoured those with first-hand experience. Third, the literature tends to describe partner recruitment practices that were more restrictive than our own; this tends to produce more selective representation of consumers. (The RAs we hired spanned the full spectrum of 'functioning' and made for more inclusive ranks.) Finally, although often written about as static and durable, power differences should shift and reconfigure in the course of truly participatory research – else what's the point of embracing capacity-building? In our case, enhancements of capacity occurred on both side of the (blurred) divide. In practice, power – with the exception of formal institutional accountability (mentioned above) – reflected the needs of the task at hand and the vagaries of expertise available to deal with it.

At the same time, it's important to note that we did encounter what the capabilities literature sometimes alludes to as damaged or stunted agency, though not incorrigibly so (Sayer, 2005; Nussbaum, 2000). Specifically, many of the people with MHARN had been excluded from decision-making and denied power and authority so frequently and for so long, that they did not seek or demand what our academic and state health department partners 'naturally' saw as the perquisites of full participation. Early cross-trainings deliberately covered all of the tasks and decisions in a research process in order to give people an overview of the participatory possibilities that would be shaping up. In addition, each partner group conducted trainings in its own area of expertise – for example, issues of importance to parents of people with MHARN. In this way, we meant to 'de-privilege' the research or academic claim to exclusive knowledge. While these trainings were initially intended to 'cross-train' community members and academics – with community members sharing their lived experience and researchers their research knowledge and skills – in fact, the transfer of knowledge was not always limited to these expected discrepancies. For instance, when NAMI members trained the group to better understand the work they do, it became clear that NAMI's experience and efforts with recruiting community participants for a number of advocacy efforts could usefully inform our efforts in recruiting research participants. Similarly, understanding how the advocacy group mobilized their network turned out to facilitate our own research efforts.

How to deal with the complex relationship between research and advocacy?

Discrepant agendas are the last problem we'll address. Getting it right in research is a slow crawl (research is a 'poor parallel-parker', to use Richard Powers' phrase, 1992), and CBPR is among the slowest types of research. The advocacy world moves quickly and often in response to specific events and deadlines. This can make for an awkward match of agendas and timetables. So while CBPR facilitates the movement of findings into policy and practice more efficiently than other research processes, by advocacy's reckoning *publicly sharable* results are slow to come and, worse, subject to a host of vetting procedures (e.g., for some purposes, peer review). Also, effective research in public mental-health often requires access to venues that can be tricky to secure, dependent upon slowly evolving (and easily destabilized) relationships of trust. Unless explicitly acknowledged and worked through as part of the ground rules of a joint enterprise, such contingencies can make for abrasive misunderstandings.

We have received calls, for example, asking us if we have any 'smoking guns' related to psychiatric emergency room services as the state develops legislation related to such care. Often these calls come from advocates working to push through specific pieces of legislation – sometimes the same advocacy groups involved in the research. So there can be a good deal of tension and disagreement over what to provide, and under what auspices (formal, informal, not for attribution) in the service of our collective cause. Without clear agreement on products (or deliverables) and timetables, we risked disappointing our allies and scuttling our hopes for collectively-informed results.

Our strategy for managing this tension has been to work from the beginning to develop research guidelines that indicate when dissemination activities can occur and, importantly, to agree that at a minimum each partner must sign off to each activity, even if they choose not to be directly involved. In practice, of course, things proved more complicated. Partners routinely write about the partnership, for example, when reporting on the agency's outreach and collaboration efforts. The reality is that a central committee can only manage disseminating activities and findings to the extent that each partner is committed to a shared agenda, while recognizing that the shared agenda inevitably represents only a portion of more encompassing individual agency/academic efforts.

CONCLUSION

For medicine to be personal – integrated into individual life circumstances and plans (Deegan, 2005) – the working premise must be that an illness is embedded in a life rather than the other way around. If one is interested and equipped, participating in the protected precincts of mental health services research can be its own reward; it may even have spill-over effects elsewhere. Participation is not only good discipline but social practice as well. It introduces self to others, teaches one to voice one's own position and to listen to that of others, instills self-confidence, builds the mutual currency of respect that we all depend upon. And although we are mindful that participation be engaged, described and gauged as a domain-specific achievement (Ibrahim and Alkire, 2007), we are also struck by the general-purpose proficiency that participation fuels.[4] Like working, deliberation, aspiration and other agency-infused faculties, participation is a competency that feeds on practice (Joas, 1997).

This doesn't mean that participation is a panacea, is right for all users, or is immune to fraud. The annals of disillusionment in international development projects are thick with

---

[4] As so to the caveat about domain-specific contingencies of agency should be added this more encompassing definition of empowerment, in the (somewhat surprising) words of the World Bank: 'enhancing the capacity of poor people to influence the state institutions that affect their lives, by strengthening their participation in political processes and local decision-making ... [and] removing the barriers – political, legal, and social – that work against particular groups and building the assets of poor people to enable them to engage effectively in markets' (World Development Report, 2000–2001, p39).

accounts of counterfeit invitations to participate, re-assertions of traditional authority relations, and coy hedging through the simple expedient of deliberately keeping the terms and conditions of participation ambiguous (Alkire, 2004; Abraham and Platteau, 2004). In public mental health, the most scrupulously documented account of state-level 'transformative' reform (so often called for in the US today) found that real service user participation was restricted (by oversight? by intent? by dint of uncorrected technical deficiencies?) to the actual design and practice of services – an important, but structurally secondary and derivative field of action, one far removed from the grittier discussions of reimbursement strategies and institutional realignment (Jacobson, 2004). And although difficult to calibrate, the costs of token participation – in further disillusionment with an already-suspect system, in disgust with the academic enterprise, in rekindled feelings of betrayal, in reinforced cluelessness among researchers – are doubtless formidable.

But all of this is only to recognize that real participation – like any power-sharing agreement – will be difficult and contentious. In a system too often characterized by bold reforms that leave lives unchanged, and by promises that somehow come up short on follow-through, that may be a welcome development.

REFERENCES

Abraham, A. and Platteau, J.-P. (2004) Participatory development: Where culture creeps in. In: V. Rao and M. Walton (Eds) *Culture and Public Action*, Palo Alto: Stanford University Press, pp 210–233.

Alkire, S. (2002) *Valuing Freedoms*. New York: Oxford University Press.

Alkire, S. (2004) 'Culture, poverty and external intervention'. In: V. Rao and M. Walton (Eds) *Culture and Public Action*, Palo Alto: Stanford University Press, pp 185–209.

Alkire, S. (2007) Measuring freedoms alongside wellbeing. In: I. Gough, J.A. McGregor (Eds.) *Wellbeing in Developing Countries*, New York: Cambridge University Press, pp. 93–108.

Alsop, R., Bertelsen, M.F. and Holland, J. (2006) *Empowerment in Practice*, Washington, D.C.: World Bank.

Anand, S., Peter, F. and Sen, A. (Eds) (2006) *Public Health, Ethics, and Equity*, New York: Oxford University Press.

Bourdieu, P. (1977) *Outline of a Theory of Practice*, New York: Cambridge University Press.

Castells, M. (2004) *The Power of Identity*, 2nd edition, Malden, MA: Blackwell.

Chamberlin, J. (1979) *On Our Own: Patient-Controlled Alternatives to the Mental Health System*, New York: McGraw-Hill.

Clay, S. (2005) (Ed) *On Our Own Together*, Nashville: Vanderbilt University Press.

Colton, C.W. and Manderscheid, R.W. (2006) Congruencies in increased mortality rates, years of potential life lost, and causes of death among public mental health clients in eight states, *Preventing Chronic Disease*, 3, 1–14. Available online at: http://www.cdc.gov/pcd/issues/2006/apr/05_0180. htm, accessed 25/10/08.

Davidson, L. (2003) *Living Outside Mental Illness*, New York: New York University Press.

Deegan, P.E. (2005) The importance of personal medicine: A qualitative study of resilience in people with psychiatric disabilities, *Scandinavian Journal of Public Health*, **33**, 1–7.

Favret-Saada, J. (1990) About participation, *Culture, Medicine and Psychiatry*, **14**, 189–199.

Fraser, N. (1998) Social justice in the age of identity politics: redistribution, recognition, and participation, *Tanner Lectures on Human Values*, **19** (Ed) Grethe Peterson, Salt Lake City, University of Utah Press.

Goffman, E. (1956) The nature of deference and demeanor. *American Anthropologist*, **58**, 475–499.

Goffman, E. (1961) *Asylums*, New York: Doubleday.

Goffman, E. (1963) *Stigma*, New York: Doubleday.

Hopper, K. (2006) Redistribution and its discontents: On the possibility of committed work in public mental health and like settings, *Human Organization*, **65**, 218–226.

Hopper, K. (2007) Rethinking social recovery: What a capabilities approach might offer, *Social Science & Medicine*, **65**, 868–879.

Ibrahim, S. and Alkire, S. (2007) Agency and empowerment: A proposal for internationally comparable indicators, *Oxford Development Studies* **35**, 379–403.

Jacobson, N. (2004) *In Recovery*, Nashville: Vanderbilt University Press.

Joas, H. (1997) *The Creativity of Action*, Chicago: University of Chicago.

Lewis, D., Shadish, W. and Lurigio, A. (1989) Policies of inclusion and the mentally ill: Long-term care in a new environment, *Journal of Social Issues*, **45**, 173–186.

Link, B.G., Struening, E.L. and Rahav, M. *et al.* (1997) On stigma and its consequences: evidence from a longitudinal study of men with dual diagnoses of mental illness and substance abuse. *Journal of Health and Social Behavior*, **38**, 177–190.

Luhrmann, T.M. (1989) *Persuasions of the Witch's Craft*, Cambridge: Harvard University Press.

Mizruchi, E.H. (1987) *Regulating Society* (Revised edition), Chicago: University of Chicago.

Nussbaum, M.C. (2000) *Women and Human Development*. New York: Cambridge University Press.

Olson, K. (2001) Distributive justice and the politics of difference. *Critical Horizons*, **2**, 5–32.

Powers, R. (1992) *The Gold Bug Variations*, New York: Harper.

Rawls, J. (2001) *Justice as Fairness*, Cambridge: Harvard University Press.

Rosenfield, S. (1997) Labeling mental illness: The effects of received services and perceived stigma on life satisfaction. *American Sociological Review*, **62**, 660–672.

Sayer, A. (2005) *The Moral Significance of Class*. New York: Cambridge University Press.

Scull, A. (1977) *Decarceration: Community Treatment and the Deviant – A Radical View*, Englewood-Cliffs: Prentice-Hall.

Sen, A. (1977) Rational fools: a critique of the behavioural foundations of economic theory, *Philosophy and Public Affairs*, **6**, 317–344.

Sen, A. (1985) Well-being, agency and freedom: The Dewey Lectures 1984, *The Journal of Philosophy*, **82**, 169–221.

Sen, A. (1992) *Inequality Re-examined*, Oxford: Clarendon.

Sen, A. (1993) 'Capability and Well-being'. In: M.C. Nussbaum and A. Sen (Eds) *The Quality of Life*, Oxford: Oxford University Press, pp 44–55.

Sen, A. (1999) *Development as Freedom*, New York: Knopf.

Smith, A. (1776) *An Inquiry into the Nature and Causes of the Wealth of Nations*. New York: Modern Library (1994).

Stastny, P. and Lehmann, P. (Eds) (2007) *Alternatives Beyond Psychiatry*, Berlin: Peter Lehmann Publishing.

U.S., Department of Health and Human Services (1999) *Mental Health: A Report of the Surgeon General—Executive Summary*, Rockville, MD. U.S. Department of Health and Human Services, Substance Abuse and Mental Health Services Administration, Center for Mental Health Services, National Institutes of Health, National Institute of Mental Health.

Wade, D.T. and de Jong, B.A. (2000) Recent advances in rehabilitation. *British Medical Journal*, **320**, 1385–1388.

World Health Organization (2001) *International Classification of Functioning, Disability and Health*, Geneva: WHO.

World Bank (2001) *World Development Report, 2000–2001: Attacking Poverty*, Washington, D.C.: World Bank, p39.

CHAPTER 7

Purposes and Goals

Purposes and Goals of Service User Involvement in Mental Health Research

**Larry Davidson, Priscilla Ridgway,
Timothy Schmutte and Maria O'Connell**
*Program for Recovery and Community Health,
Yale University, New Haven, CT, USA*

This chapter outlines the reasons why there is a particular need in mental health research for involving people with first-hand experience, as compared to other medical fields. It goes on to discuss in detail the primary purposes of such involvement, i.e. improving the quality, relevance and utility of research, and impacting on the lives of service users, with specific reference to the recovery movement. In relation to the first purpose, the authors explain how involving people with lived experience of mental health conditions in research can improve the quality of research which uses existing conventional approaches, designs and methods as well as involving them in order to develop new approaches. Examples are given for the application of both strategies. In relation to the second purpose, to impact on lives, the authors discuss service user involvement as a means of protecting human rights and assuring the ethical conduct of research as well as providing an opportunity for service users to take an active and central role in the setting of research priorities and the development of research questions. Implications are outlined and practical examples are provided.

INTRODUCTION

> ...the silenced are not just incidental to the curiosity of the researcher but are the masters of inquiry into the underlying causes of the events in their world. In this context research becomes a means of moving them beyond silence into a quest to proclaim the world.
>
> (Paulo Freire on participatory research, 1993, px)

Handbook of Service User Involvement in Mental Health Research   Edited by Jan Wallcraft, Beate Schrank and Michaela Amering
Copyright © 2009 John Wiley & Sons, Ltd

We take our charge for this chapter to be to answer the seemingly simple question of *why* include service users in the mental health research enterprise. Other chapters have dealt with the context, history, and principles of this movement which, taken together, have led to a situation in which the 'why' question may be in danger of being overlooked. In other words, we have come to a point at which we include service users in research as a matter of course, because it is the 'right' thing, the fashionable or politically correct thing, to do. To derive optimal benefit from this innovation, however, we think it important to keep in mind why we are doing it. Especially given some of the challenges described in previous chapters, it may be useful to remind ourselves of what we are hoping to accomplish by this concerted – and, we suggest, ultimately political – act of inclusion.

We suggest that there are at least two different and distinct agendas we are trying to accomplish by involving service users in mental health research. In this chapter, we describe each of these agendas, indicated as purposes 1 and 2, and under each of these we describe two specific goals or objectives (i.e. 1a, 1b, 2a, and 2b). Taken together, we suggest that these agendas highlight challenges that, if met, will serve to change and enhance both sides of the research spectrum:

- the research itself and those who seek to understand the experience and improve the care of service users
- the lives of the persons who have first-hand experiences of the phenomena we seek to understand.

As 'traditional' research (i.e. research that has not involved service users) also claims to share both of these agendas, we would like first to point out how user-involved research may approach these same agendas differently.

In traditional research methodology, researchers are typically seen as the experts – the keepers of knowledge. In typical scenarios, researchers design the protocol, based on what they think is pertinent (or what has been commissioned by funders), interview their 'subjects,' and then return to their ivory towers to analyse and interpret the findings. All the while, the funders and those with the lived experience wait eagerly on the sidelines for the final report – at times only to hear what service users may have been able to tell them in the first place. It is this perceived hierarchy of knowledge acquisition and dissemination that separates traditional researchers from those who are truly in the know and, as a by-product, also accounts for the fact that it takes on the average 25 years for medical breakthroughs to make their way into and transform routine care. By keeping people at a distance through complex methodologies, jargon, and uncommunicated agendas, the power associated with knowledge remains primarily in the hands of individuals with the research expertise, and secondarily in the hands of their funders and the policy makers who use the research, and not with the people who are (supposed) to be most benefited from such understanding. Moreover, the findings themselves may not accurately reflect the issues that are of most concern to the people most directly impacted by the conditions of interest (i.e. the service users), since they were not involved in the articulation of the 'problem' in the first place (see Humphreys and Rappaport, 1993 for discussion of the definition of social problems).

It is quite a different scenario in which service users are involved in all aspects of research design and implementation, and in which the power and knowledge are thereby shared among researchers and service users. In participatory research methodologies, those with lived experience become essential to the formulation of research questions, identification of target populations, design of protocols, collection and analysis of data, and interpretation and sharing of the study findings. While both traditional and service-user-guided research have the goal of *understanding* in hope of eventually curing or preventing disease and refining practices to enhance the lives of the people of concern, service user-guided research has *change* as an explicit goal in and of itself. This change comes about through the *immediate impact* of shared power and knowledge, the development of new valued social roles, and the enhanced quality, relevance, and utility of research.

Due to limited space and the introductory nature of this volume, we limit ourselves in this chapter to these two primary purposes of impacting the quality of research (#1), and impacting the lives of service users (#2), with two goals or objectives under each. We welcome others to add to this beginning list; we acknowledge that what we offer here is a preliminary draft and represents our collective first efforts to forge new research partnerships that we hope will contribute to the transformation of mental health services.

Purpose 1:

The involvement of service users will improve the quality, relevance, and utility of mental health research, as it will be informed by persons' lived experiences of illness and recovery, their perspectives on what opportunities and supports they have found helpful or harmful, and what role they have played in their own adaptation to illness and recovery

It would seem to be obvious to suggest that including people with first-hand experiences of a certain condition would be advantageous to a research team investigating that condition. This suggestion loses its obviousness, however, when we pause to recognize that it has not yet been adopted in any other branch of medicine as a matter of principle. That is, a researcher in oncology may have had, or may develop, cancer as a matter of coincidence or as a matter of deriving a sense of mission out of adversity (i.e. to prevent others from having to go through what one went through, or to overcome it). But there has not yet been a concerted effort to attract into cancer research investigators or staff who themselves have had the condition being studied. Such an approach to involving patients or service users in research may be just beginning to emerge slowly in some branches of medicine and health-related research (e.g. Boote, Telford and Cooper, 2002; Pickard *et al.*, 2007), but the most concerted efforts thus far have been in the area of mental health. We suggest that there are several reasons why the need for involvement of service users may be more pressing in mental health, many of which speak to the importance of improving the quality, relevance, and utility of mental health research.

That our research needs to be improved should not require explanation or justification. That we take as a given. There are, however, multiple reasons that mental illnesses specifically require a first-person perspective, including the following:

1. These are poorly understood conditions about which we know little, and for which we need to establish a more accurate descriptive base grounded in experience, both first-hand and through the lens of family members, practitioners, and others (Strauss, 1994).

2. These are conditions in which the person is able to play an active role beyond adhering to a prescribed medication regimen, and understanding the nature of this role requires consideration of that person's perspective (Davidson, Stayner and Haglund, 1998; Strauss *et al.,* 1987).
3. These are conditions from which many people are able to recover over time, but in ways and through means not accounted for by the current mental health system (Davidson, Harding and Spaniol, 2005).
4. These are conditions which have been complicated and perhaps even obfuscated by the problematic social conditions within which people afflicted with them have been confined (i.e. first the asylum and now stigma, poverty, homelessness or substandard housing, unemployment, social isolation).

We suggest that first-hand experience of the terrain would be one strategy among several that would be useful for teasing apart these different influences. Sample relevant questions emerging from first-hand experience would be: What do mental illnesses look like? How do they interfere with people's everyday lives? What factors impacting people's lives have nothing to do with the illness per se, but with secondary consequences of having the illness? What helps people get better, and/or get their lives back, once ravaged by a mental illness? What practices actually exacerbate the person's difficulties and present their own iatrogenic effects? What can the person do to actively cope with and manage these conditions? We suggest also that there are two primary vehicles for answering such questions:

- first (Goal 1a), by including people with lived experience in research projects that use existing, conventional approaches, designs, and methods
- second (Goal 1b), by involving people with lived experience in development of new approaches, designs, and methods expressly tailored to the subject matter of mental illness and recovery.

We describe each below.

Goal 1a:

To improve the quality, relevance, and utility of the implementation of conventional research approaches, designs, and methods by ensuring that the perspective of individuals with the conditions of interest is incorporated

It may be obvious, but it needs to be stated: Asking service users to evaluate a program or rate their satisfaction with services they have used is not the same as service user involvement in research. On the other hand, it also should be noted that involving service users in research does not necessarily require restructuring an entire research agenda or protocol. Service user involvement in research does require re-conceptualizing the role of the service user from simply rater, subject, or participant (primarily passive or reactive roles) to one of partner, co-researcher, collaborator, or principal investigator (active roles). A ready example of how the involvement of users can increase the quality, relevance, and utility of existing research methods is provided by user-led and/or staffed service-satisfaction teams. Within the US, several states (including Colorado, Kansas,

Pennsylvania, Ohio, New York, New Mexico, and Georgia), many counties, and some local mental-health authorities actively engage teams of service users as evaluators in the ongoing monitoring and assessment of the quality of services, service satisfaction, and other program audits. User-focused program monitoring has also taken place in England (Rose *et al.,1998*) and Australia (Malins *et al.,* 2006). In these cases, users are not only responding to survey questions administered by others (typically practitioners), but are themselves the ones developing, administering, analysing and reporting data from surveys, audits, and other assessment tools.

The methods used by these teams may be quite conventional, but the addition of service users is thought to generate many benefits, including:

- the development of more relevant outcome indicators, more sensitive process and service-use measures, and more user-friendly formats for collecting data (Campbell, 1997)
- improving the quality of the information attained from service recipients, who are more likely to be open and forthcoming when questioned by peers than by program staff who serve them (Polowszyk *et al.*, 1993)
- increasing the freedom service recipients have to advance and resolve grievances or to seriously critique the services they receive, without fear of reprisal, thereby improving accountability to the primary stakeholders
- suggesting practical change strategies to improve service provision and monitoring change efforts (Linhorst and Eckert, 2002)
- over time, increasing the potential for enhancing program performance and the quality of services and care provided, thereby ensuring that services are effective and responsive to service user needs and expressed preferences (Linhorst and Eckert, 2002), thereby improving the lives of those served by the service system.

Other examples range from service users being members of steering committees for projects, and being researchers or staff on projects (Beresford and Evans, 1999; Linhorst and Eckert, 2002; Rapp, Shera and Kisthardt, 1993), to the development of entirely user-run projects. Of particular interest are participatory action research approaches which involve service users in all phases of the research enterprise, from framing the initial questions, selecting the instruments, and collecting and analysing the data, to deciding which findings are relevant and how these relevant findings will be shared and with whom (Rogers and Palmer-Erbs, 1994; Ochocka, Janzen and Nelson, 2002). As the extensive involvement of service users in such studies has often led to the development and use of innovative approaches, designs, or methods, these studies also fall under Goal 1b, and are described in more detail below.

Goal 1b:

To improve the quality, relevance, and utility of mental health research through the development of new approaches, designs, and methods that are well-suited, if not explicitly tailored, to the nature of the subject matter of interest

Two examples of participatory-action research projects that involved service users from conception illustrate how involving users can often result in the development of innovative approaches and methods as well. In a first series of initiatives led by Barbara Schneider in Calgary, Canada, service users came together with academic researchers to conduct interviews and focus groups with individuals with serious mental illnesses. Their aim was to generate policy and practice recommendations regarding strategies for assisting individuals to exit homelessness; and for improving communication and relationships between people with schizophrenia and their medical professionals. While the methods used in collecting and analysing these data may have been conventional, the impact of the findings and the perspectives of the user researchers led to innovations in how the findings were interpreted and disseminated. Wanting to convey the power and poignancy of the participants and their narratives, the user researchers not only participated in writing the usual research reports but also chose to compose a performance piece in which they directly, immediately gave voice to the insights they gained from their interviews and focus groups. Reading dramatically from verbatim transcript passages, the users were able to convey the relevance of their findings to a professional audience in a vivid, personal, and persuasive way that would be hard to imagine emanating from an academic or magazine article. They also produced a DVD of this performance, so that it could be used as a vehicle for disseminating study findings beyond their local community.

Perhaps even more importantly, and impressively, though, was what they decided to do with their findings in relation to their 'other' audience; i.e. individuals with schizophrenia. The academic–user collaborative decided that the study findings needed to be fed back not only to the usual audience of academics and practitioners/policy makers, but also to those individuals for whom the study held perhaps the most promise. To this end, they produced a very creative and useful small book/large pamphlet full of pictures and stories about ways to resolve what they describe as 'dilemmas of care and control'. As they explain on the overleaf:

> People who care for us want to help us, but they also have authority and power over us. A relationship intended to be positive, enabling, and empowering is at the same time controlling and disempowering.
>
> (Schneider et al., 2007)

What they then offer in the book/pamphlet are descriptions and illustrations of the strategies that their participants had found to be useful in navigating the various dilemmas in which care and control come into conflict. Written from the perspective of the participants (/user researchers), what results is an extremely useful and effective self-help tool for people with schizophrenia seeking to make the most of the mental health services they currently are being offered.

A second example is provided by a study currently underway involving a member of our own team. While in the previous case the academic researcher initiated the partnership with users, in this case it was the reverse. In this case, an academic researcher was approached by a grassroots advocacy organisation made up of service users, family members, and other advocates. The members of the organisation were dissatisfied with the degree of influence they felt they were able to exert on their state mental health authority through their usual channels of conducting programme evaluations and issuing reports – at times lengthy – that they were convinced no one ever read. They sought consultation on how they might do their research and evaluation differently so that it would be more engaging and have more impact, rather than simply sit in someone's filing cabinet (as so many mental health reports seem to do). As one principle, they decided not to duplicate the efforts of any other body, so that their evaluations should not merely repeat those of the state mental-health authority or the various accrediting and regulatory bodies, each of which conducted its own evaluation or program audits. They also decided that they wanted their research to be grounded in and reflect their own concerns, which had less to do with program performance per se (and with concepts such as 'access,' 'attrition,' or 'connect-to-care rates') and more to do with whether or not (or the ways in which) recipients of services were benefiting from their contacts with the mental health system. Did receiving a service or, more commonly, a package of services, from the mental health system actually make a difference in people's lives? How could they tell? And what would they do with such information should they be able to collect it? These questions formed the basis for a collaboration between service users, advocates, and researchers which was in everyone's interests and promised to be mutually beneficial.

In consultation with the academic researcher, the users and advocates decided to focus directly and explicitly on people's everyday lives – as that was their primary interest – and to obtain training in carrying out qualitative interviews in order to access data on this topic. They then came up with the key questions they wanted to ask, including – at the end of the interview – the novel question of:

> If you could buy your own mental health services and supports, what would you spend the money on?

A total of twelve service users expressed an interest in being trained to conduct interviews, and, following the training, eight users conducted a total of 80 interviews on what they came to call 'a day in the life'. The excitement and interest generated by the interviews made the user-interviewers reluctant to turn the data over to anyone else, so they then asked to be trained in how to analyse the qualitative data. Currently, they are in the process of analysing the 80 interviews and developing creative ways to share their findings once completed. Like the Calgary group, they are developing new and innovative means for conveying the importance of their work, as their entire initiative has been driven by their desire to influence policy and practice in ways which they were unable to do by giving didactic presentations or issuing reports.

As suggested by these examples, the benefits of participatory research methodologies not only serve to enhance the research itself, but also to extend to the intra-personal realm. Researchers and policy makers are afforded opportunities to work with individuals in a new manner: no longer just as 'patient' or 'service user' but as 'colleague,' 'researcher,' or 'collaborator'. These new roles have added benefits for the user (described further in the next section), but also for those traditionally holding the power of knowledge. Not only are there opportunities for service users to be seen in new roles and to identify strengths and other areas of competencies, but the presence of service users in research serves as a constant reminder of just who services are accountable to (Byas *et al.*, 2002).

Purpose 2:

To enable persons with psychiatric disabilities to establish their claim to one of the fundamental social and cultural institutions intended to serve them as an important step in the overall process of the restoration of their full citizenship in society

It is possible to view the recovery movement within mental health as a broad-scale quality or performance improvement initiative, in which case the goals and objectives described above would be sufficient to warrant service user involvement in research. From our perspective, however, the introduction of recovery into mental health has represented first and foremost a civil rights movement (Davidson, 2006). It is for this reason that we think it important to include an additional purpose and additional goals and objectives related to the civil rights dimension of recovery. That is, involving service users in research not only improves the quality of the research carried out but also improves the lives of the service users involved – not only as researchers who are employed, and not only as the subjects of, participants in, or indirect beneficiaries of the improved research that is conducted; but also, as one vehicle among many to reclaiming their broader membership in society. Research and evaluation remain major vehicles for changing practice, preventing diseases, and discovering cures. People in recovery are also entitled to have access to these social and cultural institutions to ensure that they conduct their business in ways that are most beneficial to the people they are intended to serve. Empowerment comes about in part when people lay claim to, and exert control over, the resources they view as rightfully theirs. In mental health, these claims extend beyond the boundaries of the service system to those institutions which influence and shape the service system, including but not limited to the enterprises of research and evaluation. (Other examples include governmental agencies responsible for funding or monitoring care, the pharmaceutical industry, etc.)

In this case, we also envision two primary ways that service users can go about staking their claims and exerting control over the research and evaluation enterprises in which society invests considerable resources. The first way (Goal 2a) involves protecting the rights of research participants, while the second way (Goal 2b) involves the participation of service users in setting the research and evaluation agenda. Each of these is described below.

Goal 2a:

To ensure protection of the rights of individuals with psychiatric disabilities as participants in research through their participation in design, implementation, and human subjects/ethics review of research protocols

One important purpose for involving users in research is to advance the interests of the user community through the protection of human rights and the assurance of ethical conduct in the research enterprise. Service users have been involved on some local and federal research review panels or as consultants to large-scale research projects since the late 1980s in the US. More recently, service users in the US have articulated research issues and demanded user-oversight and involvement in every stage of publicly funded research projects (Campbell, 2001). The issues they identified included: human subjects protection and avoidance of unethical research through the advancement of choice, true informed consent and the avoidance of coercion; the minimization of risk through provision of a variety of supports and safeguards; respect for culturally and otherwise diverse populations; and the education of the user community in research methods and models.

Further, they oppose the misuse of research and the use of coercion in research activities, and support research that addresses issues of relevance to the user community. Their active participation in discussions, critique of research issues and processes, and input into decision-making provides advocacy and acts as a watchdog protecting the rights and needs of the user community.

Given the history of abuse of minority populations in the US, it has been a persuasive argument within this context to suggest, for example, that the Tuskegee syphilis experiments (in which African American patients determined to have syphilis were denied treatment and were not even informed of their condition) would never have been conducted had African Americans been involved in research or oversight capacities. Not limited to the US context, of course, user involvement in research has also been the object of recent broad policy mandates in Great Britain and Australia (Boote, Telford and Cooper, 2002; Happell and Roper, 2007; Telford and Faulkner, 2004) – perhaps in part due to their own histories of colonialism.

Goal 2b:

To offer opportunities for persons with psychiatric disabilities to take an active and central role in the determination of what research questions will be asked and in the setting of priorities in relation to which of those questions will be answered, using which approaches, designs, and methods, and to what ends

If the entities identifying the research problems (and potential research questions) are those in power (i.e. those who release the funding and control the means of research), there will be an inherent bias in the research findings that emerge. The questions may not have been the most relevant to the population of concern, they may not be framed in a manner that is culturally responsive, or the format may not allow for a broad enough range of responses. When problems are defined by those in power, rather than by those with lived experience, there is a risk not only of producing inaccurate or invalid research, but also of producing research that serves to further perpetuate the marginalization of those with less power (Humphreys and Rappaport, 1993).

Service user-guided and other forms of participatory research, on the other hand, can be a mechanism for gaining power, enhancing rights, and increasing self-determination. Service user involvement in research, in the words of Freire (1993), capitalizes on the

> *potential of women and men to know, to value, to establish limits, to choose, to imagine, to feel, to create, to decide, to formulate an action and direct it toward a goal, to refine and evaluate that action in order to humanize the world, reshaping or re-creating it... [through] participatory research they promote a politico-pedagogic instrument for moving women and men to such transformative action.*
>
> (Freire, 1993, pix)

This 'transformative action' includes amplification of the user voice in knowledge generation under the recovery paradigm. As suggested by Hall (1993 pxvii):

> *Participatory research fundamentally is about the right to speak.*

An important component of reclaiming their citizenship is for users to reclaim and exercise their voice, both collectively and individually, in order to influence (reshape or re-create) reality. The individual user-perspective or standpoint is crucial for building theoretical sensitivity in order to develop a holistic understanding of complex phenomena, such as the experiences of rebound and resilience after prolonged psychiatric disability. But the reclamation and exercise of the user voice is also integral to taking back and occupying valued social roles which may have been lost through illness, discrimination, or a combination of both.

One groundbreaking early consumer-led study on recovery conducted in the US was entitled the Well-Being Project (Campbell and Scraibner, 1989). Another example of such research involved continuous user involvement in designing, conducting, building grounded theory, and interpreting knowledge about the experience of hope and recovery (Ridgway, 2005). The service user perspective was crucial in constructing an in depth understanding of what helps and what hinders recovery (Onken *et al.*, 2002), how one lives with mental distress (Faulkner and Layzell, 2000), and how one self-manages a psychiatric condition (Martyn, 2002). Research may have as its dual goals the creation of knowledge and the simultaneous creation of research processes that liberate, emancipate, or empower the user community (Beresford and Evans, 1999). In the days when an emphasis on 'evidence-based practices' is in vogue, this includes increasing respect for research based on direct experience, as exemplified by the user slogan: 'We are the evidence.'

A final aspect of this objective of user involvement in research is the advancement of valued employment opportunities. Moving from being a full-time service recipient to part-time or full-time employment as a researcher has many benefits associated with employment in general, such as improved social status, sense of accomplishment, and increased personal income. The role and status of researcher is a respected one in society in general, and such a role provides an important and valued opportunity for people in recovery to 'give back' to others who encounter mental health issues. Employment as a mental health researcher also is meaningful in terms of personal development, self-esteem, empowerment, and skill-building (Morrell-Bellai and Boydell, 1994). People need opportunities for training, skill development and support in their role, and a certain amount of stress and role strain is to be anticipated. Benefits of such work, as identified in qualitative research, include: personal growth, development of relationships, learning, gaining valued experience and perspectives, becoming actively engaged, and, as we described above, personal and political empowerment (Malins, 2005).

CONCLUSION

The involvement of service users in mental health research has parallels in emancipatory, liberationist, or empowering approaches to research and education developed by other oppressed groups. We suggest that it is important to remain mindful of this political agenda as we go about improving the quality, relevance, and utility of our research, as much more is at stake, and much more is to be gained, through this concerted act of inclusion. The involvement of service users may interfere with the conduct of research if our expectation is that the business of research will go on as usual. It would only be possible for the business of research to go on as usual, however, were the 'transformative' power of service user inclusion to be sacrificed in the name of rigor, efficiency, or some other, often implicit, agenda. And at this point in the evolution of mental health services, it is precisely 'business as usual' which can no longer be considered adequate to the challenges at hand.

REFERENCES

Beresford, P. and Evans, C. (1999) Research note: research and empowerment, *British Journal of Social Work*, **29**, 671–677.
Boote, J., Telford, R. and Cooper, C. (2002) Consumer involvement in health research: a review and research agenda, *Health Policy*, **61**, 213–236.

Byas, A., Hills, D. and Meech, C. *et al.* (2002) Co-researching consumer experiences of child and adolescent mental health services: reflections and implications, *Family, Systems, and Health*, **20**, 75–89.

Campbell, J. (1997) How consumer/survivors are evaluating the quality of psychiatric care, *Evaluation Review*, **21**, 357–363.

Campbell, J. (2001) *Alternatives Research Plank*, Available online at: www.mhselfhelp.org/gateway. php?type=publication&publication_id=132, accessed 7/11/08.

Campbell, J. and Scraibner, R. (1989) *In Pursuit of Wellness: The Well-being Project*, Sacramento: California Department of Mental Health, Office of Prevention.

Davidson, L. (2006) What happened to civil rights? *Psychiatric Rehabilitation Journal*, **30**, 11–14. Translated into Swedish as: 'Vad hande med de medborgerliga rattigheterna?' In: A. Topor, K. Brostrom and R. Stromvall (Eds) *Vagen vidare: Verktyg for aterhamtning vid psyhisk ohalsa*, Stockholm: Forfattarna, RSMH.

Davidson, L., Stayner, D. and Haglund, K.E. (1998) Phenomenological perspectives on the social functioning of people with schizophrenia. In: K.T. Mueser and N. Tarrier (Eds) *Handbook of Social Functioning in Schizophrenia*, Needham Heights, MA: Allyn and Bacon Publishers, pp. 97–120.

Davidson, L., Harding, C.M. and Spaniol, L. (2005) *Recovery from Severe Mental Illnesses: Research Evidence and Implications for Practice, Volume 1*, Boston, MA: Center for Psychiatric Rehabilitation of Boston University.

Faulkner, A. and Layzell, S. (2000) *Strategies for Living: A Report of User-Led Research into People's Strategies for Living with Mental Distress*, London: Mental Health Foundation.

Freire, P. (1993) 'Foreword'. In: P. Park, M. Brydon-Miller, B. Hall and T., Jackson (Eds) *Voices of Change: Participatory Research in the United States and Canada*, Bergin and Garvey, Westport, CT, pp. ix–x.

Hall, B. (1993) 'Introduction'. In: P. Park, M. Brydon-Miller, B. Hall and T., Jackson (Eds) *Voices of Change: Participatory Research in the United States and Canada*, Bergin and Garvey, Westport, CT. pp. xii–xxii.

Happell, B. and Roper, C. (2007) Consumer participation in mental health research: articulating a model to guide practice, *Australasian Psychiatry*, **15**, 237–241.

Humphreys, K. and Rappaport, J. (1993) From the community mental health movement to the war on drugs: a study of the definition of social problems, *American Psychologist*, **48**, 892–901.

Linhorst, D.M. and Eckert, A. (2002) Involving people with severe mental illness in valuation and performance improvement. *Evaluation and the Health Professions*, **25**, 284–301.

Malins, G.L. (2005) *Mental Health Consumers Becoming Evaluation Researchers*. Unpublished thesis. University of Wollongong, Australia.

Malins, G., Morland, K. and Strang, J. *et al.* (2006) A framework for mental health consumers to evaluate service provision, *Australasian Psychiatry*, **14**, 277–280.

Pickard, S., Marshall, M. and Rogers, A. *et al.* (2002) User involvement in clinical governance, *Health Expectations*, **5**, 187–198.

Martyn, D. (2002) *In collaboration with 48 people with a schizophrenia diagnosis. The Experiences and Views of Self-management of People with Schizophrenia Diagnose*, London: The National Schizophrenia Fellowship,

Morrell-Bellai, T.L. and Boydell, K.I. (1994) The experience of mental health consumers as researchers. *Canadian Journal of Community Mental Health*, **13**, 97–110.

Ochocka, J., Janzen, R. and Nelson, G. (2002) Sharing power and knowledge: Professionals and mental health consumer/survivor researchers working together in a participatory action research project, *Psychosocial Rehabilitation Journal*, **25**, 379–387.

Onken, S.J., Dumont, J. and Ridgway, P. *et al.* (2002) *Mental Health Recovery: What Helps and What Hinders? A National Research Project for the Development of Recovery-facilitating Systems Performance Indicators*, Alexandria, VA: National Technical Assistance Center for State Mental Health, Planning/National Association of State Mental Health Program Directors.

Polowszyk, D., Brutus, M., Orvieto, A.A. *et al.* (1993) Comparison of patient and staff surveys of consumer satisfaction, *Hospital and Community Psychiatry*, **44**, 589–591.

Rapp, C.A., Shera, W. and Kisthardt, W. (1993) Research strategies for consumer empowerment of people with severe mental illness. *Social Work*, **38**, 727–735.

Ridgway, P.A. (2005) *Hope and Recovery: Co-constructing theory for the Recovery Paradigm. Unpublished dissertation.* University of Kansas, Lawrence, KS.

Rogers, E.S. and Palmer-Erbs, V. (1994) Participatory action research: implications for research and evaluation in psychiatric rehabilitation, *Psychosocial Rehabilitation Journal*, **18**, 3–12.

Rose, D., Ford, R., Lindley, P. *et al.* (1998) *In Our Experience: User Focused Monitoring of Mental Health Services Kensington and Chelsea, and Westminster Health Authority*, London: Sainsbury Centre for Mental Health.

Schneider, B., McDonald, C., Calderbank, C. *et al.* (2007) *Schizophrenia: Hearing [our] Voices, Dilemmas of Care and Control*, Calgary, Canada: Times Press.

Strauss, J.S. (1994) Is biological psychiatry building on an adequate descriptive base? In: N. Andreasen (Ed) *Schizophrenia: From Mind to Molecule*, Washington, D.C.: American Psychiatric Association Press, pp. 31–44.

Strauss, J.S., Harding, C.M., Hafez, H. and Lieberman, P. (1987) The role of the patient in recovery from psychosis. In: J.S. Strauss, W. Boker and H. Brenner (Eds) *Psychosocial Treatment of Schizophrenia: Multidimensional Concepts, Psychological, Family, and Self-Help Perspectives*, New York: Hans Hube Publishers, pp. 160–166.

Telford, R. and Faulkner, A. (2004) Learning about service user involvement in mental health, *Journal of Mental Health*, **13**, 549–559.

CHAPTER 8

Topics

Identifying Critical Outcomes and Setting Priorities for Mental Health Services Research

Paulo Del vecchio
Center for Mental Health Services, Substance Abuse and Mental Health Services Administration, U.S. Department of Health and Human Services, Rockville, MD, USA
Crystal R. Blyler
Center for Mental Health Services, Substance Abuse and Mental Health Services Administration, U.S. Department of Health and Human Services, Rockville, MD, USA

This chapter raises the vital issue of what topics are chosen for mental health research and how outcomes are measured. Clearly, these aspects determine not only the direction of research but also its implications for practice and service development. The authors examine the different views held by service users and traditional researchers on priorities for research and the desired outcomes of services, as well as the history and background of their diverging opinions. The writers offer the example of a multi-site research project with strong emphasis on collaboration between researchers with a traditional background and researchers with the experience of service use. This example shows how disagreements arose between the two groups regarding outcome domains, the reasons for conflicting perspectives, and how these were resolved. Challenges arising from different concepts of what should be measured and how, are related in this chapter to the concept of recovery as an evolving new paradigm in mental health service-provision and research. This highlights the difference between concepts generated by traditional medicine and service user

Handbook of Service User Involvement in Mental Health Research   Edited by Jan Wallcraft, Beate Schrank and Michaela Amering
Copyright © 2009 John Wiley & Sons, Ltd

researchers and the subsequent problems related to measurement, the comparability of outcomes and their implications for practice.[1]

INTRODUCTION

Over the past decade, evidence-based practice has become an increasingly critical concept underlying discussions and decision-making regarding funding of mental health services (Leff, 2004). Despite the growing popularity of the concept, however, the evidence-based practice movement has not been without detractors (Essock *et al.*, 2003). To the surprise of some who might have expected users of mental health services (referred to in the United States as 'consumers') to be among the strongest supporters for services that have been proven effective, consumers have been among those who have expressed reservations (Caras, 2001; Marzilli, 2002; Ralph *et al.*, 2002). Objections raised by consumers include two overarching concerns: 1. lack of consumer involvement in the development, evaluation, selection, and service delivery of practices being implemented and, consequently; 2. disagreement with the type and nature of practices being promoted. At the root of such dissension lies the divide between the mental health research world and the consumer movement.

The concept of evidence-based practice and its strength as a motivator for funding is based on the notion that mental health services, like all medical services, should be firmly grounded in science so that consumers can be assured that the services offered have been proven to be effective for achieving the intended outcomes. Unfortunately, however, a serious limitation arises in that only those services that have been subjected to rigorous research can be designated as evidence-based practices. The reality of this limitation brings into question which services become the focus of rigorous research and how such priorities are decided. Even more fundamental is which outcomes services being researched should address.

In this chapter, we will examine differences between consumers and researchers in terms of desired outcomes and priorities for research, providing specific examples from one research project in which consumers were heavily involved. Following this, we will discuss differing ways of defining and measuring one particular outcome that consumers have identified as critical: recovery.

DIVERGENT VIEWS ON RESEARCH PRIORITIES AND OUTCOMES

To be a mental patient is to be a statistic.

(Rae Unzicker, 1984)

The stark differences between consumers and researchers on research priorities and outcomes can be attributed to the chasm in perception between consumers and mental health providers.

Ridgway (1988), in a meta-analysis of studies on priority needs, concluded that these groups 'often see the world from very different perspectives'. Professionals, she noted, tend

---

[1] The views expressed in this chapter are those of the authors and do not necessarily represent the opinions of the US Department of Health and Human Services, Substance Abuse and Mental Health Services Administration, or the Center for Mental Health Services.

to focus on individual pathology and incapacities and the need for specialized interventions, while consumers are most concerned with day to day needs.

Lynch and Druzich (1986) compared provider and consumer perceptions of barriers to mental health service utilization. Providers identified 'client resistance' as the greatest barrier and cited a high need for professional services – especially medication monitoring and individual therapy. Consumers rated financial problems as the biggest obstacle along with a need for transportation and other services.

The main governmental funding for mental health research in the United States is the National Institute of Mental Health (NIMH) located within the National Institutes of Health. In their most recent strategic plan, NIMH (2007) identified the following research priorities:

- Advancing the integrative science of brain and behaviour science which provides the foundation for understanding mental disorders and their treatments
- Developing more reliable, valid diagnostic tests and biomarkers
- Defining the genetic and environmental risk architecture for mental disorders
- Developing interventions to prevent occurrence and/or reduce relapse of mental disorders
- Developing more effective, safer, and equitable treatments that have minimal side-effects, reduce symptoms and improve daily functioning
- Conducting clinical trials that will provide treatment options to deliver more effective personalized care across diverse populations and settings
- Creating improved pathways for rapid dissemination of science to mental healthcare and service efforts.

On an international level, Khandelwal (2005) reported that surveys conducted by the Global Network for Research in Mental and Neurological Health identified the following common priorities identified by researchers throughout the world:

- epidemiological studies
- efficacious and cost-effective studies
- locally relevant interventions
- awareness programmes
- stigma and discrimination
- war, conflicts, and natural disasters
- child and adolescent mental health
- depression
- epilepsy
- suicide and self-harm
- HIV and Aids
- substance abuse.

Consumer views, however, stand in contrast to these priorities. In their presentation 'From Lab Rat to Researcher', Campbell *et al.* (1993) cited recommendations from the Consumer/Survivor Mental Health Research and Policy Work Group (C/SRPWG):

- Alternative approaches to treatment (holistic, safe-houses, self-help, support groups, nutrition, etc.) and patterns of healing/recovering
- The damaging effects of treatment – from program models to medication side-effects
- Involuntary treatment

- Cultural issues
- Qualitative as well as quantitative research methods
- Community surveys, customer satisfaction, and consumer needs and preferences.

The C/SRPWG (1992) also cited the following basic values that should guide services and research:

- choice/voluntariness
- self-respect and de-stigmatization
- access to information
- self-determination
- individuality
- client-control over services
- holistic approaches to health
- informed consent
- independence.

Pertaining to outcomes, the National Committee for Quality Assurance in the United States developed the Health Employer Data Information Set (HEDIS) to assess mental health performance. As reported by Druss *et al.* (2002), HEDIS focuses on the following five mental healthcare quality measures:

1. Percentage of members hospitalized for a mental disorder who had an ambulatory visit with a mental healthcare provider within seven days of hospital discharge
2. Percentage of members hospitalized for a mental disorder who had an ambulatory visit with a mental healthcare provider within 30 days of hospital discharge
3. Effective treatment in the acute phase (ongoing medication treatment in the three-month period after a new depressive episode)
4. Effective continuation treatment (ongoing medication treatment in the 6 months after a new depressive episode)
5. Optimal practitioner contacts (at least three follow-up mental healthcare visits in the three months after a new depressive episode).

As is apparent, such measures solely address traditional mental health-service access and utilization.

Again, consumer views are quite different. The Consumer/Survivor Research and Policy Work Group (CSRPWG) (1992) identified the need to measure outcomes that address the concepts of liberty, quality of life, empowerment and recovery. A concept mapping process examining consumer perspectives on mental health outcomes (Trochim *et al.*, 1993) revealed similar findings.

One of the earliest consumer-directed research efforts, the *Well-being Project* (Campbell, 1997), identified that consumers value the following mental health services performance measures: perceived coercion; availability of choices in services and providers; sense of personhood (feeling listened to, validated, and respected by staff); and accessibility to information relevant to their care plan. Later, consumer-researchers have examined consumer-indicated priorities such as peer-operated services (Van Tosh and del Vecchio, 2001); quality of life (Delman, 2003); empowerment (Chamberlin, 1997); crisis alternatives (Dumont and Jones, 2002); outcomes (Wallcraft, undated), and recovery (Ralph, 2000).

The Mental Health Statistics Improvement Project (MHSIP) Report Card developed by the US Center for Mental Health Services (CMHS, 1996) is one example of a merge of consumer and provider performance measures.

Unfortunately, consumer perspectives have too often been ignored by researchers due to the paternalism and stigma and discrimination endemic in mental health service and research systems. A recent study conducted by the California Network of Mental Health Clients (Brody, 2007) found that consumers rated mental health professionals as the greatest purveyors of stigma and discrimination. This was manifest via disregard for consumer goals/choices, paternalism, and other factors.

Further, the Institute of Medicine (2005), in their landmark study of improving the quality of mental health and addiction services, highlighted that such stigma and discrimination – often based on false assumptions of consumer incompetency – impedes patient-centred care while fostering greater coercive interventions.

These views also permeate the research community. Scott (1993) likened these value conflicts as a 'turf war' over controlling human beings. Too often, consumer views have not prevailed. As an example, she cites Campbell and Schraiber's (1989) finding that 'freedom' was never examined as an outcome on any traditional research instrument to measure quality of life. She goes further to note that 'this selective blindness shows the extent to which traditional researchers regard their research subjects as 'other' when defining their basic needs.'

Funders of research also dictate mental health research priorities. In the US, in addition to the NIMH cited above, a major source of research funding has been pharmaceutical corporations. Such funding reinforces a medical-model orientation to mental health issues. Such funding has raised serious concerns regarding the ethics and validity of such research (Silverman, 2008; see also Chapter 16 on the influence of the pharmaceutical industry on research and its publication).

One example of the conflicts between consumer and researcher/provider perspectives is illustrated below.

THE CONSUMER-OPERATED SERVICES PROGRAM MULTI-SITE RESEARCH INITIATIVE

In 1998, the U.S. Substance Abuse and Mental Health Services Administration (SAMHSA) embarked on the first ever multi-site study of consumer-operated services (http://www.cstprogram.org/consumer%20op/index.html; Rogers *et al.*, 2007). Eight sites were selected through a competitive peer-reviewed process to engage in the development and implementation of a research protocol that randomized consumers to receive either consumer-operated services combined with traditional mental health services, or traditional services alone. As specified in the funding request for applications (Center for Mental Health Services, 1998), each site paired an evaluation team with a local consumer-operated service program. Explicit among the goals of the Consumer Operated Service Program multi-site research initiative (COSP) was the expectation of creating

> strong and productive partnerships among consumers, service providers and services researchers that demonstrate to the field that these groups are capable of complementing each other's strengths and that their joint efforts will yield the most effective service delivery models possible.

(p4)

In order to develop a cross-site research protocol that would best characterize the interventions and outcomes of all sites involved, Substance Abuse and Mental Health Services Association (SAMHSA) established a Steering Committee comprised of the principal investigators from each site; one consumer from each site, who was to be selected by a local consumer advisory panel; one SAMHSA staff collaborator; and the principal investigator for a cross-site Coordinating Center (CMHS, 1998, p10). For decision-making purposes, each member of the Steering Committee possessed a single vote. Because several of the principal investigators were also consumers, the Steering Committee was comprised of more consumers than non-consumers. Further consumer involvement in the design and implementation of the study came about through establishment of cross-site and local consumer advisory panels, as well as through participation of the Executive Directors of the programs being evaluated in Steering Committee discussions.

Working in close collaboration on this complex study, the varying priorities of the consumer and research communities were apparent from the outset. The earliest meetings of the Steering Committee focused on selection of domains to be assessed through the common research protocol. The grant announcement had mandated assessment of empowerment, housing, employment, social inclusion, satisfaction with services, and costs, but disagreement quickly arose about outcome domains that might be added to this core set. In keeping with the traditions of mental health services research, several researchers proposed including assessment of symptoms and diagnosis as a matter of course. Consumer service-providers objected on the grounds that their programs were not designed to reduce symptoms but, rather, were aimed at increasing hope, providing a place of comfort and safety, facilitating recovery, and improving well-being. Some consumer providers further objected that asking program participants about their diagnoses was antithetical to the very principles on which the consumer-operated services were based; that is, in contrast to traditional mental health services, consumers are ensured that when entering a consumer-operated service program, 'you leave your diagnosis at the door' – participants in these services are seen and treated as peers and not as diagnostic labels.

Unexpectedly confronted with this vastly different conception of the critical outcomes of interest, researchers in the project were doubly challenged. First they were challenged by the need to operationalize (that is, to figure out how to measure) such seemingly fuzzy concepts as empowerment, recovery, and hope. Fortunately, some previous work had been conducted on such concepts and pre-existing scales were found that could reliably capture the outcomes on which these programs focused. The second challenge to researchers in the project was to their ability to justify the study's results to colleagues in the research and traditional mental health services fields if they did not measure the primary outcomes on which these fields had been built. Through extended discussion, the Steering Committee reached agreement that although symptoms would not be considered a primary outcome, their measurement would be included in the common protocol for the explicit purpose of demonstrating the comparability of populations served to potential detractors and as a possible moderating variable that might explain why some consumers benefit more or less from the services in particular ways than others. To obtain diagnoses without violating the principles of the consumer-operated service programs, the researchers, rather than the service providers, would ask research participants for permission to obtain diagnostic information from their traditional mental health records.

Although some disagreements within the COSP Steering Committee regarding measurement of outcome domains could be resolved through compromise, others could not because appropriate measurement instruments for domains of importance to consumers had not yet been developed. In one striking example, consumers proposed that a critical difference between consumer-operated and traditional services was in the level of coercion involved in delivering the services. In response, researchers were quick to produce the well-regarded (by researchers) MacArthur Perceived Coercion Scale (Gardner *et al.*, 1993; Swartz *et al.*, 2002) as a potential instrument for consideration by the group. After examining the items of the inpatient and outpatient versions of the scale, consumers felt that the scales did not adequately get at the coercive behaviours and attitudes of staff once a person enters a program. Satisfaction-type items from the Well-being Study (Campbell and Schraiber, 1989) and the Mental Health Statistics Improvement Project scale (CMHS, 1996) were considered but also found lacking. In a further attempt to explain what was being sought, one of the consumers in the group, Vicki Fox Wieselthier (now Smith), crafted the following items that reflected her view of the concept:

1. I feel pressured by staff to do what they want me to do.
2. I feel like staff will get back at me if I do not do what they want me to do.
3. I have to butter up staff to get what I want.
4. I have to butter up staff to get what I need.
5. I have to do something staff wants to get something I want.
6. Staff threatens me with the loss of my housing.
7. Staff threatens me with the loss of my spending money.
8. Staff threatens me with hospitalization.
9. Staff threatens to make me take medication I do not want.
10. Staff threatens me in other ways.

The items of what came to be known within COSP as 'the Vicki Scale' were met with universal acclaim by other consumers involved in the COSP. Unfortunately, however, the program was not in a position to adequately validate this newly proposed scale in time to use it within the common research protocol (Note: Some psychometric testing of the renamed 'Felt Coercion Scale' was later completed as part of the Peer Outcomes Protocol developed by Campbell *et al.*, 2004). The need for such a scale to capture a concept of great importance to consumers and the lack of the existence of a well-developed measure to do so point to the need for consumers to be involved not only in determining priorities for what will be studied, but also in the creation and development of critical measurement instruments.

A third example from COSP of differences between the perspectives of consumers and researchers regarding measurement tools arose in a discussion of the response categories used across scales and items. Standard practice in psychiatric research dictates that response categories be included for items in which missing data might be expected, in order to code the reason for unanswered questions. In standard parlance, the response categories provided for such purpose are 'don't know' and 'refused' (to answer). While so common as to go unnoticed by researchers in COSP, the consumers involved in the program found both response codes troublesome. Examples of the 'don't know' category were pointed out among personal items that consumers felt anyone would know about themselves; to the consumers, therefore, such coding would imply some kind of cognitive incapacity that was not truly present. The category 'refused' evoked strong visceral reactions due to negative associations to the word within the mental health services context—as one consumer stated, 'The last time I 'refused' something, I was slapped into four-point restraints.'

Upon further discussion, the group determined that the primary reason for these response codes was to distinguish whether the item had been inadvertently skipped or whether it had been asked but not answered. Having specified such and accepting that the specific way these response categories were coded was unlikely to affect the research results, the researchers agreed to change the response codes for missing answers across items and scales to 'not asked' and 'not answered'.

The final prioritization of outcome measures to be included in the COSP common protocol was determined through a consensus-driven process that gave equal value to the scientific merit and 'consumer integrity' of the scales. The principal investigators from each site were asked to rate final candidate scales for scientific merit on the basis of psychometric properties, as well as use in and results from previous research. The consumer representatives to the Steering Committee from each site were asked to rate the scales for consumer integrity on the basis of relevance of the scale to all consumer-run programs in the study, sensitivity to consumer values, and use of language that was understandable and unobjectionable to consumers. With the means and standard deviations from both sets of ratings of the prospective scales before them, the Steering Committee was able to engage in negotiations to select the set that would best meet the needs of the study from both perspectives.

RECOVERY

In the example above, consumers were active and numerous participants in all phases of conducting the research. This close interaction in carrying out a common project necessitated a coming together of researchers and consumers in prioritizing outcome measures for the research. In typical research endeavours, however, consumers are absent from the conversation. This has led to a gap between the outcomes on which research has focused and those that consumers are increasingly striving to achieve. The growing emphasis on recovery as the overarching aim of mental health service systems in the United States (New Freedom Commission on Mental Health, 2003) has thrown a spotlight on this disconnection.

In keeping with the New Freedom Commission's (2003) definition of recovery as 'the process in which people are able to live, work, learn, and participate fully in their communities,' some researchers have proposed adding vocational functioning, independent living, and peer relationships to operational criteria for recovery from schizophrenia (Liberman et al., 2002; Nasrallah et al., 2005). Although an improvement over prevailing outcome definitions that focus almost exclusively on clinical symptoms, Liberman et al. themselves found that 'a higher proportion of researchers than consumers . . . endorsed our operational . . . approach to defining criteria for recovery' (p259).

Other researchers, despite recognizing that 'in recent years there has been an appropriate increase in emphasis on clinical outcomes that are meaningful to patients, families, and clinicians, as well as a greater focus on functional recovery' (Andreasen et al., 2005, p442) have chosen to spend their efforts operationalizing older concepts of symptom remission (Andreasen et al.) or functioning (Bellack et al., 2007). In choosing to exclude recovery as a focus of their endeavors, Bellack et al. asserted that 'self-perceptions of recovery are determined by so many diverse factors that it will often not be suitable as an outcome in clinical trials' (p809). Andreasen et al. shied away from defining criteria for recovery because 'recovery...is a more demanding and longer-term phenomenon than remission' (p442). They went on to explain that

> *Consensus regarding operational criteria for recovery, which might include improvements in cognition or psychosocial functioning, was considered outside the scope of the working group, because more research is needed on this topic.*

(p442)

In contrast to researchers, consumers have put substantial effort in recent years into exploring individual concepts of recovery (Ridgway, 2001; Young and Ensing, 1999), developing consensual definitions (CMHS, 2005; Jacobson, 2004), and developing and testing instruments to measure these concepts and definitions (Allott *et al.*, 2002; Ralph, 1998). The definitions of recovery derived from consumer-driven initiatives are considerably richer than the outcomes that have been the primary focus of research. Recovery, as consumers define it, comprises hope, empowerment, social connectedness, meaning/purpose, aspirations, contributions to society, satisfaction with life, building on personal strengths and resources, well-being, positive sense of self, roles and life beyond the mental health system, respect, connections, self-determination, and spiritual development. It is a process/journey, way of life, attitude, or way of approaching the day's challenges rather than a point-in-time outcome; the journey is nonlinear in nature. Not synonymous with cure, mental health recovery may involve ongoing symptoms, treatment, or supports.

The complexity of consumer definitions of recovery makes operationally defining the concept a challenge. Fortunately, however, considerable developmental work on recovery measurement instruments has already been completed. The first attempt to collect instruments that could be used to assess recovery as defined by consumers yielded a collection of instruments that measured only certain aspects of recovery and/or content related to, but not synonymous with, recovery (Ralph *et al.*, 2000). By 2005, however, numerous endeavours to measure the broader concept of recovery had ensued, and Campbell-Orde, Chamberlin, Carpenter, and Leff collected nine instruments for measuring individual recovery in a Compendium of Recovery Measures; in addition, four instruments were found that measure recovery-promoting environments. Two years later, two additional instruments measuring recovery-promoting environments were identified (Evaluation Center at the Human Services Research Institute, 2007).

The development of instruments to measure recovery-promoting environments is an important addition to the mental health services and research fields, as the definition of recovery that one uses will greatly influence the factors that research finds to be most effective in promoting recovery. Based on the research literature that used older outcome definitions related to symptoms and functioning, Liberman *et al.* (2002; Table 2) found the following factors to be associated with 'recovery':

- supportive family or other caregivers
- absence of substance abuse
- shorter duration of untreated psychosis
- good initial response to neuroleptics
- adherence to treatment
- supportive therapy with a collaborative therapeutic alliance

- good neurocognitive functioning
- absence of the deficit syndrome
- good pre-morbid history
- access to comprehensive, coordinated, and continuous treatment.

These factors stand in stark contrast to factors found by consumer-led, qualitative research efforts to be most helpful to consumers in promoting recovery (Dumont et al., 2006; Mental Health Foundation, 2000), which include:

- person-centred decision-making and choice
- personhood
- self-care and wellness
- basic life resources, such as money
- meaningful activities and roles
- peer advocacy
- physical exercise
- religious and spiritual beliefs
- hobbies and interests
- information
- acceptance
- shared experience
- peace of mind and relaxation
- security and safety
- pleasure.

With differences in measured outcomes leading to such divergent research results, the utility of measures of recovery-oriented services based on consumer definitions of recovery is apparent.

Liberman et al. (2002) found that practitioners, like consumers, tended to view recovery as 'better defined by an indefinite coping and striving process rather than attaining a particular endpoint or goal' (p259). The support of service providers for the consumer-driven concept of recovery is reflected in the position statement on the concept of recovery issued by the American Psychiatric Association (2005) and in the guidelines for recovery-oriented services issued by the American Association of Community Psychiatrists (Sowers, 2005).

As mental health service providers embrace the concept of recovery, they recognize the importance of providing services that support individual recovery goals. Consequently, communities are selecting and promoting services, including evidence-based practices, that they increasingly tout as being recovery-oriented or contributing to recovery. Because instruments to measure consumer concepts of recovery have only recently been developed, however, such claims are not supported by the nascent recovery science (Anthony et al., 2003; Bellack, 2006; Ralph et al., 2002). To remedy this dearth, Ralph et al. recommend that

> empirical studies of recovery, its components, and their relation to traditional and consumer mental health services (process and outcome) should be funded. This funding should include studies where recovery is the major research objective, and studies where traditional mental health services are the primary research focus and inclusion of recovery measures is required.
> (p25)

They further recommend that

traditional measures of mental health treatment should be broadened to include recovery issues and perspectives.

(p26)

Heeding these recommendations would play a significant role in narrowing the gap between researchers and consumers regarding outcomes of interest.

CONCLUSION

The differences between consumers and researchers in priorities for research and outcome measurement highlight the need for consumers to be involved in all phases of research. Consumer involvement is especially critical at the beginning phases of research when priorities are set and outcome measures are selected, although involvement at the analysis phase is also necessary to ensure that interpretations are consistent with consumer experience. Because consumers have so long been absent from research administration, considerable work may be required initially to develop instruments to measure concepts that are important to consumers but for which measurement instruments currently do not exist.

The controversies that have emerged due to the simultaneous rise of the evidence-based practice and consumer recovery movements exemplify the historic discordance between research and consumer cultures. The current confluence of these two movements opens up exciting new opportunities for consumers and researchers to work together to develop recovery-oriented evidence-based practices (Farkas *et al.*, 2005) and to forge a new science, based on consumer priorities and concepts of recovery. Ultimately, to transform mental health systems to become both evidence-based and recovery-focused, we must first transform the science on which the system is based.

REFERENCES

Allott, P., Loganathan, L. and Fulford, K.W.M. (2002) Discovering hope for recovery: a review of a selection of recovery literature, implications for practice and systems change, *Canadian Journal of Community Mental Health*, **21**(2), 13–34.

American Psychiatric Association (2005) *Use of the Concept of Recovery: Position Statement* [Online]. Arlington, VA: APA. Available online at: http://www.psych.org/Departments/EDU/Library/APAOfficialDocumentsandRelated/PositionStatements/200504.aspx, accessed 25/10/08.

Andreasen, N.C., Carpenter, W.T. and Kane, J.M. *et al.* (2005) Remission in schizophrenia: proposed criteria and rationale for consensus, *American Journal of Psychiatry*, **162**(3), 441–449.

Anthony, W., Rogers, E.S. and Farkas, M. (2003) Research on evidence-based practices: future directions in an era of recovery, *Community Mental Health Journal*, **39**(2), 101–114.

Bellack, A.S. (2006) Scientific and consumer models of recovery in schizophrenia: concordance, contrasts, and implications, *Schizophrenia Bulletin*, **32**(3), 432–442.

Bellack, A.S., Green, M.F. and Cook, J.A. *et al.* (2007) Assessment of community functioning in people with schizophrenia and other severe mental illnesses: a white paper based on an NIMH-sponsored workshop, *Schizophrenia Bulletin*, **33**(3), 805–822.

Brody, D. (2007) Strategies for transformation: identifying, reducing and ending discrimination and stigma in mental health and primary care settings. In: *Improving Provider Attitudes, Behaviors, and Practices Toward People with Mental Illness* [Online archived teleconference]. Rockville, MD: Substance Abuse and Mental Health Services Administration, Resource Center to Address Discrimination and Stigma. Available online at: http://www.promoteacceptance.samhsa.gov/archtelPDF/June_StigmaProviders2.pdf, accessed 25/10/08.

Campbell, J., Einspahr, K., Evenson, R. and Adkins, R. (2004) *Peer Outcomes Protocol (POP): Psychometric Properties of the POP* Chicago, IL: U. of Illinois at Chicago, National Research and Training Center on Psychiatric Disability. Available online at: www.cmhsrp.uic.edu/download/POP.Psychometrics.pdf, accessed 25/10/08.

Campbell, J., Ralph, R. and Glover, R. (1993) From Lab Rat to Researcher: The history, models, and policy implications of consumer/survivor involvement in research, *Proceedings: Fourth Annual National Conference on State Mental Health Agency Services Research and Program Evaluation*, pp 138–157, Alexandria, VA: National Association of State Mental Health Program Directors Research Institute.

Campbell, J. and Schraiber, R. (1989) *In Pursuit of Wellness: The Well-Being Project: Mental Health Clients Speak for Themselves*, Sacramento, CA: California Department of Mental Health.

Campbell, J. (1997) How consumers/survivors are evaluating the quality of psychiatric care, *Evaluation Review*, **21**, 357–363.

Campbell-Orde, T., Chamberlin, J., Carpenter, J. and Leff, H.S. (2005) *Measuring the Promise: A Compendium of Recovery Measures: Vol. II* (Publication No. 55), Cambridge, MA: Human Services Research Institute.

Caras, S. (2001) *It's Time for a New Paradigm* [Online]. Available online at: http://www.peoplewho.org/readingroom/caras.newparadigm.htm accessed 25/10/08.

Center for Mental Health Services (2005) *National Consensus Statement on Mental Health Recovery (Publ. No. SMA05-4129) [Brochure]*. Rockville, MD: Substance Abuse and Mental Health Services Administration, US Department of Health and Human Services.

Center for Mental Health Services (1998) *Cooperative Agreements to Evaluate Consumer-Operated Human Service Programs for Persons with Serious Mental Illness* (Guidance for Applicants No. SM 98-004) Rockville, MD: Substance Abuse and Mental Health Services Administration, U.S. Department of Health and Human Services.

Center for Mental Health Services (1996) *The MHSIP Consumer-Oriented Mental Health Report Card. The Final Report of the Mental Health Statistics Improvement Program (MHSIP) Task Force on a Consumer-Oriented Mental Health Report Card* (Publication No. MC96-60) Rockville, MD: Substance Abuse and Mental Health Services Administration, U.S. Department of Health and Human Services.

Chamberlin, J. (1997) A working definition of empowerment, *Psychiatric Rehabilitation Journal*, **20** (4), 43–46.

Consumer/Survivor Research, Policy Work Group (CSRPWG) (1992) *Focus Group Meeting on Client Outcomes*, Ft. Lauderdale, FL: Mental Health Statistics Improvement Project Ad Hoc Advisory Group.

Delman, J. (2003) *CQI Quality of Life Needs Assessment Report*, Roxbury, MA: Consumer Quality Initiatives.

Druss, B.G., Miller, C.L. and Rosenheck, R.A. *et al.* (2002) Mental healthcare quality under managed care in the United States: A view from the Health Employer Data and Information Set (HEDIS), *American Journal of Psychiatry*, **159**, 860–862.

Dumont, J. and Jones, K. (2002) Findings from a consumer/survivor-defined alternative to psychiatric hospitalization, *Outlook*, 4–6. (A joint publication of the Evaluation Center at Human Services Research Institute and the National Association of State Mental Health Program Directors Research Institute.)

Dumont, J.M., Ridgway, P., Onken, S.J. *et al.* (2006) *Mental Health Recovery: What helps and what hinders? A National Research Project for the Development of Recovery Facilitating System Performance Indicators.* Alexandria, VA: National Association of State Mental Health Program Directors, National Technical Assistance Center for State Mental Health Planning.

Essock, S.M., Goldman, H.H., Van Tosh, L. *et al.* (2003) Evidence-based practices: setting the context and responding to concerns, *Psychiatric Clinics of North America*, **26**(4), 919–938.

Evaluation Center at the Human Services Research Institute (2007) Addendum to Measuring the Promise: A Compendium of Recovery Measures, Volume II, Cambridge, MA: HSRI.

Farkas, M., Gagne, C., Anthony, W. and Chamberlin, J. (2005 April) Implementing recovery oriented evidence based programs: identifying the critical dimensions, *Community Mental Health Journal*, **41**(2), 141–158.

Gardner, W., Hoge, S., Bennett, N. *et al.* (1993) Two scales for measuring patients' perceptions of coercion during hospital admission, *Behavioral Sciences and the Law*, **20**, 307–321.

Institute of Medicine (2005) *Improving the Quality of Healthcare for Mental and Substance Use Conditions*, Washington, DC: National Academies Press.

Jacobson, N. (2004) *In Recovery: The Making of Mental Health Policy*, Nashville, TN: Vanderbilt University Press.

Khandelwal, S. (2005) *Mental Health Research Priorities in Developing Countries*. Paper presented at the Global Forum for Health Research, Forum 9, Mumbai, India. Available online at: http://www.globalforumhealth.org/filesupld/forum9/CD%20Forum%209/papers/Khandelwal%20S.pdf, accessed 25/10/08.

Leff, H.S. (2004) A brief history of evidence-based practice and a vision for the future, In: R.W. Manderscheid and M.J. Henderson (Eds) *Mental Health, United States, 2002* (pp 224–241). (DHHS Publication No. SMA 3938) Rockville, MD: Substance Abuse and Mental Health Services Administration, U.S. Department of Health and Human Services.

Liberman, R.P., Kopelowicz, A., Ventura, J. and Gutkind, D. (2002) Operational criteria and factors related to recovery from schizophrenia, *International Review of Psychiatry*, **14**, 256–272.

Lynch, M.M. and Druzich, N.M (1986) Needs assessment of the chronically mentally ill: practitioner and client perspectives, *Administration in Mental Health*, **4**, 237–248.

Marzilli, A. (2002) Controversy surrounds evidence-based practices, *The Key, National Mental Health Consumers' Self-Help Clearinghouse Newsletter*, **7**(1), 5.

Mental Health Foundation (2000) *Strategies for Living: A Summary Report of User-led Research into People's Strategies for Living with Mental Distress*. London: Mental Health Foundation.

Nasrallah, H.A., Targum, S.D., Tandon, R. *et al.* (2005, March) Defining and measuring clinical effectiveness in the treatment of schizophrenia, *Psychiatric Services*, **56**(3), 273–282.

National Institute of Mental Health (2007) *Strategic Planning Reports: Overview of priorities*, Rockville, MD. Available online at: http://www.nimh.nih.gov/about/strategic-planning-reports, accessed 25/10/08.

New Freedom Commission on Mental Health (2003) *Achieving the Promise: Transforming Mental Healthcare in America. Final Report* (DHHS Pub. No. SMA-03-3832), Rockville, MD: NFCMH.

Ralph, R.O. (2000) *Review of Recovery Literature: A Synthesis of a Sample of Recovery Literature*. Alexandria, VA: National Association of State Mental Health Program Directors, National Technical Assistance Center for State Mental Health Planning.

Ralph, R.O. (1998) *Recovery: Background Paper for the Surgeon General's Report on Mental Health*, Portland, ME: University of Southern Maine, Edmund S. Muskie School of Public Service.

Ralph, R.O., Kidder, K. and Phillips, D. (2000) *Can We Measure Recovery? A Compendium of Recovery and Recovery-Related Instruments* (Publication No. 43), Cambridge, MA: Human Services Research Institute.

Ralph, R.O., Lambert, D. and Kidder, K.A. (2002) *Recovery Perspective and Evidence-based Practice for People with Serious Mental Illness: A Guideline Developed for the Behavioral Health Recovery*

Management Project. An Initiative of Fayette Companies, Peoria, IL; Chestnut Health Systems, Bloomington, IL; and the University of Chicago Center for Psychiatric Rehabilitation. Available online at: http://bhrm.org/guidelines/mhguidelines.htm, accessed 28/10/08.

Ridgway, P. (2001) Restorying psychiatric disability: learning from first person recovery narratives, *Psychiatric Rehabilitation Journal*, **24**(4), 335–344.

Ridgway, P. (1988) *The Voice of Consumers in Mental Health Systems: A Call for Change – a literature review*, Burlington, VT: University of Vermont, Center for Community Change through, Housing and Support.

Rogers, E.S., Teague, G.B., Lichenstein, C. *et al.* (2007) Effects of participation in consumer-operated service programs on both personal and organizationally mediated empowerment: results of multi-site study, *Journal of Rehabilitation Research and Development*, **44**(6), 785–800.

Scott, A. (1993) Consumers/survivors reform the system bringing a 'human face' to research, *Resources*. **5**(1).

Silverman, E. (2008, June 25) *Senate targets Stanford psychiatrist over conflicts*. Available on-line at: http://www.pharmalot.com/2008/06/senate-targets-stanford-psychiatrist-over-conflicts/, accessed 28/10/08.

Sowers, W. (2005) Transforming systems of care: the American Association of Community Psychiatrists Guidelines for Recovery Oriented Services, *Community Mental Health Journal*, **41**(6), 757–774.

Swartz, M.S., Wagner, H.R., Swanson, J.W. *et al.* (2002) The perceived coerciveness of involuntary outpatient commitment: findings from an experimental study, *Journal of the American Academy of Psychiatry and Law*, **30**, 207–217.

Trochim, W., Dumont, J. and Campbell, J. (1993) *Mapping Mental Health Outcomes from the Perspective of Consumers/Survivors*, Alexandria, VA: National Association of State Mental Health Program Directors, Research Institute.

Unzicker, R. (1984) *To Be a Mental Patient* [Online]. Available: http://www.disabledinaction.org/activist/2001–05/index. html#rae, accessed 29/01/09.

Van Tosh, L. and del Vecchio, P. (2001) *Consumer/Survivor-operated Self-help Programs: A technical report* (Publication No. SMA01-3510). Rockville, MD: Substance Abuse and Mental Health Services Administration, U.S. Department of Health and Human Services.

Wallcraft, J. (2008) *Clinical Outcomes v Patient Outcomes: Is There a Disparity?* Facilitated Workshop at the Second National Conference of Measuring and Monitoring Clinical Outcomes, 30 April 2008, Portland Place, London, UK.

Young, S.L. and Ensing, D.S. (1999) Exploring recovery from the perspective of people with psychiatric disabilities. *Psychiatric Rehabilitation Journal*, **22**(3), 219–231.

CHAPTER 9

Methods

'We Are the Evidence,' an Examination of Service User Research Involvement as Voice

Jean Campbell
Missouri Institute of Mental Health, Saint Louis, USA

This chapter introduces the concept of mental health service user 'voice' as an approach to defining an authentic research methodology and to implement empirical studies guided by service user perspectives. It explains the concept, explores the dynamics of 'voice' in the research process and comes to some conclusions about the value service user researchers bring to the production of knowledge. Issues connected with the methodology of 'voice' are then reflected in the light of real world research experience. Selected studies that involved mental health service users in research roles are examined, and barriers to and best practices for successful service user involvement identified.

INTRODUCTION

'We are the evidence,' has become a clarion call for persons diagnosed with mental illness as evidence-based practices increasingly take a dominant role in guiding mental health policy and service provision throughout the modern world. The US President's New Freedom Commission on Mental Health, *Achieving the Promise: Transforming mental health care in America, Final Report* (2003), the driving force towards transformation in mental health care in America, states that

> *research activities must include a serious science-to-services endeavour resulting in delivering the very best evidence-based practices to consumers in a timely way.*
>
> (p72)

This report also observes,

In the past decade, mental health consumers have become involved in planning and evaluating the quality of mental health care and in conducting sophisticated research to affect system reform.

It recommends

Local, state and federal authorities encourage consumers and families to participate in planning and evaluating treatment and support services.

(p37)

Although in theory increasing availability of services and supports with demonstrated effectiveness should be a priority, there is growing concern that privileging select practices through dissemination and funding initiatives limits service user[1] choice by narrowing the range of available services (Anthony, 2001; International Association of Psychosocial Rehabilitation Services, 1998; Essock, Goldman, Van Tosh *et al.*, 2003). In particular, service users worry that focusing on evidence-based practices neglects other factors service users use in selecting mental health services (Frese, Stanley, Kress *et al.*, 2001; Marzilli, 2002). These factors include how well program and service user goals coincide: the kindness, respect, and co-operation experienced by the service recipient, and overall comfort with the program.

Service users question the consistency of many evidence-based practices with recovery-based, person-directed practice. They view the focus on evidence-based practices as paternalistic, following a 'top-down' medical model that is not congruent with the recovery vision articulated by users. Most evidence-based research supports the status quo because it looks at recovery through the lens of symptoms, recidivism, and treatment outcomes and not the promotion of wellness outcomes such as empowerment, self-efficacy, meaning in life, and hope (Marzilli, 2002). Similarly, Fisher and Ahern (2002) note

Currently, the benchmark for evidence-based practice is maintenance: symptom reduction and medication compliance. However, when community integration is used as the outcome measure, the recovery model is clearly more evidence based than the medical model.

(p633)

The focus on effectiveness and the efforts to define mental health outcomes has historically reinforced a

kind of turf war over controlling human beings in a landscape that includes an entire array of service options and widely different goals and definitions of mental health and quality of life.

(Scott, 1993, p1)

In the wake of this tension, a vibrant service user research methodology has emerged based on the values of meaningful input and inclusion from the lived experience of persons diagnosed with mental illness.

---

[1] 'service user' – for ease of reading, the term 'service user' will be used throughout this chapter, but other terms are implied. For more on terminology, please see Chapter 1 of this Handbook.

Service users lay claim to insider knowledge of service user expectations for services and supports and the ways the mental health service system meets or fails to meet their needs and preferences (Campbell, 1996). I suggest that the introduction of mental health service user perspectives within research is a type of collective voice of persons who have received mental health services but for decades were denied input into the design, delivery, or evaluation of such services (Kaufmann and Campbell, 1995).

By developing participatory ways for constructive dialogue to occur about research results, and for shared decision-making to take place in the development and implementation of research initiatives, service users have begun to speak for themselves through mental health services research (Campbell, 1996; 1997). In the following chapter I explore the roots of service user involvement in research and evaluation through voice and social action, identify common themes and methods, and discuss best practices in the implementation of empirical studies guided by service user perspectives.

WHAT IS VOICE?

Science is a social construction: partial, colluded, and inscribed with power, bias and stereotype. It is seldom an innocent process of discovery. Rather, it obscures its origins in social values, the commitment to methodological rigor, and resistance to critical self examination. In the modern world, the dominant biomedical epistemologies take material and ideological form in the questions that are asked, the methods of inquiry, the units of analysis and the interpretation of results. This has "profound impact on what we study, how we study it, and how we relate to people or 'subjects' and what actions may be taken on the basis of findings" (Chesler, 1991, p758).

Persons who experience mental illness and the professionals who study them and try to treat them see the world from very different perspectives (Ridgway, 1988). Mental health professionals assume authority through the delivery of mental health treatments and services. For the service recipients, a diagnosis often comes with an assault on identity and sense of self. Persons diagnosed with mental illness often draw on metaphors of degradation, anger, and sadness when they speak about their experiences as psychiatric patients. We are largely excluded from the circle of talk that produces theories and constructs of clinical psychiatry and mental health service delivery. If we are admitted at all, it is by special invitation, and persons other than service users decide whom to invite.

These experiences stand as a robust critique of biomedical psychiatry and the mental health services delivery system (Blaska, 1991; Chamberlin, 1978; Colom, 1981; Deegan, 1988; Leete, 1989; Lovejoy, 1984; Nide, 1990; Susko, 1991; Unzicker, 1989; Zinman *et al.*, 1987). In an interview with service user researchers, Scott (1993) quotes Judi Chamberlin:

Controlling symptoms and behavior of consumers and maintaining the effectiveness of the service system are expressed priorities of mental health professionals, while consumers ask, 'What does this do for my life?'

(p4)

The defining role of our experience within a scientific methodology illustrates the power of service user research to humanize people in a significant way. Simply by collecting and publishing our stories, a fundamental challenge to psychiatric stereotypes is mounted. This has both personal implications in terms of validating how we think about ourselves and it has political consequences by challenging how others think about us as a social group.

I begin with the concept of 'voice' to explore the dynamics of the research process and to come to some conclusions about the value mental health service user researchers bring to the production of knowledge. As a point of departure, I offer my own testimony as a mental health service user and researcher:

> *Mental health professionals subsume our identity with a global sentence of illness and disability. It is often presumed that we do not know what is in our own best interests. Our feelings of anger and joy are scrutinized for signs of pathology and violence. Our needs and desires are imputed for us, as if we were mute. Studies of our everyday lives are routinely emptied of quality, hope, and dignity.*

> (Campbell, 2005, p17)

Voice is more than an academic short-hand for a person's point of view. It is an expression of individuality in the face of negative social stereotypes: an act of self-validation that can be examined as metaphor for protest. This feature of voice is well understood among feminist researchers, as Belenky and others (1986) explain:

> *In describing their lives, women commonly talked about voice and silence: 'speaking up, speaking out, being silent, not being heard, really listening, really talking, words as weapons, feeling deaf and dumb, having no words, saying what you mean, listening to be heard, and so on in an endless variety of connotations all having to do with sense of mind, self worth, and feeling of isolation from or connection to others. We found that women repeatedly use the metaphor of voice to depict their intellectual and ethical development; and the development of a sense of voice, mind, and self were intricately intertwined*

> (p18)

The very existence of voice presents a profound argument that we are conscious human beings rather than disease entities. By coming to voice we reclaim dominion over our mental subjectivity and create a social identity. Voice as the presentation of our experience provides an understanding of the dehumanized role that we are obligated to play in society and illuminates the transformative power of our experience when cast within an evolving drama of social awareness. When one looks beyond the immediate expression of experience to the concept of voice, you immediately find that persons diagnosed with mental illness have a narrative talent that undermines the idea that we are in some way incapable of interpreting our own world and desires.

The methodological traditions from feminist epistemology rely on the need for unmediated voice (Rheinharz, 1992) or direct subjectivity (Marcus, 1986). As Rheinharz notes,

> *the more subjective the voice... the greater the potential that the material will dissolve differences between the reader and the speaker.*

> (p228)

Marcus takes the voice of 'women mental patients' as testimony of the victim:

> *The less the victim speaks, the less the value of her text for subversion of an oppressive social regime. Our curve of discourse on female [madness] begins in the most subjective mode, autobiography, and moves on to fiction, (or poetry); the case study... and the literary-critical*

analysis of text [about madness]. . .Crucial in this distinction is the authority of the narrator of
each story, from victim to expert.

(p3)

Giving voice reveals the orientation points which organise an individual's sense of self,
while comparison permits the construction of social consciousness. As Misztal (1981)
suggests, such experiences are

. . .the way of building visions of the surrounding world, the building of a picture of one's own
self, the problem of presenting the identity of oneself in the outer world, and the understanding
of the identity of others.

(p184)

Among mental health service users, expressions of our experiences take a variety of forms
spanning a range of media from oral commentary to computer networks. There are
numerous autobiographies, first-persons accounts, newsletters, in-house publications, local
speeches, poetry, renegade journals, and computerized electronic bulletin boards where
service users communicate directly with others about their experiences. These media
provide a forum for thought, interpretation, and learning ways of talking about mental
illness. Through such communications our stories have become central to an emerging
culture of resistance, recovery and resilience (Campbell, 1993; Sommer and Osmond,
1983). I draw on feminist methodology for a fuller understanding of this process:

[w]e maintain that personal narratives are particularly rich sources because. . .they illumi-
nate both the logic of individual courses of action and the effects of system-level constraints
within which those courses evolve. . . . [They] allow us to see lives as simultaneously individual
and social creations, and to see individuals as simultaneously the changers and the changed.
(Personal Narratives Group, 1989, p6)

Social consciousness is a living thing, always a work in progress. We revise our images of
the present as we narrate our experience. By telling our stories there is 'a surfacing of
meaningfulness that binds past and present together' (Schrager, 1983, p77).

The act of public testimony changes the message and intent of personal experience,
building a social consciousness through knowing that we are not alone. The sharing of
our stories, the formation of our perspectives, the taking of a point of view and making it our
own is part of an unending reservoir of correspondences that have the potential for being
held in common. In a personal correspondence a service user related (Campbell-
Skillman, 1991):

My first conference in San Francisco in 84 just blew me away. I was in shock and ecstasy
watching the speakers one by one, speak eloquently of their experiences in the system – I never
thought I would see the day when ex-mental patients would stand up in public and talk about
what they had been through in the system. It was truly a spiritual experience.

(p371)

From our experience we write or talk to communicate meaning and opinion. This is
obvious. However, when the audience interprets the message as a valid request for change,
the message also entails a call for action. In discussing the purposeful nature inherent in the
production of native knowledge, Bertaux-Wiame (1985) observed

Native knowledge is not developed for the sake of contemplation, but learned the hard way and synthesized in view of action.

(p31)

Mental health service users gather and organise. The telling, listening and recording of our experiences and insights establishes dominion over the public, private, and interior realms of our consciousness critical to the transformation of a victim sensibility or patienthood to one of entitlement, unity of purpose, and validation as worthwhile persons. We are reclaimed through coming to voice as experts by experience.

In a qualitative study that examines first-person accounts of recovery from psychiatric disability, Ridgway (2001) shows how narrative accounts of recovery challenge the mental health field to critically examine institutional structures and processes that focus on the inevitability of chronic disorder, a downwardly spiraling course and life-long disability. Rather, recovery stories 'open new pathways and present positive trajectories for a life course of discovery and personal growth after the experience of prolonged psychiatric disability' (p340).

Over the past thirty years, mental health service user experiences have pressed forward a participatory research methodology that captures both the form and content of individual experience and social consciousness rendered silent by biomedical science and public prejudice. Our experiences have raised overlooked but important questions, and whatever pertains to our subjectivity can no longer be treated as impalpable, ineffable, and unknowable.

FROM LAB RAT TO RESEARCHER

Since the 17th century and the dawn of scientific methods, persons diagnosed with mental illness were involved in research as objects to be observed by scientists for changes in reactions or functioning as a result of some bio-medical 'treatment'. With the rise of survey research in the 1950s, they were also used as subjects who responded to questions posed by scientists to measure their subjective physical and mental states. In the past 30 years, service users around the globe have taken on empowered roles as part of the mental health research enterprise: as employees such as an interviewer or research assistant; as partners involved in some aspect of the planning, designing, and conducting of the research project with professional researchers in control; and as independent researchers designing, conducting, analyzing data, and publishing the results of research projects (Campbell *et al.*, 1993).

One finds great similarities between mental health service user struggles and other ethnic minorities, women, homosexuals, and people with physical disabilities who have been labeled, dismissed and denied control and responsibility for their own lives. Traditionally disempowered and stigmatized groups in society have protested, organised self-help groups and civil organisations, and become involved in research as part of a civil rights movement.

In the 1980s, the first American service user researchers looked to the work of Dr. Kenneth Clark who had compiled the social science evidence that segregation had an impact on black schoolchildren's mental status cited in the landmark U.S. Supreme Court's ruling in Brown v. Board of Education of Topeka, 347 U.S. 483 (1954) which ended centuries of segregation in US schools (Guthrie, 1993). They also studied the actions of the members of Act-Up, a gay activist group, who challenged AIDS researchers at professional meetings, and encouraged people participating in clinical trials of HIV medications to break the research protocols in order to compel the Federal Drug Administration to begin distributing these life extending drugs before the research studies were completed (Eigo *et al.*, 1988). Most notably, they were informed by women scientists who resisted traditional research methodologies by developing a feminist epistemology that was both emancipatory and participatory based on the principles of cooperation (Shepherd, 1993).

The Hill House Project in Cleveland, Ohio (1979) was one of the earliest efforts to involve service users in the design of the research instruments and data collection of efforts in the United States. The professionals who directed the research demonstrated that Hill House members had the expertise to identify and classify their feelings (Prager and Tanaka, 1979). The investigators proclaimed,

> *Representing the consumer's perspective on the meaning of mental illness and the correlates of 'getting better', the process of client involvement in evaluation design and implementation is not only realistic and feasible; it is, we feel, a professional necessity whose time is overdue.*
>
> (p51)

In 1986, the California Network of Mental Health Clients wrote a successful research proposal to the California Department of Mental Health to investigate what factors promote and deter the well-being of people with severe mental illness in California (Campbell and Schraiber, 1989). They believed that social science held out the possibility of improving the quality of life for people with psychiatric diagnoses in California. The investigators insisted that it was essential to the project that mental health service users conduct the research. The participants needed to speak for themselves through research about the quality of their everyday lives.

The Well-Being Project was the first survey research project in history that was developed, administered, and analyzed entirely by persons diagnosed with mental illness. It began informally with a group of service users telling their life stories. As they came upon experiences that triggered questions for the surveys that were to be developed, they wrote them down on colored index cards and piled them in the middle of the room. In the end, the group had generated over 400 cards with questions about what factors promote or deter our well-being. Most of the questions developed had never been asked before. The survey questionnaires that evolved from that process were very different from those developed by mental health professionals. The questions asked produced very different results that challenged the common assumption that experts knew what was in the best interest of persons with mental illness.

Using a mixed method approach, The Well-Being Project surveyed over 500 mental health service users, family members, and service providers and collected over 40 hours of recorded testimony. The subsequent findings were presented in two volumes, a 56 minute video documentary, and a compendium book of testimony, poetry, prose and art. The project contributed both new knowledge about the power of personhood in promoting well-being and new understandings of the importance of service user perspective in conducting research and evaluation. Campbell and Schraiber (1989) understood that:

> *Well-being is not a neutral category or set of variables impinging on everyday life from the outside. It is composed of experiences and relationships which not only determine particular choices and decisions at particular times, but also structures experientially how those choices are defined.*
>
> (p3)

Mental health researchers did not recognize the extent to which an individual's identity, psyche, and sense of self derive from social context. In order to get inside this dynamic, a social science that could capture the fullness of experience, the richness of living was crafted. The point of departure was the focused points of human experience – individual perceptions, beliefs, and feelings. These constituted the most important units of analysis. However, in order for this approach to succeed, it also had to empower all project participants by valuing individual insight, work and knowledge. Most decisions involving the development and execution of The Well-Being Project were made by consensus.

Ultimately, The Well-Being Project was about people coming to voice. This was the critical lesson for the service user researchers that were to follow. Biomedical research ignores the meaningful human aspects that encompass personal and social needs and all the factors that differentiate people from symptoms, brains, or molecules. This effort never was intended to be a survey on 'mental illness,' or for that matter, on emotional or psychological problems. Rather, by not categorizing people under psychiatric labels, and by focusing on the promotion of wellness, it underscored the basic humanity and uniqueness of the individual through its research protocol and in the content of its findings.

Further, the incongruities identified in the survey results between the perceptual and experiential framework of those that managed and delivered mental health services, and those that received such services, brought into question the appropriateness of the opinions and studies of mental health professionals when contrasted with the insights and preferences of service users and their families.

In the ongoing years, the concept of the 'consumer perspective' and the need to develop multi-stakeholder approaches within program evaluation began to gain currency among progressive forces in state and federal government agencies and in the mental health field in general (Campbell, 1996). In 1989 the National Association of State Mental Health Program Directors (NASMHPD) approved a position paper that recognizes that former mental patients/mental health consumers have a unique contribution to make to the improvement of the quality of mental health services in many areas of the service delivery system. The paper recommended that consumer contributions should be valued and sought in areas of program development, policy formation, program evaluation, quality assurance, systems designs, education of mental health service providers, and the provision of direct services.

Growing numbers of professionals and policymakers responded to service user demands by redesigning professional roles and creating opportunities for people who receive services to provide input and perspective (Blanch et al., 1993; Kaufmann, 1994; McCabe and Unzicker, 1995). Rapp, Shera and Kisthardt (1993) observed that research concerning the care and treatment of people with mental illness has not been consonant with an emphasis on empowerment and argued that 'research should amplify 'the voice of the consumer' by attending to the context of research, the vantage point, the process of formulating research questions, the selection of interventions to be tested, the selection of outcomes and measures, and the dissemination of research results' (p727). Many professional efforts to accommodate service user participation failed to include persons diagnosed with mental illness at all key stages of the research and data collection process. However, there has also been broad experimentation in participatory styles of research and evaluation that have led to empowering service user roles (Delman, 2007; Fenton et al., 1993; Leff et al., 1997; Loder and Glover, 1992).

Service users as researchers, administrators and providers began to apply sophisticated data and health informatics strategies to public policy debates, peer-run services, and the conduct of science itself (Campbell, 1997). In a series of focus group sessions supported by the Center for Mental Health Services (CMHS), the Mental Health Consumer/Survivor Research and Policy Work Group, a coalition of service user leaders and researchers, began a systematic articulation of outcomes of mental health services and supports from a service user perspective (1992). Concept-mapping, a computerized software program that facilitated the organisation and analysis of focus group interactions (Trochim, 1989; Trochim and Linton, 1986) was used in the inquiry because the methods were structured and replicable on the one hand, and participatory and democratic on the other hand. Further, Jeanne Dumont, a service user researcher was one of the developers of the program (Dumont, 1989).

From the brainstorming, sorting, and ranking sessions, 'maps' were generated that identified domains and performance indicators (Trochim *et al.*, 1993). According to participants, traditional mental health services pathologised problems in living, held low expectations of consumer achievement, were paternalistic, offered a limited range options, and defined anger as symptomatic. The most frequently identified concerns were:

1. Mental health provider threats of involuntary treatments
2. Subtle forms of coercion
3. Lack of respect
4. Debilitating side-effects of psychotropic medications.

Recovery, personhood, well-being and liberty were identified as valued outcomes (Mental Health Consumer/Survivor Research and Policy Work Group Task Force Reports, 1992). It was noted by participants that traditional researchers seldom developed measures of detrimental effects of treatment and care (negative outcomes) and positive psychological outcomes such as recovery were missing from most research studies. Building on these preliminary studies, service users advocated for a value-based Consumer-Oriented Mental Health Statistics Improvement Program Report Card which included the performance indicators they had identified (Teague *et al.,* 1997).

Key to development of a peer-support services evidence-base in the United States was the continued support of the federal government to promote self-help alternatives, generally known as peer-run services, as part of a broader policy effort to reform psychiatry through patient self-advocacy. Consumer involvement in mental health services was mandated by federal law and actively promoted by projects at the federal and state levels (Parrish, 1989; National Institute of Mental Health, 1991). With federal and state support through block grants and other federal funding such as research demonstration initiatives, the number of peer-run service models continued to expand throughout the 1990s and evaluation of these efforts produced a wealth of descriptive and quasi-experimental data from service users who directed or were involved in key research project on peer-run programs. Most notably, the Community Support Program (CSP) in the Center for Mental Health Services funded 14 projects designed to implement and evaluate peer-run services during the period from 1988–1991. Although only one evaluation project was headed by a service user (Kaufmann *et al.*, 1993), a review of these programs was conducted by Van Tosh and del Vecchio (2000), well-known service user professionals, and published by the federal government.

Service users in the United States also identified the needs and preferences for housing and supports (Collaborative Support Programs of New Jersey, 1991; Tanzman, 1993; Ralph and Campbell, 1995), profiled state mental-health systems (Campbell, 1998), introduced the consumer satisfaction team (Fricks, 1995), and promoted the use of focus groups (Abramczyk, 1995; Midgley *et al.*, 1994). Today, service users are beginning to partner with professionals or to initiate independent efforts to develop positive psychological measures of well-being, empowerment and recovery (Campbell-Orde *et al.*, 2005; Ralph *et al.*, 2000; Rogers *et al.*, 1997), and to conduct rigorous quantitative studies of peer-run services (Clay *et al.*, 2005; Dumont and Jones, 2002; Campbell *et al.*, 2006).

The Peer Outcomes Protocol (POP) Project developed, field-tested, and disseminated an evaluation protocol to measure service and programmatic outcomes for mental health community-based peer support programs (Campbell, 2002). Funded as part of the 1995–2000 University of Illinois at Chicago's (UIC) National Research and Training Center (NRTC) on Psychiatric Disability, it was largely designed, directed, and implemented by researchers, advocates, and providers who had a diagnosis of mental illness. The POP is a modularized instrument, each outcome domain measured with objective as well as subjective items. Self-report items ask specifically about the effects of peer support on the particular outcome in question. A manual describing how to administer the POP, a question-by-question guide, the survey instrument, a set of response cards, and a report on the psychometric properties of the protocol are available on the NRTC website (http://www.psych.uic.edu/uicnrtc/pophome.htm, accessed 28/10/08).

Mental Health Recovery: What Helps and What Hinders? (Onken *et al.*, 2002) was a national research project for the development of recovery facilitating system performance indicators that evolved from collaborative efforts among a team of service user and non-service user researchers, state mental health authorities, and a consortium of sponsors. The project involved a grounded theory inquiry concerning the phenomenon of recovery, creation of prototype systems-level performance indicators, and pilot testing. Structured focus groups and grounded theory qualitative research methods were used in nine states with a diverse cross-section of 115 service users to gain knowledge on what helps and what hinders mental health recovery. The research team then used a process of qualitative coding and member checks to develop a single set of emergent themes and findings that informed a conceptual paradigm for organising and interpreting the phenomenon. Two sets of performance indicators were developed with small scale prototype testing involving eight state mental health authorities and approximately 200 service users. The final combined set of indicators was incorporated into a stand alone recovery orientation systems level measure that is rapidly becoming a standard in the field.

The growing evidence base of the effectiveness of peer-run services (Davidson *et al.*, 1999) and the high quality of the evidence encouraged policy efforts to expand peer supports within the continuum of community care. In an experimental research demonstration project, Dumont and Jones (2002) discovered that access to a crisis hostel program produced healing/recovery and greater sense of empowerment than traditional hospital-based services. Campbell and others in the Consumer-Operated Service Program (COSP) Multi-site Research Initiative (2006) found that COSPs (peer-run service programs) are effective as an adjunct to traditional mental health services in improving the outcomes of adults diagnosed with serious mental illness and established a significant link between the service elements of peer-run programs and positive psychological functioning.

The COSP Multisite Research Initiative (Clay *et al.*, 2005; Campbell *et al.*, 2006) represented a major advance in bringing the voice of persons with mental illness into dialogue with researchers to deepen the understanding of the programs and services that consumers have developed for themselves to promote their wellness. It was the largest and most rigorous study of consumer-operated services ever conducted and one of the most participatory involving significant numbers of service users at all levels of the project in meaningful research roles (Campbell *et al.*, 2006). Funded by the Substance Abuse and Mental Services Administration, it utilized a randomized, controlled trail design with an optimized, common *a priori* hypothesis and an intent-to-treat analysis. Analysis of over 1600 participants revealed that those offered consumer-operated services as an adjunct to their traditional mental health services showed significant gains in hope, self-efficacy, empowerment, goal attainment and meaning of life in comparison to those who were offered traditional mental health services only. Further, the greatest gains in well-being were found for the group of participants who actually used the peer services the most and variations in well-being effects across sites were unrelated to formal COSP models of peer service delivery.

Funded by the Ontario Ministry of Health and Long Term Care, a similar longitudinal study of four consumer-run organisations was conducted in Canada to evaluate the impacts on both individuals and systems of consumer/survivor initiatives (CSIs) or consumer-run alternatives to mainstream mental health services using participatory action research (Nelson *et al.*, 2006). The research was guided by a Steering Committee composed of professional researchers and service users who met quarterly to discuss, review, and approve all of the research activities. Service users were also hired and trained to recruit study participants, conduct interviews, and attend research team meetings. Information about study results were disseminated to the service user community as they became available. The participatory-action research approach challenged traditional assumptions of how to conduct research as roles and relationships were re-examined by both professional and consumer/survivor researchers. Reflections on the research process and outcomes of service user involvement led professional researchers to observe the importance of building relationships as a means to share power and knowledge (Ochocka *et al.*, 2002).

In the United Kingdom mental health policy, research and the role of mental health service users was contested throughout the past decades. In the 1990s, the main thrust of quality assurance policy appeared to be more concerned with service priorities than service user issues (Lewis and Glennerster, 1996), although patient satisfaction had long been a central part of quality assurance (McIver and Carr-Hill, 1989). Evidence provided by Vouri (1991) argued that the focus should be on outcomes rather than service users' perceptions of outcomes (Shaw, 1997). However, the government white paper, *The New NHS: Modern, Dependable* (Department of Health, 1997), stated the 'the Government will take special steps to ensure the experience of service users and carers is central to the work of the NHS' (p66).

Service user researchers observed

If it can be difficult to see that users of mental health services are people first and foremost, it may be equally difficult to accept that users of psychiatric services can play a central part in service evaluation, by taking the role of interviewers and site visitors

(Rose et al., 1998, p5)

Service user research was supported by voluntary organisations such as Mind, the Mental Health Foundation, and the Sainbury Centre for Mental Health (Wallcraft, 2007). For example, the Sainbury Centre for Mental Health developed a long-term co-research relationship with a group of psychiatric service users to evaluate community mental health services (Bereford and Wallcraft, 1997). In the final report, Beeforth *et al.* (1994) made an argument for service user led research:

> *It was strongly believed that users, who can demonstrate their common experience with other users, could get at the truth much better because they could persuade others of their independence from the service. . . . In particular the issue of independence from the service provider is very difficult for non-user researchers. Their background, presentation and links with service agencies make it difficult for users to believe that their views will not get back to hose who provide the service directly . . . The perceptions that (user-led research) seeks are those that users would want to tell each other, not what they have been told is good for them.*

(p4)

The partnership between Kensington, Chelsea and Westminster Health Authority and the Sainsbury Centre for Mental Health demonstrated that 'people with severe and enduring mental illness can have a voice in decisions about the mental health services they receive' (Rose *et al.*, 1998, p3) by participating in the development and implementation of a service user-focused monitoring system. The User-Focused Monitoring Team, staffed by mental health service user researchers, established that when they received appropriate training and support they could elicit the views of others diagnosed with severe mental health problems. Their instruments were based on the experiences of local service users so the questions asked would really matter to service users. The interviewers and site visitors were local service users of mental health services who were trained, supported, and paid to carry out face-to-face interviews and site visits. In *Getting Ready for User-Focused Monitoring (UFM): A Guide for Mental Health Service Providers, Users and Purchasers* (Sainsbury Centre for Mental Health, 1998), the benefits of service user feedback of their mental health service delivery were identified as 'improved information about what matters to service users, better targeted services based on identified needs, better working relationships between staff, service users and carers, and, a greater sense of service user 'ownership' (p2).

In another evaluation effort, the Mental Health Task Force User Group, composed of current and former service users representing three service user organisations in England, was commissioned by the Department of Health to carry out consumer-satisfaction research as services were transferred to the community with the closure of a large psychiatric hospital. Based on this research, a set of rights and principles on which persons diagnosed with mental illness specified they wanted services to be based were identified (Mental Health Task Force User Group, 1994).

In assessing early service user led research, Beresford and Wallcraft (1997) concluded,

> *While the findings of orthodox research generally point to incremental changes within the existing paradigm, user-led research posits more radical shifts of control, rights, knowledge and resources to service users and their organisations.*

(p80)

In an examination of the evidence for a range in alternative therapies in mental health, Wallcraft (1998) found clear evidence that service users wanted alternatives and valued them when they received them. They called for more open, equal and holistic approaches to both existing ideas and services in the United Kingdom based on first hand accounts of service user experiences (Pembroke, 1992;1994).

Wallcraft (2007) described the Strategies for Living service user program at the Mental Health Foundation as the 'biggest and most influential project' of research alternatives to psychiatry (p345). With funding from the National Lottery, research was managed by service users and overseen by an advisory group of service users. One study conducted by this project was *Knowing Our Own Minds* (Faulkner, 1997), a large survey of over 400 people diagnosed with mental illness about their thoughts on mental health treatments and therapies and what kinds of personal self-help strategies they found useful. Results from the study emphasized alternative supports and coping strategies which offered opportunities for empowering interpersonal relationships such as being accepted and sharing experience, finding meaning and purpose, ways to take control over one's life, and achieving peace of mind (Faulkner and Layzell, 2000). A survey of 56 persons' experiences with losing employment due to mental health problems was also undertaken (Tibbs *et al.*, 2003).

In Amsterdam, Holland, Harrie van Haaster founded the Dutch organisation Instituut voor Gebruikersparticipatie en Beleid (IGPB) in 1995 to provide support for service user groups seeking to make their own assessments of the quality of service provision or to conduct research from a service user perspective. The service user-run research company continues to be engaged in a wide range of research and development projects including assessment, management, and writing a life story, as well as offering 'Experts by Experience' training courses. The Institute stresses the importance of systematizing patients'/ service users' knowledge acquired through experience – only in this way can it provide trusted input into the management and development of health care systems. Harrie van Haaster (psychminded.co.uk, 2007) commented on the importance of making experiential knowledge of service users explicit:

> ...there is all the knowledge gained through the self-help movement. It may not be written, evidence-based knowledge, but self-help is full of knowledge... And while it is important that knowledge is connected with individual stories, it is also important to find the 'inter-subjective' knowledge...'we-knowledge'...and develop our own validation strategies...It is not about being against professionals, but about building our self esteem.

The IGPB model of research participation supports service user involvement at all stages of a project: service users design and implement the study and professional researchers provide support as needed. Therefore, the responsibility for initiating research lies with service user organisations. This model ensures that the issues studied are appropriate, the service user perspective is represented, and participating organisations achieve an effective voice in policy-making.

In a related effort, long-term mental-health care service users in the Netherlands in collaboration with Trimbos Institute developed the TREE program (Boevink, 2007). The underlying principle of this program is to produce and pass on narratives in order to recover a sense of self. By exchanging experiences service users support each other, recover, become empowered, and gain experiential expertise. Participants craft collective stories from the transformation of individual narratives to build experiential knowledge base and to make it available to fellow service users, mental health professionals and others.

In Australia, in order to better align health and medical research with community need, and improve the impact of research, the National Health and Medical Research Council joined with the Consumers' Health Forum of Australia to release a Statement on Consumer and Community Participation in Health and Medical Research that supports the rights of consumers to participate in research (Saunders *et al.*, 2006). A qualitative survey of the opinions of mental health service users about research priorities for mental health in Australia rated 'involvement of mental health consumers in planning the research as of very high priority, as did carers.' (Griffiths *et al.*, 2002). However, Griffiths (2004) warned that researcher and provider attitudes served as a significant barrier to widespread participation. In response to this challenge, in 2004 a group of forty mental health and health delegates participated in the national workshop 'Promoting Consumer Participation in Mental Health Research' (Griffiths *et al.*, 2004). One outcome of this effort was the publication of aims and principles to 'improve the mental health of the community and expand and strengthen the current mental health knowledge base through increased participation in mental health research' (p100). Among the recommendations included the acknowledgement that research partnerships involving consumers 'should be adaptable and based on understanding, respect, and shared commitment,' and that budgets would 'appropriately include the cost of consumer involvement' (p105).

REFLECTIONS ON A METHODOLOGY OF VOICE

The growth and development of service user involvement in research worldwide is impressive as the descriptions of selected efforts above have clearly shown. Still, I find it problematic to take as a given that service users truly 'speak for themselves' from their own experiences as persons who have been diagnosed with mental illnesses when their voices are mediated by persons who stand outside the experience of being a person who has been diagnosed with a mental illness. Further, personal anecdotes and testimonies, regardless of sophisticated methodologies to collect and analyse such information, seldom generalise to other people in other situations with any scientific certainty. Therefore, I wonder how traditional researchers can give perspective to someone else's experience without violating that person's view of his/her experience. Do such methodological problems also apply to my own work as a mental health service user? Consider this quote from bell hooks (1989):

> In all my writing classes, I was the only black student. Whenever I read a poem written in the particular dialect of southern black speech, the teacher and fellow students would praise me for using my 'true,' authentic voice, and encouraged me to develop this 'voice,' to write more of these poems. From the onset this troubled me. Such comments seemed to mask racial biases about what my authentic voice would or should be.
>
> (p11)

The effect of professionals validating the 'raw' material of service user experience, and placing it in 'perspective' reinforces the biomedical research ideology that sees people as sources of data rather than as shapers and interpreters of their own experience.

Traditional researchers may assume a close identification between the person and the illness in an attempt to explain mental illness from the perspective of study participants. In an exploratory study by Estroff *et al.* (1991), the authors presented results from in-depth interviews with a largely in-patient sample of people with psychiatric diagnoses and treatment histories indicative of severe mental illnesses. The writers talked about 'normalisation' as a special process within identity talk among their interviewees and as a problem in identity construction in the face of psychiatric labeling. The normalisation process was presented in the title as 'everybody's got a little mental illness' and continued through a series of quotes from the transcribed texts of interviewees that, in the authors' judgment, provided examples of 'normalisation talk'. Content analysis was used to develop an empirical base from which to launch the interpretation of self-labeling. Claims to being normal were scrutinized in the verbal accounts of patients in psychiatric hospitals in an effort to understand how patients make sense of their diagnosis and the fact that they are in a mental hospital. To quote the authors:

> ...accounting for mental illness unavoidably entails giving account of oneself, so closely implicated are person and illness.

(p333)

I find the authors enmeshed in a set of social assumptions about people with mental illness that required them to account for cases that deviate from an implied stereotype. They present a young adult man named Ed who has been involuntarily hospitalized with a diagnosis of bipolar affective disorder. Ed has refused to co-operate with the interviewer, having withdrawn his informed consent to follow-up interviews. He denies he is mentally ill, is reluctant to co-operate with drug therapy and community rehabilitation programs, and is obviously a member of a well-to-do social class. Unlike his fellow patients in the psychiatric ward, Ed notes that he is better educated and more aware of the world. He recognizes the social contrasts and the social distances between his own experience as the son of a wealthy family and those of others in the hospital with less education and financial resources.

The authors discussed this as a problem with Ed, rather than one embedded in the perspective of the researchers. Ed is described with unflattering physical characteristics, though it is doubtful he would describe himself in that way. When he states, correctly, that he is not like the other patients, the authors takes this as an example of his denial of social reality and as an omen for the downward social drift his future implies. The interview confronts the participant with an uncomfortable reality: Ed's unwillingness to describe himself as having a mental illness.

However, this act may be more than a simple case of denial, but rather an attempt on Ed's part to reject the stereotype of the 'chronic mentally ill'. Viewed from Ed's perspective, it could be an act of self-validation that can be examined less as an example of one person's refusal to accept reality than a claim to more complex and varied social roles outside of the psychiatric hospital. I believe that this possibility would be entertained more easily if the researchers began the scientific inquiry from the point of view of the participant rather than the observer.

I sometimes find accounts of researchers in which their qualitative interpretation of personal narratives or empirical analyses of interviews have not conformed either to their assumptions or the individuals providing perspective. Martin (1987) reflects on the differences between first-hand experience and empirical generalizations drawn from a collection of experiences:

> When a researcher gathers together the talk of many individuals, organizes it around what appears to be common themes, and presents these back to those who talked in the first place,

the result is hard to predict. . . . When the streams of talk we collected are gathered together, many hard truths are also revealed. But in addition, putting together many individual voices has produced a resounding chorus . . . [that] tells us of many visions of life, different for different women, and powerfully different from the reality that now holds sway.

(p203)

In fact, I have encountered persons diagnosed with mental illnesses who learn to talk about their experiences in therapeutic terms, and refer to him/herself using terms developed within the mental health system. For example, a spokesperson for mental health service users may introduce his/herself as 'high functioning', a term used by professionals in psychosocial rehabilitation to denote a client who does well with relatively few professional supports. Such talk tends to validate the values of mental health service-providers as the primary interpreters of other people's experiences of mental illnesses.

I have found that admission-by-invitation to the spheres of empirical research and policy-making carries with it a burden to represent the hosts' idea of the social group that as the invited person I am supposed to represent. I am often expected to play the part of critic and token and to speak 'from the consumer perspective' as though people with mental illnesses shared some common views of their experiences that could be captured in the opinions of a few key people.

BEST PRACTICE OR CAUTIONARY TALE?

The opportunity as principle investigator of the Coordinating Center for the Consumer-Operated Service Program (COSP) Multisite Research Initiative to lead the effort to incorporate the methodologies of service user involvement into an important and very large randomized, controlled multisite study proved both challenging and very rewarding. Ultimately, the integration of diverse service user and professional cultures and perspectives into the conduct of research tested the limits of leadership, knowledge, experience and good intentions. Therefore, by detailing some of the social interactions among all the stakeholders within the multisite study can instruct the effort to determine best practices for service user involvement in research.

The COSP Multisite study established a national Consumer Advisory Panel (CAP) composed of service user representatives and researchers from each participating study site. Each site also had a local CAP composed of the national CAP representatives, program participants, staff and local service user movement leaders. The COSP study also employed service user personnel in many roles of the project including principle investigators, project managers, data managers, interviewers, data entry personnel and interview respondents.

In the design phase of the study, the formulation of the research questions focused on service user movement concerns from patienthood to personhood involving the constructs of hope, empowerment, meaning in life, recovery, social inclusion, self efficacy, stability of housing, movement toward work, satisfaction with services and satisfaction with life. Clinical constructs such as symptoms and diagnoses were of less interest. Measurement instruments were carefully selected, not only for validity and reliability, but also for sensitivity to the service user perspective and respectful tone. Interviewer training strongly emphasized respect for participants in the data collection process. Service user choice was emphasized within the informed consent and randomization processes. COSP policies mandated the highest standards of confidentiality in data storage and transmission in recognition of service user feelings of vulnerability when divulging private and potentially sensitive information.

Later on, knowledge dissemination plans included formats and forums that were accessible and comprehensible to lay service user readers. COSP findings were presented at state and national consumer conferences in publications with a consumer readership and through web-based consumer forums. From the beginning, the study intended that consumer-operated service programs would be able to use the study results to improve peer practices by adapting evidence-based service models to better support their members.

The empowerment of mental health service users in the administration, design, implementation, and analysis activities on the COSP study necessitated an ongoing dialogue between service users, researchers, and mental health professionals to reach common ground regarding issues of authority, expertise, and language. Values and goals that arose from culturally dissimilar experiences, tended to separate people and polarize discussion. There was no common language or set of experiences that would naturally bring people together. Further, issues of data collection became a focus in struggles for influence as the choice of measures was often contested during the development of the common protocol. Bridging differences between people on a personal level was supported through social activities at the national Steering Committee meetings in Washington DC such as formal and informal dinners, tours of the city, a talent show, and group attendance at a variety of entertainment venues.

Service user led sessions on the history of the service user movement and individual experiences with the mental health system were held at Steering Committee face-to-face meetings. Researchers also shared their life stories at another meeting.

To help service users without research experience participate fully in research discussions, the Coordinating Center familiarized them with the use of research terms through publication of a glossary for non-researchers and hosting technical assistance workshops about the nature and conduct of research. Specialists were also brought to CAP meetings to discuss issues such as hypothesis development, logic modeling, random assignment, and power analysis.

Important factors such as remuneration and power-sharing were also addressed. While some thought it might be a financial benefit to employ service users at a lower rate, it was recognized that adequate pay and reimbursement of expenses was essential for trust, cooperation, and sustained commitment.

The COSP multisite study found that 'consumer' meant many different things within the study. It embraced participants both within traditional mental health services and consumer-operated service programs. Mental health service users also served as staff or program directors within all COSPs and some of the traditional mental health programs. Thus, in addition to being 'consumers', they were also providers.

To further confuse the issue, a number of service user researchers were serving in roles from interviewers to principal investigators. It became clear that the major source of tension in the multi site was not between service users and traditional researchers as originally assumed, but rather was located within the relations of research production. Each study site had initially proposed its own study, with its own procedures and instruments, and the necessity to change these proposals in order to develop a common interview protocol with common study procedures met with resistance. Similarly, as in many other randomized clinical trials, programs – both consumer-operated and traditional – bristled in the beginning of the study as difficult issues associated with actually implementing random assignment and maintaining the values of choice became apparent. Efforts to standardize procedures by the Coordinating Center were sometimes seen as criticism at the study site level and challenged the authority of site investigators.

One area of concern expressed at key points within the study involved the fragility of some of the consumer-operated service programs participating in the study. Service user providers recognised from the outset that research involvement might stress these programs by distorting program operations, goals and outcomes. They encouraged a commitment within the research to 'First, do no harm,' and at the midway point the Steering Committee engaged in self-examination to assess the potentially negative effects of study participation on programs.

The extensive processing of research decisions and study interactions decisions slowed the expected start-up of the research, resulting in fewer study participants assigned to the COSP, elevating costs, and leading to some staff turnover and additional training requirements. Within some programs, turnover among program directors produced uncertainty and periods of turmoil. Although turnover itself is not necessarily an indicator of greater fragility, the organisational structures that allowed for the orderly succession of administrators were strained.

Due to the scope, complexity, decentralization, and problems in the execution of collaborative decision-making, the study leaders found it useful to engage formal facilitation and consultation to help the COSP multisite study remain sensitive to program and participant values and achieve research objectives. At three points, the multisite turned to organisational consultants or facilitators to study difficulties, to allow all parties within the process to have a voice in discussions, and to explore tensions. In one case, interviews by an organisational psychologist allowed for development of a clearer set of expectations that the various parties in this study (the federal representatives, the Coordinating Center, and study sites) had of one another, and produced a strategic response to better manage these expectations. In another case, a facilitator helped the Steering Committee to identify some of the potentially negative consequences of participatory methods in the multisite study, and attempted to play a role in bridging a perceived gap in the perspectives of service users and mental health professionals. In a third case, facilitators initiated a dialogue among Steering Committee members that led to the adoption of recommendations that enhanced the tone and content of communications. The COSP research experience suggested that skilled organisational consultants and facilitators can play a useful role providing a safe forum for all parties to share mutual concerns and engage in collaborative problem-solving when organisational mechanisms to resolve conflict are not clearly developed and lines of authority blurred.

The broad involvement of service users in the COSP multisite study was central to developing an appropriate study hypothesis, selecting measures of positive psychological impacts of the COSPs, and implementing research protocols that were consistent with the values of persons diagnosed with mental illness. Further, the Consumer Advisory Panel identified and organised 46 common ingredients of peer practices at the participating COSPs into an objective, structured tool called the Fidelity Assessment Common Ingredients Tool (FACIT). The FACIT was administered to both the COSPs and the traditional mental health programs at each study site by the Coordinating Center to determine the extent that they implemented the COSP model, processes, and values (Johnsen, Teague and McDonel Herr, 2005). The FACIT also identified characteristic differences between COSPs and traditional mental health programs and differences between COSP models. Analyses of FACIT and outcome results established evidence of a strong relationship between key peer practices that support inclusion, peer beliefs and self-expression and an increase in study outcomes. Such capabilities have advanced the capacity of researchers, peer providers, and mental health administrators to promote evidence-based practices in developing consumer-operated services, guided quality improvements in mature COSPs, and identified and measured 'consumer-friendly elements' of traditional mental health programs.

As the research limps towards publication of its results many years after funding was exhausted, I am still not certain if the multisite study was an example of best practices or a cautionary tale for future endeavors. The participatory approaches ate into valuable time needed for data analysis and interpretation, were expensive and added additional costs to fixed research budgets, and were emotionally draining for the Coordinating Center staff as well as many other project participants. I began to experience marginalization as a member of the service user community. Some members of the CAP attacked my work and commitment to realize the promise of the study for service users throughout the nation. In an ironic role reversal, at one point I was charged with serving research goals over the best interests of the COSPs and the service users involved as research partners in the multisite study.

All is well that ends well in this case. By expanding the evidence base of effectiveness of peer-to-peer services to promote and enhance recovery, the COSP multisite study has validated efforts to bring mental health service users into the mental health workforce within peer-run programs and as peer specialists within traditional mental health services. Many professional and service user researchers and providers who participated have expressed pride in our accomplishments and appreciation for my leadership and dedication.

FINAL THOUGHTS FOR FUTURE PRACTICE

Such disquieting experiences as a service user researcher linger below the surface of my everyday work to emerge into consciousness and confront my practice as I seek to increase the meaning and usefulness of mental health investigations through methods that utilize service user voice. Can we begin to draw some conclusions from our accomplishments and challenges over the past thirty years that can guide service users in the continued production of experiential knowledge?

Certainly, participatory methods can go beyond the statistics that record and analyze numbers to include meaningful interactions with those living with a psychiatric diagnosis when we listen to the voices of engaged and involved participants: productive, thinking, feeling, creating, honoring others' values and choices, and respectfully listening as each person understands his/her own voice.

Voice does not privilege any particular kind of research. It comes to the process of research when service users claim the right and the power to make decisions for themselves, including research decisions. Voice intrudes into the methods of qualitative studies with the collection of unmediated narratives, in-depth interviews, testimonies and the like. It finds expression in quantitative studies with the weighing of perspectives through surveys and focus groups. Voice does not speak in one language, carry one message, or have one messenger. It is diverse, multicultural, and unpredictable precisely because it is empowering and democratic. Voice calls out for skills, scholarship and individual responsibility to honor the value of the pursuit of truth and knowledge.

In general, I have found that the best features of most service user research projects include practices that incorporate the products of voice:

- grassroots accounts
- bottom-up approaches
- participants as partners
- issues of ownership and control of the findings confronted
- the research story told
- personal impact captured
- knowledge exchange an important goal.

Besides the structural relations of researchers and service users regarding the level and type of involvement, the quality of relationships between traditional mental health researchers and consumers/survivors involved in a research projects can be interrogated by assessing those research practices that protect and encourage voice or subvert and mute voice through the use of informed consent protocols, diagnostic labels and 'jargon' to refer to people being studied, the devaluation of consumer contributions to the research, the imposition of token roles, and the explicit expression of status differentials between professional researchers and consumer/survivor participants.

C. Wright Mills (1959) challenged us all to use our sociological imagination to

grasp what is going on in the world, and to understand what is happening in [ourselves] as minute points of the intersections of biography and history within society.

(p7)

It is ironic that although the mental health system exists within perhaps the most tumultuous times in history, most traditional mental health researchers do not see themselves as agents of change. Rather, persons diagnosed with mental illness are the visionaries struggling to prevail over the skepticism and despair of the mental health system and the prejudices of society at large. Speaking for ourselves, we can teach our research partners that to enslave people's dreams through biomedical science is more expensive morally and financially than to empower human beings to become the moral architects of their own destinies.

In order to integrate the diverse cultures of mental health professionals and service users into a research environment as participatory processes are established, it is necessary for all of us to pause and to encourage critical dialogue and self-reflection. We must incubate new relationships and methodologies as we consider the lessons learned from the past decades of service user research. The lived experience of mental health professionals and people diagnosed with mental illness can only enhance the quality and relevance of mental health research if our discourse is grounded in mutual respect and reciprocity as we all share our personal stories, organise and advocate for our beliefs, and help one another along the way.

By risking the comforts of an unexamined conscience, service users and professionals can 're-search' in its most literal sense the assumptions, responsibilities, and behaviours inscribed in our methods. I believe that attention to the demands of rigorous scientific methods and reconciliation of subjectivity in participatory processes remains paramount as we push forward. As one voice in the chorus who proclaimed that 'research ought to and can enhance service user choice, power and knowledge' (The Mental Health Consumer/Survivor Research and Policy Work Group, 2002), I share an optimism deepened by our learned experiences as service user researchers that the validity of our diverse perspectives depends on clarity in design, persistent attention to data quality, and respect for the power our voices bring to the scientific enterprise.

REFERENCES

Abramczyk, L. (1995) *SHARE Evaluation: Consumer perspective*, South Carolina: SHARE.

Anthony, W. (2001) Need for recovery-compatible evidence-based practices. *Mental Health Weekly*, 11(42), p 5.

Beeforth, M., Conlan, E. and Graley, R. (1994) *Have We Got Views for You: User evaluation of case management*, London: Sainsbury Centre for Mental Health.

Belenky, M.F., Clinchy, B.F. Goldberg, N. *et al.* (1986) *Women's Way of Knowing: The development of self, voice, and mind*, New York: Basic Books.

Beresford, Pand and Wallcraft, J. (1997) Psychiatric system survivors and emancipatory research: issues, overlaps and differences, In: C. Barnes and G. Mercer (Eds) *Doing Disability Research*, London: The Disability Press, pp. 66–87.

Bertaux-Wiame, I. (1985) Between social scientists: responses to Louise Tilly. *International Journal of Oral History*, 6(1), 25–31.

Blanch, A., Fisher, D. Tucker, W. *et al.* (1993) Consumer-practitioners and psychiatrists share insights about recovery and coping. *Disability Studies Quarterly*, 13(2), 17–20.

Blaska, B. (1991) What it is like to be treated like a CMI? *Schizophrenia Bulletin*, 17(1), 173–176.

Bodman, R., Davies, R. Frankel, N. *et al.* (1997) *Knowing Our Minds*, London: Mental Health Foundation.

Boevink, W. (2007) Survival, the art of living and knowledge to pass on: recovery, empowerment and experiential expertise of persons with severe mental health problems, In: P. Stastny and P. Lehmann (Eds.) *Alternatives Beyond Psychiatry*, Berlin, Germany: Peter Lehmann Publishing, pp. 105–116.

Campbell, J. (1996) Toward collaborative mental health outcomes systems. *New Directions for Mental Health Services*, 71, 68–77.

Campbell, J. (1997) How users/consumers/survivors/survivors are evaluating the quality of psychiatric care. *Evaluation Review*, 21(3), 357–363.

Campbell, J. (1998) *The technical assistance needs of consumer/survivor and family stakeholder groups within state mental health agencies*, Alexandria, VA: National Technical Assistance Center for State Mental Health, Planning.

Campbell, J. (2002) *New Studies and Tools for Consumer-operated Service Programs*, Washington, D.C.: National Conference on Mental Health Statistics.

Campbell, J. (2005) The historical and philosophical development of peer-run support programs, In: S. Clay, B. Schell, P.W. Corrigan, and R.O. Ralph (Eds) *On Our Own Together: Peer programs for people with mental illness*, Nashville, TN: Vanderbilt Press, pp. 17–64.

Campbell-Skillman, J. (1991) *Towards Undiscovered Country: Mental health clients speak for themselves*: Ann Arbor. U.M.I.

Campbell, J. and Schraiber, R. (1989) *The Well Being Project: Mental health clients speak for themselves*, Sacramento, CA: California Department of Mental Health.

Campbell, J., Lichtenstein, C. and Teague, G. *et al.* (2006) *The Consumer Operated Service Programs (COSP) Multi site Research Initiative: Final Report*, Saint Louis, MO: Coordinating Center at the Missouri Institute of Mental Health.

Campbell, J., Ralph, R. and Glover, R. (1993) 'From Lab Rat to Researcher: The history, models, and policy implications of consumer/survivor involvement in research', *Proceedings of the Fourth annual national conference on state mental health agency services research and program evaluation*, Alexandria,VA: National Association of State Mental Health Program Directors, pp. 138–157.

Campbell-Orde, T., Chamberlin, J., Carpenter, J. and Leff, S. (2005) *Measuring the Promise: A compendium of recovery measures*, Volume II Cambridge, MA: Health Services Research Institute.

Chamberlin, J. (1978) *On Our Own: Patient-Controlled Alternatives to the Mental Health System*, New York: McGraw-Hill.

Chesler, M.A. (1991) Participatory action research with self-help groups: an alternative paradigm for inquiry and action. *American Journal of Community Psychology*, **19**(5), 757–768.

Clay S., Schell B., Corrigan P.W. and Ralph R.O. (Eds) (2005) *On Our Own Together: Peer programs for people with mental illness*, Nashville, TN: Vanderbilt Press.

Collaborative Support Programs of New Jersey (1991) *Consumer Housing Preference Results and Executive Summary*, New Jersey: Freehold.

Colom, E. (1981) Reaction of an angry consumer. *Community Mental Health Journal*, **17**(1), 92–98.

Davidson, L., Chinman, M. and Kloos, B. *et al.* (1999) Peer support among individuals with severe mental illness: a review of the evidence. *Clinical Psychology: Science and Practice*, **9**(2), 165–187.

Deegan, P.E. (1988) Recovery: The lived experience of rehabilitation. *Psychosocial Rehabilitation Journal*, **11**(4), 11–19.

Delman, J. (2007) Consumer-driven and conducted survey research in action, In: T., Kroll, D., Kerr, P., Placek, J. Cyril and G. Hendershot (Eds) *Towards Best Practices for Surveying People with Disabilities*, New York: Nova Publishers, Inc, pp. 71–87.

Department of Health (1997). *The New NHS: Modern, Dependable*, London: HMSO.

Dumont, J. (1989) Validity of multidimensional scaling in the context of structured conceptualisation. *Evaluation and Program Planning*, **12**(1).

Dumont, J. and Jones, K. (2002) The Crisis Hostel: Findings from a consumer/survivor-defined alternative to psychiatric hospitalisation. *Outlook*, P. 4–6.

Eigo, J., Harrington, M. and McCarthy, M. *et al.* (1988) *FDA Action Handbook*, New York: ACT–UP.

Essock, S.M., Goldman, H.H. and Van Tosh, L. *et al.* (2003) Evidence-based practices: setting the context and responding to concerns. *Psychiatric Clinics of North America*, **26**, 918–938.

Estroff, S., Lachicotte, W., Illingworth, L. and Johnston, A. (1991) Everybody's got a little mental illness: Accounts of illness and self among people with severe, persistent mental illness. *Medical Anthropology Quarterly*, **5**(4), 331–369.

Faulkner, A. and Layzell, S. (2000) *Strategies for Living*, London: Mental Health Foundation.

Fricks, L. (1995) *Georgia Evaluation and Satisfaction Team (GEST) Handbook*, Atlanta: Georgia Division of Mental Health, Mental Retardation and Substance, Abuse.

Fisher, D.B. and Ahern, L. (2002) Evidenced-based practices and recovery. *Psychiatric Services*, **53**, 632–633.

Frese, F., Stanley, J., Kress, K. and Vogel-Scibilia (2001) Integrating evidence-based practices and the recovery model. *Psychiatric Services*, **52**(11), 1462–1468.

Griffiths, K. (2003–2004) Promoting consumer participation in mental health research in Australia: a national workshop. *The Australian Health Consumer*, **3**, 11–12.

Griffiths, K., Christensen, H. and Barney, L. *et al.* (2004) *Promoting Consumer Participation in Mental Health Research: A national workshop*, Canberra: Centre for Mental Health Research, The Australian National, University.

Griffiths, K., Jorm, A., Christensen, H., Medway, J. and Dear, K. (2002) Research priorities in mental health, Part 2: An Evaluation of the current research effort against stakeholders' priorities. *Australian and New Zealand Journal of Psychiatry*, **36**(3), 327–339.

Guthrie, R.V. (1993) *Even the Rat was White: A historical view of psychology*, Boston, MA: Allyn and Bacon.

hooks, b. (1989) When I was a young soldier for the revolution: coming to voice, in: *TalkingBack: Thinking feminist, thinking black*, Boston, MA: South End Press.

International Association of Psychosocial Rehabilitation Services (1998) *IAPSRS Position Statement: The single model trap*, Columbia, MD: International Association of Psychosocial Rehabilitation Services.

Johnsen, M., Teague, G. and McDonel Herr, E. (2005) 'Common ingredients as a fidelity measure for peer-run programs', In: S. Clay, B. Schell, P.W. Corrigan and R.O. Ralph (Eds) *On Our Own Together: Peer Programs for People with Mental Illness*, Nashville, TN: Vanderbilt Press, pp. 213–238.

Kaufmann, C.L., Ward-Colesante, C. and Farmer, J. (1993) Development and operation of drop-in centers operated by mental health users/consumers/survivors. *Hospital and Community Psychiatry*, **44**, 675–678.

Kaufmann, C.L. (1994) Roles for mental health consumers in self help group research. *Journal of Applied Behavioral Science*, **29**(2), 257–271.

Kaufmann, C.L. and Campbell, J. (1995) *Voice in the Mental Health Consumer Movement: An examination of services research by and for consumers*, American Psychological Association Annual Meeting, Washington D.C.

Leete, E. (1989) How I manage and perceive my illness. *Schizophrenia Bulletin*, **15**(2), 197–2000.

Leff, H.S., Campbell, J., Gagne, C. and Woocher, L.S. (1997) Evaluating peer providers, In: C.T. Mowbray, D. PMoxley, C.A. Jasper and L.L. Howell (Eds) *Consumers as Providers in Psychiatric Rehabilitation*, Columbia, MD: International Association of Psychosocial Rehabilitation Services, pp. 488–501.

Lewis, J. and Glennerster, H. (1996) *Implementing the New Community Care*, Buckingham: Open University Press.

Loder, A. and Glover, R. (1992) New frontiers: Pioneer dialogue between consumers/survivors and commissioners, *MHSIP Updates*, pp. 13–14.

Lovejoy, M. (1984) Recovery from schizophrenia: A personal odyssey. *Hospital and Community Psychiatry*, **35**(8), 809–812.

Marcus, J. (1986) Of madness and method. *Women's Review of Books*, **3**(11), 3.

Martin, E. (1987) *The Woman in the Body: A cultural analysis of reproduction*, Boston, MA: Beacon Press.

Marzilli, A. (2002) Controversy surrounds evidence-based practices, *The Key National Mental Health Consumers' Self-Help Clearinghouse, Newsletter* **7**(1).

McCabe, S. and Unzicker, R. (1995) Changing roles of consumer/survivors in mature mental health systems. *New Directions for Mental Health Services*, **66**, 61–73.

McIver, S. and Carr-Hill, R. (1989) *The NHS and its Consumers*, New York: Centre for Health Economics.

Mental Health Consumer/Survivor Research and Policy Work Group (1992) *Report 1 and 2. Fort Lauderdale*, Fl: The Well-Being Program, Inc.

Mental Health Task Force User Group (1994) *Guidelines for a Local Charter for Users of Mental Health Services*, Leeds: National Health Service Management Executive.

Midgley, J., Gilliland, S. and Rose, S. *et al.* (1994) *Initial development of a consumer-centered outcome monitoring system for mental health services to adults with severe mental illness, Findings and recommendations*. Baton Rouge, LA: Louisiana State University.

Mills, C.W. (1959) *The Sociological Imagination*, London: Oxford University Press.

Misztal, B. (1981) Autobiographies, diaries, life histories, and oral histories of workers as a source of socio-historical knowledge; *International Journal of Oral History*, **2**(3), 181–193.

Nelson, G., Ochocka, J., Janzen, R. and Trainor, J. (2006) A longitudinal study of mental health consumer/survivor initiatives: Part 1 – Literature review and overview of the study, *Journal of Community Psychology*, **34**(3), 247–260.

National Association for State Mental Health Program Directors (NASMHPD) (1989) NASMHPD position paper on consumer contributions to mental health service delivery systems, Alexandria, VA: NASMHPD.

National Institute of Mental Health (1991) *Caring for people with severe mental disorders: a national plan of research to improve services*, DHHS Pub. No. (ADM) 91-1762). Washington, DC: U.S. Government Printing Office.

New Freedom Commission on Mental Health (2003) *Achieving the Promise: Transforming mental health care in America, Final report*. DHHS Pub. No. SMA-03-3832. Rockville, MD.

Nicholls, V. (2001) *Doing Research Ourselves*, London: Mental Health Foundation.

Nide N. (Ed) (1990) *Yes I Can! Seven True Stories of Persons Coping with Mental and Emotional Illness*, Franklin, OH: Alliance for the Mentally Ill.

Ochocka, J., Janzen, R. and Nelson, G. (2002) Sharing power and knowledge: Professional and mental health consumer/survivor researchers working together in a participatory action research project. *Psychiatric Rehabilitation Journal*, **25**(4), 379–387.

Onken, S., Dumont, J. and Ridgway, P. *et al.* (2002) *Mental Health Recovery: What helps and what hinders? A national research project for the development of recovery facilitating system performance indicators*, Alexandria, VA: National Technical Assistance Center for State Mental Health, Planning, National Association of State Mental Health Program Directors.

Parrish, J. (1989) The long journey home: accomplishing the mission of the community support movement. *Psychosocial Rehabilitation Journal*, **12**, 107–124.

Pembroke, L.R. (1992) *Eating Distress: Perspectives from personal experience*, London: Survivors Speak Out.

Pembroke, L.R. (1994) *Self-harm: Perspectives from personal experience*, London: Survivors Speak Out.

Personal Narratives Group (Ed). (1989) *Interpreting Women's Lives: Feminist theory and personal narratives*, Bloomington, IN: Indiana University Press.

Prager, E. and Tanaka, H. (1979) A client-developed measure (CDM) of self-assessment and change for outpatient mental health services. In: *New Research in Mental Health*, Columbus: Ohio Department of Mental Health, pp. 48–51.

Ralph, R.O. and Campbell, J. (1995) Using a consumer developed housing/supports preference survey as a continuous outcome survey. In: *Proceedings: Fifth annual national conference on state mental health agency services research and program evaluation*. San Antonio, TX: National Association of State Mental Health Program Directors Research Institute.

Ralph, R.O., Kidder, K. and Phillips, D. (2000) *Can We Measure Recovery? A compendium of recovery and recovery-related instruments*, Cambridge, MA: The Evaluation Center at HSRI.

Rapp, C.A., Shera, W. and Kisthardt, W. (1993) Research strategies for consumer empowerment of people with severe mental illness, *Social Work*, **38**(6), 727–735.

Rheinharz, S. (1992) *Feminists Methods in Social Research*. New York: Oxford University Press.

Ridgway, P.A. (1988) *The Voice of Users/Consumers/Survivors in Mental Health Systems: A call for change*, Vermont: Center for Community Change through Housing and Support.

Ridgway, P.A. (2001) Re-storying psychiatric disability: Learning from first person recovery narratives. *Psychiatric Rehabilitation Journal*, **24**(4), 335–343.

Rogers, E.S., Chamberlin, J., Ellison, M.L. and Crean, T. (1997) A consumer-constructed scale to measure empowerment among users of mental health services. *Psychiatric Services*, **48**, 1042–1047.

Rose, D. (1996) *Living in the Community*, London: The Sainsbury Centre for Mental Health.

Rose, D., Ford, R., Lindley, P. and Gawith, L. and The KCW Mental Health Monitoring Users' Group (1998) *In Our Experience: User-focused monitoring of mental health services in Kensington and Chelsea and Westminster Health Authority*, London: Sainsbury Centre for Mental Health.

Sainsbury Centre for Mental Health (1998) *Getting Ready for User-focused Monitoring: A guide for mental health service providers, users and purchasers*, London: Sainsbury Centre for Mental Health.

Saunders, C., Crossing, S. and Girgis, A. *et al.* (2007) Operationalising a model framework for kconsumer and community participation in health and medical research. *Australian and New Zealand Health Policy*, **4**(13), 1–6.

Schrager, S. (1983) What is social in oral history? *International Journal of Oral History*, **4**(2), 76–98.

Scott, A. (1993) Consumers/survivors reform the system, bringing a human face to research. *Resources*, **5**, p. 1

Shaw, I. (1997) Assessing quality in mental health care: the United Kingdom experience. *Evaluation Review*, **21**(3), 364–370.

Shepherd, L.J. (1993) *Lifting the Veil: The feminine face of science*, Boston, MA: Shambhala Press.

Sommer, R. and Osmond, H. (1983) A bibliography of mental patients' autobiographies, 1960–1982. *American Journal of Psychiatry*, **140**(8), 1051–1054.

Susko M. (Ed) (1991) *Cry of the Invisible: Writings from the homeless and survivors of psychiatric hospitals*, Baltimore, MD: Conservatory Press.

Tanzman, B. (1993) An overview of mental health users/consumers/survivors' preferences for housing and support services, *Hospital and Community Psychiatry*, **44**(5), 450–455.

Teague, G., Ganju, V. and Hornik, J. *et al.* (1997) The MHSIP Mental Health Report Card: a consumer-oriented approach to monitoring the quality of mental health plans, *Evaluation Review*, **21**(3), 330–341.

Tibbs, N., Tovey, Z. and Unger, E. (2003) *Life's Labour Lost*, London: Mental Health Foundation.

Trochim, W. and Linton, R. (1986) Conceptualization for planning and evaluation, *Evaluation and Program Planning*, **9**(4), 289–308.

Trochim, W. (1989) Concept mapping: soft science or hard art? *Evaluation and Program Planning*, **12**, (1).

Trochim, W., Dumont, J. and Campbell, J. (1993) *A Report for the State Mental Health Agency Profiling System: Mapping mental health outcomes from the perspective of consumers/survivors*. Technical report series Alexandria, VA: National Association of State Mental Health Program Directors.

Unzicker, R. (1989) On my own: A personal journey through madness and re-emergence. *Psychosocial Rehabilitation Journal*, **13**(1), 71–77.

Van Tosh, L. and del Vecchio, P. (2000) *Consumer-operated self-help programs: a technical report*, Rockville, MD: Center for Mental Health Services.

Vouri, H. (1991) Patient satisfaction: does it matter? *Quality Assurance in Health Care*, **3**, 83–189.

Wallcraft, J. (1998) *Healing Minds*, London: Mental Health Foundation.

Wallcraft, J. 2007 User-led research to develop and evidence base for alternative approaches: the role of research in mental health, PStastny and PLehmann (Eds) *Alternatives Beyond Psychiatry* Berlin: Peter Lehmann Publishing, pp. 105–115.

Wilson, S.F. and Blanch, A.K. (1987) *The Role of Ex-patients and Users/Consumers/Survivors in Human Resource Development for the 1990s*, Holyoke, MA: Western Massachusetts Training Consortium.

Zinman S., Harp H.T., Budd S. (Eds) (1987) *Reaching Across: Mental Health Clients Helping Each Other*, Riverside, CA: California Network of Mental Health Clients.

CHAPTER 10

Service Users as Paid Researchers

Service Users as Paid Research Workers: Principles for Active Involvement and Good Practice Guidance

Jonathan Delman

Executive Director, Consumer Quality Initiatives, Inc., Boston, MA, USA

Alisa Lincoln

Associate Professor of Health Sciences and Sociology, Northeastern University, Boston, MA, USA

Service users working in academic and other institutional settings can be a major asset to both the team and the research itself, with the potential to improve research relevance quality, and dissemination. However, without proper preparation and planning, there is great potential for the project to be derailed by tension existing between and among academics and service users. Hence, in order for this kind of service user involvement to achieve its full potential, some basic principles should be taken into account.

This chapter starts out with a discussion of the benefits that active involvement of service user research employees can bring to different aspects of a research project, as well as to others involved, including academic researchers and the service users. Common problems and challenges to such active involvement are also considered from the perspective of both. Subsequently, drawing on the literature as well as on personal experience, a number of key principles are recommended, essential for both senior researchers and service users to overcome the barriers to success and attain maximum benefit. The chapter concludes with a concise and practical step by step guide for senior researchers to achieve the active involvement of service user research workers.

Handbook of Service User Involvement in Mental Health Research Edited by Jan Wallcraft, Beate Schrank and Michaela Amering
Copyright © 2009 John Wiley & Sons, Ltd

INTRODUCTION

Research organisations, such as academic institutions, decide to pay service users as research workers for a variety of reasons. These include a general sense of obligation to people who have been disadvantaged, the value added to the project and/or to meet a grant application requirement. Regardless of the reason, the successful employment of service users requires researchers to dedicate the time and resources to support both services users and themselves. In this chapter, we will discuss the key principles of and considerations for hiring service users as paid researchers.

The paid service user research worker

For the purposes of this chapter, we are adopting the 'service user' definition of Branfield and Beresford (2002), which is people who 'have or have had long-term experience of health and social care services or would qualify to receive such services'. Service users have in common the experience, voluntarily or involuntarily, of mental health treatment and mental health difficulties, and often the marginalization and discrimination that accompanies these experiences.

When we talk about paid service user research worker (SUR) in the chapter, we are referring to people hired, in part because they are service user, to actively participate in the research production process. The employment may only be for a particular research project or as regular staff to participate in ongoing projects, but would be over a significant time period. Thus, SURs are to be distinguished from service users hired for discrete non-analytical activities, such as data entry. SURs are also to be distinguished from academic and other experienced service user researchers, such as author Delman (Griffiths *et al.,*2004) have an excellent discussion on this topic.) This chapter will thus focus on service user researchers who wish to have active involvement in a research project but who have little experience or education in research.

The researchers overseeing the hiring process we will refer to as 'senior' or 'academic' researchers.

Benefits of active service user involvement

In our view, the active involvement of service users in the research process will improve the relevance, quality, and impact, and thus the social value, of the research. In addition there are other powerful potential benefits for everyone involved, including stigma reduction, researcher education, and service user skill development.

Quality and relevance of research

Service users bring an experience and expertise (Deegan, 1993) that can enrich all aspects of the research process (Beinecke and Delman, 2008). Through their interactions with service users, researchers can develop a better understanding of the daily lives and hopes of service users, leading to more relevant study questions and outcomes measures.

Many service users have been 'study subjects,' and are aware of the kinds of research methods most acceptable to service users (Beinecke and Delman, 2008). Service user input here can result in survey questions that more understandable and consent forms with more user friendly language (Beinecke and Delman, 2008). In addition, SURs can be leaders in deciding how to most effectively and sensitively recruit service users, including people who are homeless and other groups difficult to reach. In this way, their presence can effectively lead to the completion of the research project in a timely and effective manner.

In addition, Clark et al. (1999) and others have found that study participants feel more free to talk openly to service user interviewers, leading to more honest and in depth data.

Dissemination, translation to policy and practice

Research results are often disseminated in lengthy documents with an overabundance of research jargon, limiting their policy impact. SURs can help motivate senior researchers to focus more on dissemination for policy impact (O'Donnell and Entwistle, 2004).

Studies have demonstrated that research findings are much more likely to have a policy impact if written up as brief summaries and without jargon and/or if delivered orally (World Health Organisation, 2004). Service users who have participated in research design, data collection and analysis, are in an excellent position to explain the research findings in a clear and thoughtful way (Israel et al., 2003). And when SURs present research results orally while citing their personal experiences, policy-makers may be more likely to take notice than if delivered by academic researchers (Delman, 2007).

SURs can effectively determine how best to disseminate findings to community stakeholders (e.g. service users), often through community forums. Many SURs have had advocacy experience and/or are connected to service user advocacy groups, an important action point for the findings.

Stigma reduction

Service users are often generalized to be lacking in judgment, unpredictable, unreliable, cognitively challenged, or any combination of the above (United States Public Health Service Office of the Surgeon General, 1999). When projects are done well, SURs are full participants in a complex and lengthy research process. Full participation is likely to have an impact on the stigmatizing views of academic researchers and perhaps the self-stigmatizing views of the SURs (see Wyatt et al., 2008). In addition, conference presentations and reports on the process and effects of involving SURs can make other community members aware of service users' potential

Researcher education

The education of senior researchers, particularly academic researchers, about the lives, experiences and knowledge of service users is an additional benefit of SUR involvement (O'Donnell and Entwistle, 2004; Wright et al., 2006). Senior researchers and SURs cross-training each other presents an additional opportunity to learn about SUR lived and learned knowledge. (See Israel *et al.*, 2004.)

Service user skill development

Service users have the opportunity to gain valuable skills, including (but not limited to) data entry, transcription, data management, research literacy, team building following protocols, and leadership.

Challenges to the active service user involvement

The hiring of service users challenges the typical way of conducting research in academic institutions.

Differing expectations and competing demands

While senior researchers and SURs may share expectations for the research process, some of their expectations are likely to be different. First, researchers and service users will probably have differing perspectives on what the highest priority research topics are (Faulkner, 2004). Second, service users tend to focus on the impact research will have on their daily lives (including provider practices). This focus conflicts with the demands of academic appointments such as timely publications in academic journals, accountability to funders, and a focus on the next potential research project (Griffiths *et al.*, 2004). Finally, some academics may be concerned that service users will introduce personal biases or a 'hidden' advocacy agenda to the study, and service users may have their own negative biases with regard to the intentions of academic researchers, creating trust issues (Beinecke and Delman 2008). All of these differences can lead to sustained tension. (Wyatt *et al.*, 2008; Faulkner, 2004).

A very good example of this misalignment of expectations relates to data dissemination. Academics tenure decisions are based largely on publication of research articles in peer-reviewed journals. In addition, successful publication in the most prestigious journals is often based on the rigor of the research. This publication focus can run in contrast to service users' focus on research for social policy change. Thus, service users are often more interested in producing documents that are written both for their fellow service users and for policy-makers. The differences here can affect plans for research design as well resources developed to writing about data.

Imbalance in knowledge, experience and resources

The imbalance in knowledge, experience and resources between academics and the service user community is substantial. Academic and other research institutions usually have a built-in infrastructure to assess funding opportunities and write grant proposals, something service user organisations usually do not have. A large majority of SURs have had little experience conducting research, and many have limited general education and/or employment experience. The research jargon used thus presents a real barrier for many SURs to intelligently discuss the research, unless researchers explain terms as they go along (Faulkner, 2005). This means that the research process must include an investment in bringing service users 'up to speed' through training and education (Wright *et al.*, 2006).

That unsteady feeling service users have working in academia

Service users signing on to be paid research workers often have an unsteady feeling related to their new employers/employment. Many service users who have answered the academic call for involvement in research in the past have found a lack of both opportunity and support/training to influence the process. Academia is often hierarchical in nature, which may present a difficult challenge to those who have not worked recently, or who have been involved in consumer organisations, which tend to have less structure (Faulkner, 2005). When service users are hired to work on a particular project (as opposed to regular employees), they may at times feel that 'that they are seen as products with limited shelf lives As a result, service users may constantly be wondering what's going to happen next' (Stevens *et al.*, 2003).

Lack of infrastructure and/or funding for bridging the gap

As will be discussed in more detail below, it is necessary for a research group or project to assign resources to achieve successful employment of paid service user researchers (Faulkner, 2005; Stevens *et al.*, 2003). If an institution takes on user involvement on a project-by-project basis, they will need to build that support into each project, which is difficult when a funding organisation does not value that level of support. The research institution may then want to reconsider their overall policy of service user involvement and hiring in order to build a mission and infrastructure that will survive individual grants. The barrier here is ongoing challenge of institutions ability to transform themselves.

Principles for the active involvement of SURs

We recommend the following nine key principles as a framework for the active involvement of paid service users working on research projects in academic and other institutional settings. An understanding of these principles for both senior researchers and service users is essential for overcoming the barriers to success noted above and to attain the substantial benefits.

1. Personal commitment
2. Inclusion
3. Clear communication
4. Respect
5. Education/training
6. Effective hiring practices
7. Individualized attention

8. Supportive infrastructure
9. Additional resources and project flexibility

These principles are based on the research literature, working guidelines for mental health service user involvement in research, and our own experience (see, for example, Faulkner, 2005). With regard to the literature, several of the articles we cite have effectively documented the experience of service users with other health difficulties (e.g. cancer); these articles reflect our experiences and are consistent with mental health literature and guidelines. Regarding our experience, author Delman has directed a not-for-profit user-led research organisation for nine years, has hired and worked with many paid service users over that time, and has consulted with universities to achieve the active involvement of service users in research (see Delman, 2007). Author Lincoln has hired SURs directly as principle investigator of a National Institute of Mental Health (US) participatory-action research project.

Personal commitment

Senior researchers *and* SURs should be committed to both active SUR involvement and learning about the other's perspective. (See Wyatt *et al.*, 2008; Faulkner, 2004.) Without that commitment, the natural frustrations that accompany the research process and the differing viewpoints on the project's direction may undermine the process.

This commitment on the researcher side is usually based on a belief that active service user involvement will add value to the research process (Wyatt *et al.*, 2008). Without that belief, there may be little motivation to commit the time and resources to develop the researcher-user working relationship. As such, when researchers are hiring SURs only because of a funding mandate, that commitment is likely to be lacking. When senior researchers would like to work with SURs for the first time, they should first consider observing or participating in such a project, attending service user involvement trainings, and hiring an experienced consultant (see Faulkner, 2004).

When hiring SURs, an important consideration is the service user applicant's belief in the importance of the research topic and the potential for findings to affect policy. The SUR's commitment is important since the research process does not always go according to plan, and patience is required to see the project through. In addition, researchers may be learning about SUR involvement as they go along. SURs dissatisfied with an aspect of the project should not assume that researchers are aware of this, and should attempt to address it with them directly.

Inclusion

The SUR should have a sense of belonging to the research team. Thus, SURs should have the opportunity to be involved in all aspects of the research process, from issue determination to dissemination (Wright *et al.*, 2004; Wyatt *et al.*, 2008). (If not so included, the reasons should be made explicit – Faulkner, 2005). For this involvement to be active, the service user's contributions will need to be valued, encouraged and acknowledged (Faulkner, 2005). Regular (eg., weekly) meetings of the research team, including users, are critical to build camaraderie and the sharing of updates and plans. Regular group emails can buttress the meetings.

In order to provide a basis for SURs to trust researchers, the differences in experience, background and expectations between the groups should be openly acknowledged early in the project (Faulkner, 2005). This allows SURs to openly discuss their support needs and senior researchers to clarify their expectations.

Wyatt *et al.* (2008) found that physical proximity of senior researchers to SURs is important and can result in off-line 'get to know you' conversations; these events are important because the researcher and service user begins to see the other as a human being. 'Social bonding and fun' can also result from attending conferences, trainings and site visits together (Faulkner, 2004).

Inclusion also requires that materials and meeting locations be made accessible to people with different disabilities and other needs. For example, for someone who has difficulty climbing stairs, it is important to have meetings at a location's first floor or have lift access.

Clear communication

As noted by Faulkner (2005), senior researchers need to be clear with service users on what they wish to accomplish with the research project, their reasons for paying service users, and 'the roles and responsibilities of all parties' (including limits to their involvement). This includes clarity on compensation, training, support, and supervision (Faulkner, 2004).

A major challenge for researchers when collecting data is the ability to stay true to the projected time frame. As noted above, the researchers should clearly communicate this and keep SURs updated on changes.

SURs should be clear with the senior researchers on what their needs and expectations are. This clarity is not a one time event, but must be maintained on a regular basis to avoid misunderstandings. And if not feeling well or dissatisfied, SURs should address their concerns directly with the research director and/or leaders to attempt to negotiate a satisfactory solution, instead of just dropping out.

A contract stating the participants' respective rights and responsibilities may provide more clarity (Faulkner, 2004).

Respect

All parties should respect the others' right to present their own, perhaps opposing, point of view (Wyatt *et al.*, 2008). With the potential for discussions to become heated, there should be at least one participant, such as a project director/co-ordinator, who is seen as a moderating influence. That person will need the caring support of the senior researchers to be able to address needs and resolve difference (Faulkner, 2004).

Senior researchers need to have respect for the hard earned expertise of SURs, and SURs for the academic experience of the researcher (Beinecke and Delman, 2008). While the SUR's expertise may be in recruiting people for a study, a researcher may have much more experience getting a research protocol through a human subjects review board (see Wright *et al.*, 2006). That means listening to opposing points of view, considering them as a reasonable approach to a situation, and at times deferring to expertise.

Education/training

Effective training is a critical element for successful SUR involvement in the research production process. When people lack familiarity with research terminology and processes, they quickly become discouraged from participating (Stevens *et al.,*2003). A good training program not only builds knowledge, but also generates excitement about the research process and the potential policy implications of the work.

Preparing new researchers to engage in the research process is best done through a combination of didactic learning, observation, role-playing and feedback (Elliot *et al.*, 2002). The initial training should present at a minimum an introduction to research, research ethics, information on the subject matter (including previous research) of the research, and research interviewing. Interview guide and analysis training is best addressed as that work is actually being carried out.

The training should have a strong cross training component (Israel *et al.*, 2003). SURs can present to senior researchers on their relevant areas of expertise; we have had SURs present on strengths-based care, person-first language, and the advocacy work of the user group to which they belong. Senior researchers should also take a flexible approach to the training schedule (Wright *et al.*, 2006). When one of our service users missed several trainings in a row, we caught her up on a one-to-one basis.

The training should include sessions on the practice and policy context of the research. We have had governmental policy-makers discuss with service users their own roles in policy-making, and the benefits research findings will have to them. And we've had providers discuss the specifics of how a particular service works. These discussions provide an additional impetus for the SURs to carry on the research, as they know there will be an audience for the findings.

The training should include a team-building process to create a mutually supportive atmosphere (Israel, 2003). We have also found it advantageous on several levels to have service users demonstrate their new competencies through an exam process.

Effective hiring practices

The service user hiring process should be carried out carefully. Clear job descriptions should be developed based on the essential job functions and minimum qualifications. To attract a diverse group of candidates, the job description should be distributed widely, including to service user groups, vocational programs and universities. Oral presentations by researchers to these groups can boost recruitment.

Upon the receipt of expressions of interest and resumes, researchers should examine the application to detect an interest in the research topic and a desire to work in research. It is best for researchers to interview in teams to counteract possible prejudices (e.g. race, class); a service user ideally should be one of the interviewers.

And as explained in the "support" section, it is beneficial to hire in groups (Faulkner, 2005). There are some service users who would prefer not to work full-time, and it's likely that at least one SUR will leave (see O'Donnell and Entwistle, 2004). In our work we aim for diversity with regard to at least age, gender, race/ethnicity, and experience with the mental health care system.

Individualized attention

SURs bring different interests, skills and needs to the table, and it is important to attend to that individuality for the purpose of motivating SURs whose commitment is wavering (Delman, 2007).

SURs may go through periods of poor health during the course of their employment, and the research leaders should make every attempt accommodate these special needs (Beinecke and Delman, 2008). People who are depressed and having difficulty attending meetings may require extra encouragement and/or 'reminder' calls. Some people may need to work fewer hours or take a break from the process to maintain their mental health; this can often be accommodated when there are other service users to pick up the slack.

If a SUR is not performing essential job functions well, the supervisor should work with him/her to consider a reasonable accommodation, such as extra training or a job coach (Beinecke and Delman, 2008). If a person is unable to perform essential tasks with accommodations, it may make sense for the employment to end until the SUR's health improves.

Building on a SUR's strength is also important, particularly when his/her interest in the project is wavering. One way we do this is by matching the SUR's strengths to a particular research stage. I (Delman) employed a SUR who was most interested in the political implications of the research, so we had him meet with policy-makers to discuss the research and to present the findings. Another SUR was particularly interested in 'creative writing'. Thus, we secured a small grant for her to develop a booklet containing first-person accounts of women ageing out of the adolescent system.

Supportive infrastructure

Several reports have noted that practical, emotional and research supports are critical ingredients of success (Faulkner, 2004; Wright *et al.*, 2006). This support should happen on an individual basis and in groups. The practical support may relate to transportation, accessible space, regular supervision, and an 'open door' communication policy with senior researchers and the project director (Faulkner, 2004).

The emotional support is necessary to build the SUR's confidence and to address triggering experiences that may occur because of the research (Faulkner, 2004). Active listening and encouragement are important aspects of support. SURs may develop their own emotional support network, working through challenging issues together. They are also likely to each bring in new types of knowledge, enhancing SUR researcher capacity.

Additional resources and project flexibility

The employment of SURs for active involvement requires resources in addition to what's ordinarily provided for a research project. Training, team building, supportive infrastructure and the establishment of clear communication channels will require additional funding, extra time, and flexible deadlines (Faulkner, 2005). If SURs' input is to be taken seriously, there will need to be flexibility with regard to research methodology and methods (Faulkner, 2005).

The project's budget should take into account SUR wages, including training time. Other considerations for a budget include a user involvement consultant, a portion of the project director's time, additional computers, job coaches, and accessibility items for people with physical disabilities.

Good practice guidance

Below are some basic steps that senior researchers can take to achieve the active involvement of SURs.

Researcher preparation

1. Develop relationships with service user groups well in advance of hiring paid service users in order to identify key community issues and to identify service users interested in research.
2. If inexperienced in the active involvement of SURs, attend a relevant training, observe or participate in such a project, and hire an experienced consultant to help develop the project.
3. Work internally and with funders to develop a flexible budget and timeline for the hiring of SURs.
4. Identify the concerns the human subjects board may have with SUR involvement (particularly as interviewers), and be prepared to defend that involvement.

Hiring service users

1. Develop a clear job description, highlighting the essential job functions and minimal qualifications necessary.
2. Hire SURs in small groups and from diverse backgrounds.
3. Distribute the job notice widely; include user groups and different multicultural groups.
4. Interview job applicants in teams.

Compensation

1. Pay SURs the prevailing market wage for their time, consistent with other project/ organisational staff.
2. Communicate clearly to the SURs the activities for which they will and will not be paid, particularly if the person is paid hourly (this should include the training time). Relevant out of pocket expenses should be reimbursed promptly.
3. Co-ordinate early on with the finance department.
4. Prepare to connect SURs to a public benefits counsellor.

Training

1. Focus the training on a specific project to provide trainees with a clear goal.
2. The training should be interactive, with discussion, role plays, and visits to relevant programmes.
3. SURs and senior researchers should cross train each other.
4. Develop presentations and materials that use clear language, with jargon minimized but defined if used.
5. Be flexible and prepared to adjust the training in response to the expressed needs of the SURs as a group, as well as to an individual SUR, based on informal feedback and formal evaluations.

Supervision

1. Clearly communicate to SURs the reasons for including them and the manner by which the research topic was chosen.
2. Develop an individual and group supervision process Supervisors and SURs should discuss their respective roles, responsibilities and expectations.
3. Provide to the SUR *at least* one direct supervisor, often a project director or research co-ordinator. That person should have the support of and regular contact with senior researchers.
4. Provide direct supports for aspects of the research process a SUR finds particularly challenging.
5. Group supervision should include regular group meetings involving SURs, the project director *and* the senior researchers. The project director should not serve as the sole connector between SURs and researchers. Supplement the meetings with written communications (e.g. email) on research progress issues and other updates.
6. Extra supervisory attention should be given to research activities that happen outside group processes and/or which could be triggering, such as research interviewing. This could include the review of interview transcripts.

Support

1. Provide emotional, practical and research support.
2. Make every effort to accommodate service user's needs, particularly in relation to health difficulties. When a SUR returns after taking time off, senior researchers and the project director should take the time to bring him/her 'up to speed' and to assess the need for job accommodations.
3. Encourage SURs to communicate clearly to their supervisors the need for an accommodation.
4. Identify the strengths and desires of each SUR; encourage SURs (particularly those who are discouraged) to focus on the research stages that excite them most.
5. Openly appreciate and acknowledge the SUR efforts and contributions. Consider group celebrations for significant achievements (e.g. completing a research report).

6. Provide SURs the space and equipment (e.g. computer) to accomplish their work.
7. Encourage and nurture peer-support among the SURs.
8. Make meetings and materials accessible to all SURs, including assistance with transportation, flexibility with locations of the meetings (including the use of teleconferencing and Internet forums) and large print text.
9. Work with user-led organisations to support SURs.

Team building

1. Create a 'space' for participants to acknowledge the differences in experience and backgrounds between SURs and senior researchers.
2. Engage in several team-building exercises so that research participants can begin to know one another beyond their labels/diagnoses ('service user' or 'researcher').
3. Develop with the SURs a conflict-resolution plan.
4. Work in close physical proximity to the SURs at least some of the time.

Opportunities for involvement at all stages

1. Build connections to user-led organisations.
2. Prepare the SURs to be primary presenters of the findings to policy-makers and community members.
3. Create opportunities for SURs to be a primary or co-author on a research paper and/or to present at conferences.
4. Do not require that SURs participate at every stage of the project.

Additional resources (time, funding)

1. Assess the types and costs of the additional resources required.
2. Negotiate with the funding agency for additional funding, a realistic project completion time-period, and flexibility with both budget and timeline.
3. Other budgetary line items will include:
   - training for senior researchers on SUR involvement
   - SUR involvement consultant to project
   - accessible training materials
   - a portion of the project director's time to co-ordinate and supervise SURs
   - service user compensation costs
   - physical resources, such as computers and tape recorders.

REFERENCES

Beinecke, R. and Delman, J. (2008) Commentary: Client involvement in public administration research and evaluation, the innovation journal, *The Public Sector Innovation Journal*, **13**(1), Article 7.
Branfield, F. and Beresford, P. (2006) *Making User Involvement Work: Supporting Service User Networking and Knowledge*, York: Joseph Rowntree Foundation.

Deegan, P.E. (1993) Recovering our sense of value after being labeled mentally ill. *Psychosocial Nursing and Mental Health Services*, **31**(4), 7–11.

Delman, J. (2007) *Consumer Driven and Conducted Survey Research in Action in Towards Best Practices for Surveying People with Disabilities* (Volume 1). Edited by T. Kroll, D. Keer, P. Placek, J. Cyril, G. Hendershot, Hauppauge, NY: Nova Publishers.

Elliot, E., Watson, A.J. and Harries, U. (2002) Harnessing expertise: involving peer interviewers in qualitative research with hard-to-reach populations, *Health Expectations*, **5**, 172–178.

Faulkner, A. (2004) *Capturing the Experiences of those Involved in the TRUE Project: a story of colliding worlds.* Available online at: http://www.invo.org.uk/All_Publications.asp, accessed 28/10/08.

Faulkner, A. (2005) *Guidance for Good Practice: Service user involvement in the UK Mental Health Research Network*, London: Service user Research Group.

Griffiths, K., Jorm, A.F. and Christensen, A.H. (2004) Academic consumer researchers: a bridge between consumers and researchers, *Australian and New Zealand Journal of Psychiatry*, **38**, 191–196.

Israel, B.A., Schulz, A.J. and Parker, E.A. *et al.* (2003) Critical issues in developing and following community based participatory research principles. In: M. Minkler and N. Wallerstein (Eds) *Community Based Participatory Research for Health*, San Francisco: Jossey Bass, pp. 53–76.

O'Donnell, M.O. and Entwistle, V. (2004) Consumer involvement in research projects: the activities of research funders. *Health Policy*, **69**(2), 229–238.

Stevens, T., Wilde, D., Hunt, J. and Ahmedzai, S.H. (2003) Overcoming the challenges to consumer involvement in cancer research. *Health Expectations*, **6**, 81–88.

United States Public Health Service Office of the Surgeon General (1999) *Mental Health: A Report of the Surgeon General*, Rockville, MD: Department of Health and Human Services, U.S, Public Health Service.

World Health Organisation (2004) *World Report on Knowledge for Better Health*, Geneva: WHO.

Wright, D., Hopkinson, J., Corner, J. and Foster, C. (2006) How to involve cancer patients at the end of life as co-researchers. *Palliative Medicine*, **20**(8), 821–827.

Wyatt, K., Carter, M. and Mahtani, V. *et al.* (2008) The impact of consumer involvement in research: an evaluation of consumer involvement in the London Primary Care Studies Programme. *Family Practice*, **25**, 154–161.

CHAPTER 11

Consultation

Virginia Minogue
*West Yorkshire Mental Health Research
and Development Consortium, Leeds, UK*

The consultation of service users is a fundamental element of public involvement and engagement in healthcare and research. Consultation is the most frequently used level of involvement and is often the point at which many professional researchers start the process of involving service users. This chapter deals with the question of what consultation means and what its purposes may be. It examines different levels of involvement within consultation and their implications and potential. Different points in the research process at which service users can be consulted are outlined, methods for such consultation are proposed and potential consultees are suggested. Furthermore, the potential values and benefits of consultation as a means of service user involvement are discussed, as are the limitations, barriers and pitfalls related to it. Finally, recommendations for good practice are offered in order to help researchers render their consultation endeavours meaningful and successful.

INTRODUCTION

Service users have moved a long way from being passive subjects of the research process and there are many examples of how individual and groups of service users have been involved in mental health research as active participants in consultation, collaboration, and as service user researchers (Faulkner and Morris, 2003; Rose, 2004; Trivedi and Wykes, 2002; Minogue *et al.*, 2005; Staley and Minogue, 2006). The level of involvement ranges from consultation to user-led research and reflects the broader changes in service user involvement activity within health services since the 1980s. Service user involvement in health service delivery has been a policy directive in the National Health Service for over a decade (National Health Service, 1999, 2000; Department of Health, 2000, 2001a. 2001b, 2004, 2005a, 2005b) and is crucial to ensuring health services reflect the needs of those they serve. Undoubtedly, mental health services have experienced a significant increase in service user involvement both in service delivery and in research, as evidenced by the number of collaborative and user-led projects, particularly in research.

Handbook of Service User Involvement in Mental Health Research Edited by Jan Wallcraft, Beate Schrank and Michaela Amering
Copyright © 2009 John Wiley & Sons, Ltd

The debate about the validity of service user involvement has moved away from whether service users should be involved to trying to determine which are the most effective methods, and the impact and value, of involvement. Service user involvement already takes place in a number of areas including education and training of mental health and social care clinicians and practitioners, through Patient Forums, Patient Advice and Liaison Services (PALS), staff recruitment, Local Partnership Boards, audit, evaluation and research. As a result, there are many skilled service users, and carers, bringing their expertise and experience of being in receipt of health and social care services to assist in developing practice and service delivery. A key aspect of this is active involvement in the research process in order to ensure that evidence-based healthcare is inclusive of the knowledge and experience of service users, that research funding and resources are used effectively, and that outcome measures reflect the concerns and interests of service users not just NHS researchers.

There are many examples of active service user involvement in service planning, delivery and research within mental health services and roles have been created to facilitate the increased inclusion of service users and carers e.g. service user development workers, Support, Time and Recovery (STR) workers, public involvement departments, PALS, and service user researchers. However, service user involvement remains patchy with an emphasis on consultation rather than influence, partnership or control. Whilst the legitimacy of the service user voice in mental health service-development and organisation, and by association research, is accepted, barriers to involvement remain. These barriers include lack of information, financial and time costs, professionals' concerns over the representativeness of service users and resistance to the idea of service users as experts. Many mental health service users lack the information to facilitate choice or are excluded from involvement (Sainsbury Centre for Mental Health, 2006; Tait and Lester, 2005; Rethink, 2003). This can be particularly true for hard-to-reach groups, for example: Black and minority ethnic communities, people with physical and learning difficulties, and older adults, who may not know where to access information about available services.

Simpson et al. (2002) advocate the recognition of service users as stakeholders and put forward the premise that mechanisms for involving users can be seen as health technologies. One such technology is consultation, which can be utilised by encouraging feedback to service providers, for example, through consulting service user, ex-user, or carer organisations, or setting up user discussion and focus groups. Consultation is a fundamental element of public involvement and engagement in healthcare and in health services research. Even if the intended level of engagement is higher i.e. more participatory or empowering, consultation may be the first stage of the process. Consultation is necessary in order to engage in a dialogue to determine the level of participation the 'public' – users of health services – wish to have and may precede collaboration or user-controlled work.

CONSULTATION AND ITS ROLE IN SERVICE USER INVOLVEMENT

At this stage, in order to understand the role of consultation in service user involvement in mental health research, it is useful to examine both what it means and its purpose. Definitions of consultation variously describe it as:

- procedures for assessing public opinion about a plan or proposal
- a conference for two or more people to consider a particular issue or question
- a two-way flow of information.

Consultation is also described as a process for exchanging thoughts and information with individuals, groups or the wider public. It may be used for collecting or disseminating information, identifying issues, seeking advice, hearing views and opinions. It will be noted from many of these definitions and descriptions that the process of consultation may be limited to information receiving and giving and may not involve those consulted being involved in decision-making or necessarily impacting on the process of change. Consultation can mean that professionals hold onto their power, and power relationships are maintained, as those who are consulting retain the ability and control to make decisions rather than the process being shared. Consultation within the research process may be limited to low level involvement where service users are asked to provide their view of a survey or project outline.

Other levels of involvement, such as collaboration and user-control, suggest a much greater degree of empowerment is lodged with the service user. Collaboration assumes a partnership approach and a more equal distribution of power (see also Chapter 12 on collaborative research); user control represents a significant shift in power (see also Chapter 13 on user-controlled research). Consultation usually involves a greater degree of passivity than collaboration. Beresford (2005) identifies two approaches to service user involvement, the managerial/consumerist vs. the democratic approach. The managerial/consumerist approach focuses on the organisational system with the service user informing services through, for example, information-gathering and consultation, thus, the organisation retains rather than cedes power. Does consultation within the research process therefore have any value and can it be described as 'active' involvement? The widely utilised Arnstein's 'ladder of participation'[1] draws the distinction between the extent to which people participate at each level and suggests that consultation does not constitute genuine participation and is representative of a more tokenistic than inclusive approach and delegates little or no power to the service user (Arnstein, 1969). Consultation can feel tokenistic to service users and be perceived as a 'tick box' exercise driven by political imperative. It does not necessarily lead to service users feeling any sense of ownership of the research process, particularly if there is no requirement on the part of those leading the consultation to feed back to those who have been consulted or communicate the outcome.

LEVELS OF CONSULTATION

Although Arnstein (1969) regards consultation as low level, possibly tokenistic, involvement, the ladder of participation presents a very linear framework which does not take into account the changes in policy and thinking, in relation to public and service user involvement in mental health services, that have occurred over the subsequent four decades. The

---

[1] Arnstein's ladder of participation has 8 rungs: 1 – manipulation, 2 – therapy, 3 – informing, 4 – consultation, 5 – placation, 6 – partnership, 7 – delegated power, 8 – citizen control. Rungs 1and 2 of the ladder correspond to non participation, rungs 3, 4, and 5 degrees of tokenism, rungs 6, 7 and 8 degrees of citizen power.

focus of Arnstein's model of participation on power also fails to recognise the complexities of service user involvement in health services research (see also Chapter 3); the different motivations people bring to the process (see also Chapter 2); their capacity to get involved whilst managing their mental health and related issues, and also their wish to make a choice about when and how they get involved. Collins and Ison, (2006) and Tritter and McCallum (2006) argue for a re-think of the ladder of participation and development of a model that recognises the interdependency of a number of factors, such as relationships between groups and individuals, processes, and desired outcomes.

In addition to the different levels of participation outlined by Arnstein and others (Arnstein, 1969; Collins and Ison, 2006; Tritter and McCallum, 2006), there are, arguably, different levels of service user involvement within consultation. The four levels of consultation outlined at Figure 11.1, below, allow for those initiating in consultation to invite varying degrees of involvement by service users. Although the level of consultation may be determined by the type and design of the research project, it will also depend on the person leading the consultation and their preferences in terms of the extent of service user involvement. As Figure 11.1 demonstrates, each level of consultation implies different degrees of engagement, empowerment, and potential for future involvement, for service users.

SERVICE USER INVOLVEMENT IN RESEARCH AND THE ROLE OF CONSULTATION

Service user involvement in research takes place at three levels:

- consultation
- collaboration
- user controlled.

(Involve, 2004; see also Chapter 3)

Involvement may take place at one or more of the various stages of the research process (see Figure 11.2). It may also take place at different levels ranging from involvement simply as a subject of research, to control of the process as a service user researcher on a user-led or user-controlled project. Consultation is a level of involvement which may encompass a greater or lesser degree of engagement, motivation, and investment on the part of the consulter and the consultee. Motivation to get involved is clearly critical to the level of involvement and, as Tarpey (2006) points out, there are varied reasons why service users or carers may choose to get involved in research as consultees or more active participants. The reasons may be intrinsic or extrinsic and range from the personal benefits to be realised, their experience of mental health services (positive or negative), to more altruistic expectations of improving services for others (find more on motives for involvement in Chapter 2). A legacy of the survivor movement, and experiences of participatory research, may have resulted in some mental health service users in particular also seeking to use the research process to challenge perceptions of service delivery, and to use their experiences to lead to improvements and changes to services and treatment. Tarpey also suggests that motivation to get involved in research develops over time and can be facilitated through membership of existing groups or organisations whose expertise

Level of consultation	Degree of service user involvement
Seek views	Information-gathering exercise that may be viewed as tokenistic Service users: • unlikely to be fully informed about project • views may not be acted upon • may not have knowledge of outcome of consultation • little sense of ownership of project • low level of empowerment.
Seek views, engage in discussion	Information-gathering exercise that may be viewed as tokenistic Opportunity to engage in discussion about project May be a level of co-creation of knowledge between consulter and service users Service users: • views may not be acted upon • may not have knowledge of outcome of consultation • little sense of ownership of project • moderate level of empowerment.
Seek views, engage in discussion and feedback	Opportunity to engage in discussion about project May be a level of co-creation of knowledge between consulter and service users Service users: • views more likely to be acted upon • outcome of consultation known • further involvement beyond initial consultation unlikely • some ownership of project • moderate level of empowerment.
Seek views, engage in discussion and feedback, actively seek further collaboration at different stages of project	Service users: • fully informed of process • involved in more than one stage of consultation • may be a level of co-creation of knowledge and convergence of goals • views acted on and taken seriously – clearly developed action plan • active involvement in decisions • higher level of interest of project and • willingness to participate.

Figure 11.1   Levels of consultation.

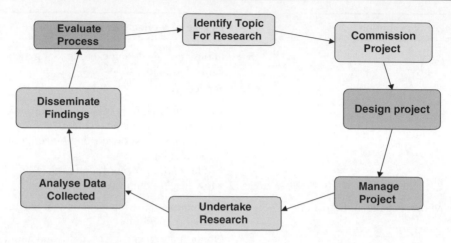

Figure 11.2   The research process.

and experience are then utilised by researchers. One of the most important aspects of motivation in the consultation process is the receipt of feedback. Lack of feedback may have a negative impact on the motivation of service users and also impact on their confidence in those who are leading the research and willingness to engage in further activity.

Consultation is the most frequently used level of involvement as this is potentially the most straightforward means of entering into a dialogue with service users and carers. Engaging in collaboration or partnership – providing adequate time and support is devoted to it – increases the empowerment of the service user and carer but is likely to be more resource- intensive. Service user-led initiatives allow the service user or carer to take full control of the research process. Consultation is the point at which many professional researchers start the process of involving service users or carers in research. It can be seen as a less demanding level of involvement in terms of time, support and resources that need to be expended. It can also mean less investment in the outcome of engagement by the professional as consultation does not necessarily imply acting on the outcomes of the consultative process.

Consultation restricts the role of the person consulted and limits the choices they make. To overcome the potential to further disempower service users within the research process, mental health researchers intending to consult service users need to recognise that any form of participation should be a two -way process. However, this can mean a significant shift in perception for some considering involving service users as they may fear negativity, i.e. the expression of critical views of either the research and/or services. Researchers may also be concerned about their own eventual disempowerment by service users if they become more involved in the research project and increase their level of ownership and control.

In terms of the research process, consultation could take place at any point in the research cycle (see Figure 11.2) – i.e. identification of topic, commissioning, design, management, undertaking the research and analysis, dissemination – but may in reality be limited to certain aspects of a project, such as design. Service users have undertaken a consultative role at national, strategic, and local NHS Trust level. At a national level, service users have informed the selection of research topics and identification of research questions through consultation exercises conducted by, for example, the Health Technology Assessment programme part of the National Institute for Health Research (NIHR)[2] research programmes (Samele et al., 2007). The NIHR also invites service user consultation through commissioning groups and peer review of research proposals and applications for funding through its research programmes. Involve[3] are funded by the NIHR to support service user involvement in the research process. Mental health research is led by the Mental Health Research Network (MHRN) with service user involvement supported by the Service User Research Group England (SURGE) and a network of regional MHRN hubs.

The centrality of the service user in the research process is clearly stated by the UK Department of Health in its research strategy 'Best Research for Best Health' (2006) where one of the stated objectives is to develop effective patient and public engagement initiatives to facilitate involvement at all levels of the research process. This is to be welcomed as one of the issues service users have faced in being asked to take part in consultations about choice of topic, or included in the process of putting together a bid for funding, has been the limitation of not being involved in shaping the research beyond that stage. Collaboration suggests a rather more inclusive and longer term relationship than a potentially one-off consultation exercise. Consultation, therefore, may be more concerned with involving service users in the process of research rather than the outcomes. However, consultation is a useful tool in order to hear the service user perspective and could be the first stage in building collaboration.

Many research and development departments in NHS Trusts across the UK have actively sought to involve service users in their activities to improve and enhance research governance procedures but also because of the perceived value of that involvement in the conduct of research. Different points of consultation where service users can be engaged in the research process, and how they might be engaged, are outlined at Figure 11.3.

The benefits of consultation as a means of involving service users in research

Consultation is one means of bringing the service user perspective into the research process. Although it is clearly less empowering than other forms of involvement, it presents a starting point and even this level of involvement can lead to challenges to stereotypical views of the user experience or perception of services. It is also a step in the direction of making research accessible to those people who experience mental health services and allowing service improvement to be shaped by the experience of those who receive

---

[2] The National Institute for Health Research is a virtual organisation that provides the framework for the Department of Health to deliver the different elements of NHS research. It provides management for the main research programmes and funding for NHS research through a central commissioning facility. It also coordinates various research centres, topic specific networks, and units.

[3] Involve is a national advisory group, which is funded by the Department of Health. It promotes and supports active public involvement in health and social care research in the belief that this leads to research that is more relevant to people who use services and is more likely to be utilised.

Point of consultation	Method of consultation	Potential consultees
Identification of research priorities	Undertake consultation exercise e.g. survey Commissioning groups Topic specific research networks R&D committees Liaison with service user groups Use of relevant websites	• Service user members of NIHR commissioning and peer review groups • Service users involved in MHRN hubs • Service user members of NHS Trust R & D Committees • Service user groups • Individual service users
Decisions about use of R&D funding	Commissioning groups Invite participation or views of service user stakeholders through: • consultation exercise • topic specific research networks • R&D committees	• Service user members of NIHR commissioning and peer review groups • Service users involved in MHRN hubs • Service user members of NHS Trust R&D Committees • Individual service users
Fomulating a research strategy	Liaison with stakeholders including service user groups Consultation exercise Focus groups to develop strategy Use of relevant websites	• Service user members of NIHR commissioning and peer review groups • Service users involved in MHRN hubs • Service user members of NHS Trust R&D Committees • Service user groups • Individual service users
Recruitment of research staff	Liaison with service user groups who are potential stakeholders re: job description and person specification	• Service user groups • Individual service users
Selection of topics for research, identification of research questions, design and focus of research	Seek expert opinion on a topic or research design to improve research proposals though the following: • Commissioning groups • Topic specific research networks • R&D committees • Seek advice and opinion of service user-led peer review panels	• Service user members of NIHR commissioning and peer review groups • Service users involved in MHRN hubs • Service user members of NHS Trust R&D Committees • Service user groups • Individual service users

Figure 11.3   Points of consultation in the research process.

Point of consultation	Method of consultation	Potential consultees
	• Liaison with service user groups • Involvement of service users on research project management groups to oversee design and conduct of research • Use of relevant websites	
Preparation of bids for funding	Invite participation of, seek advice of or request review of bids by: • Commissioning groups • Topic specific research networks • R&D committees • Liaison with service user groups • Use of relevant websites	• Service users involved in MHRN hubs • Service user members of NHS Trust R&D Committees • Service user groups • Individual service users
Advice on involving or recruiting service users in the project or programme	Seek expert opinion through: • Liaison with service user groups • Involvement of service users on research project management groups to oversee design and conduct of research • Use of relevant websites	• Service users involved in MHRN hubs • Service user members of NHS Trust R&D Committees • Service user groups • Individual service users
Provision of views or advice on research findings	Seek expert opinion through: • Liaison with service user groups • Involvement of service users on research project management groups to oversee design and conduct of research • Feedback to research participants	• Service users involved in MHRN hubs • Service user members of NHS Trust R&D Committees • Service user groups • Individual service users
Writing for publication	Seek expert opinion through: • Liaison with service user groups • Involvement of service users on research project management groups to oversee design and conduct of research • Feedback to research participants	• Service users involved in MHRN hubs • Service user members of NHS Trust R&D Committees • Service user groups • Individual service users

Figure 11.3   (*Continued*)

Point of consultation	Method of consultation	Potential consultees
Advice about appropriate methods of dissemination	Seek expert opinion through: • Liaison with service user groups • Involvement of service users on research project management groups to oversee design and conduct of research • Consultation with research participants	• Research sponsors and funders • Service users involved in MHRN hubs • Service user members of NHS Trust R&D Committees • Service user groups • Individual service users

Figure 11.3   (*Continued*)

services. Service users have a vast amount of experience of health services, expertise, knowledge, and can contribute their views to the process without necessarily requiring specific training for their involvement. Intimate knowledge of services generally means that service users will know the 'right' questions to ask as part of the research process and not the assumed questions asked by researchers. They can also provide a useful check for the use of appropriate and understandable language in the development of data collection tools which can in turn increase the response and participation rate. Service users and carers' links with other service users, and service user or interest groups, can be invaluable to researchers in knowing how to recruit or involve participants. They can contribute to the design of user focused outcomes and user friendly research design. Service users have been shown to influence the design of mental health research projects through the consultation process and Boxes A and B outline ways in which this might occur. Other examples of the diversity and range of service user consultation in research can be seen in research projects involving areas as diverse as psychiatric intensive care, older adults, and forensic services (Trivedi and Wykes, 2002; Faulkner and Morris, 2003; Joseph Rowntree Foundation, 2004).

Involvement in the research process through consultation provides opportunities for service users to share their experience, gain knowledge and skills, increase their self-esteem and confidence. However, a key issue mental health service researchers need to address within the research process is diversity. Accessibility of services can be an issue for some minority and marginalised groups – such as Black and minority ethnic people, those with dual diagnosis, asylum seekers, those with learning difficulties and mental health problems. To understand the needs of those groups researchers need to involve them in the research process. This may be to identify the appropriate research questions or design the project and in order to do so there is a need to engage in consultation. Groups such as asylum seekers or those with learning difficulties can present communication problems and are often excluded because of this. They may also lack the structures through which to engage with health service or academic researchers. Lack of visibility, disenfranchisement and disempowerment also contribute to low involvement but are barriers that must be overcome in order to promote open dialogue. The challenge for the researcher is to be pro-active in seeking user involvement and to develop innovative methods of consultation in order to engage such communities of interest.

BOX A: EXAMPLE OF SERVICE USER CONSULTATION IN PRACTICE

Examples of consultation

Peer review panels

The Research Governance Framework for Health and Social Care (Department of Health, 2005b) requires NHS organisations to ensure that an independent scientific and ethical review of research proposals is undertaken. This is to ensure the quality, relevance and value of the research. The West Yorkshire Mental Health Research and Development Consortium has two parallel systems in place for undertaking such reviews. These systems ensure that review of applications to carry out research by employees of the constituent organisations within the Consortium, or by those who wish to undertake research within the constituent organisations, is undertaken by appropriately qualified peers (i.e. clinicians, academics, experienced research personnel) and by service users and carers. Three panels made up entirely by service users and carers, with appropriate training, meet on average once a month to review research applications. The panels are supported by a Research Governance Manager who also reviews the application, provides any additional information required and coordinates the feedback to the applicant. The feedback from all the peer reviewers is given equal weighting.

The panels require a high level of commitment on the part of the service user and carer as they are time consuming due to the amount of preparation and reading required. Training and ongoing support is crucial as the format of the applications to the National Research Ethics Service (NRES) is complex and not always 'user friendly'. The variety of applications also means that the members of the panels are likely to be scrutinising some topic areas that are outside their own interest and experience. Recompense for time and involvement should be offered wherever possible.

The role of the service user and carer review-panels has been particularly useful in providing an opinion on the relevance of research questions, appropriate methodologies, the clarity and readability of information sheets, questionnaires and interview schedules. It has also been possible to identify the potential for service user involvement within projects that have not considered this and suggest consultation with service user groups to an applicant. Although service users and carers would like to experience interaction with clinical and academic reviewer colleagues, this process allows all members to express their views and minimises the power dynamics that might be present in a multi-professional group.

How effective can consultation be as a method of involving service users in research?

Although the evidence base for the effectiveness and value of service user involvement in the research process is still developing, organisations such as Involve, the NHS Centre for Involvement, and the Royal College of Nursing are broadly supportive of this activity and

BOX B: EXAMPLE OF SERVICE USER CONSULTATION IN PRACTICE

Examples of consultation 2

Service user research group

In 2001, a group of service users and carers from the South West Yorkshire Mental Health NHS Trust set up a service user and carer research group. The original aims of the group were to:

- ensure that the views and experiences of people receiving mental health services (either directly or indirectly as carers) influence local research and development at all levels
- be a resource for local research and development in mental health and managers may approach the group for their advice and input
- advise on and develop research that is led by people with mental health needs and their carers.

The group meet monthly to share their interests, plan research projects and share progress on ongoing research projects they lead or are collaborating in. Researchers from the Trust or partner organisations regularly attend those meetings to consult the group on their research idea, project design, methodology, or advice on the provision of information for research participants. The group have also been asked to review bids for funding and are often asked to join project teams and act as consultants throughout the research process. Members of the group also act as specialist advisers and consultants in other research fora and project groups such as the Trust wide research forum, research committees, and topic specific research groups such as ageing and mental health.

believe it adds value to the research process, to its outcomes, and also has value and benefit for the service user. Critics suggest, however, that methods of service user involvement in research frequently focus on the process and pay little attention to the outcome and whether such involvement leads to any longer term impact (Social Care Institute for Excellence, 2004). This can be particularly true of consultation as a technology for involvement as it tends to be time limited and restricted to a specific part of the research cycle. Lack of evaluation of the process and impact of involvement and absence of recorded outcomes can be a significant gap in terms of measuring the value of consultation. Power is a complex concept but it is clearly something that may be a barrier to involvement particularly in mental health where the relationship current service users have with a clinician researcher may be affected by the coercive nature of treatment.

Consultation may appear to be a relatively straightforward means of engaging service users in the research process, but the service user may question their involvement if they have not been involved in determining the focus of the research and are unable to affect the outcome. The policy and political imperative underpinning service user involvement is welcome but has also brought some difficulties as health service professionals seek ways of involvement. Sometimes consultation is inappropriate and is as negative an experience as tokenism for the service users. Moreover, frequent consultations can result in overload or consultation fatigue. Lack of coherence on the purpose or outcomes of involvement and lack of shared expectations on the part of the service user and organisation are also responsible for decreasing motivation. Those aiming to undertake consultation also need to believe in its value as lack of commitment to the process will be demonstrated through their attitude and responsiveness. There is often an assumption that researchers and clinicians know and understand the importance of involvement and how to go about it when they may not in fact have had adequate training.

Good practice requires the organisation or individual wishing to engage service users in consultation to identify different methods of involvement to suit individual needs and to approach groups or individuals within their own environment or community. This will aid the inclusion of a diverse range of people. Adequate time and resources need to be identified to make the process of consultation meaningful. The limitations imposed by restricted resources or because of the nature of the research project or methodology need to be outlined at the outset, as should the nature of the role of the people being consulted and the expectations of the process. The organisation needs to be responsive to change and to implementing suggestions and should be prepared to provide feedback to service users who have been involved. Ideally, consultation should take place as early in the research process as possible. Facilitated sensitively, preferably in collaboration with service users, consultation can lead to consensus and a smoother process of change. Practical issues that can assist in facilitating consultation include the provision of adequate training where necessary, use of jargon free accessible language, reimbursement of expenses, and offering mentoring and support for involvement.

CONCLUSION

Although there is still a lack of evidence about the impact and effectiveness of service user involvement at all levels, the consensus from NHS researchers and academics is that it is a worthwhile exercise and contributes to increasing knowledge of the service user perspective of mental health services. Consultation can play a key role as a technology for involving service users in mental health research but consulters will need to have appropriate tools to engage in meaningful consultation. It is important to recognise that consultation is part of a process and, ideally, it should be part of a continuum of involvement rather than a single exercise. Early consultation with service users can help to identify the extent of the role they can play within the whole project. It is important that service users retain control of their involvement and determine the level at which they engage. Even within low level involvement, consultation, researchers need to adopt the concept of service users as 'active partners' in the research process rather than simply stakeholders.

The Department of Health has signalled its support for the involvement of service users in the research process which is to be welcomed. The NIHR and MHRN have provided a lead by involving service users in their work but for this to be more than mere tokenism, it needs to be linked to NHS professionals and researchers wishing to involve service users in the design of bids for research funding in their desire to achieve success, consultation, along with other levels of involvement has to be supported with adequate resources. To understand the true value of consultation as a technology for user involvement in mental health research, it is important to recognise the need to evaluate both the process and the outcome. Outcomes can be in the form of personal gains for the service user (increased confidence, learning, participation, enhanced skills) but should also lead to gains for mental health services through increased knowledge of the service user perspective informing change and development.

REFERENCES

Arnstein, S.R. (1969) A ladder of citizen participation, *Journal of the American Planning Association*, **35**(4), 216–224.

Collins, K. and Ison, R. (2006) *Dare We Jump Off Arnstein's Ladder? Social learning as a new policy paradigm*, Milton Keynes: Open University.

Department of Health (2000) *Reforming the Mental Health Act*, London: DH.

Department of Health/Parliament (2001a) *Health and Social Care Act 2001*, London: The Stationery Office.

Department of Health (2001b) *Involving Patients and the Public in Healthcare*, London: DH.

Department of Health (2004) *NHS Improvement Plan*, London: DH.

Department of Health (2005a) *Creating a Patient Led NHS*, London: DH.

Department of Health (2005b) *Research Governance Framework*, Second edition, London: DH.

Department of Health (2006) *Best Research for Best Health. A new national health research strategy.* London: DH.

Faulkner, A. and Morris, B. (2003) *User Involvement in Forensic Mental Health Research and Development. National R & D Programme on Forensic Mental Health*. Published online by Involve: www.invo.org.uk, accessed 28/10/08.

Joseph Rowntree Foundation (2004) *Older People Shaping Policy and Practice*, York: Joseph Rowntree Foundation.

Minogue, V., Boness, J., Brown, A. and Girdlestone, J. (2005) The impact of service user involvement in research, *International Journal of Healthcare Quality Assurance*, **18**(2), 103–112.

NHS Centre for Involvement: www.nhscentreforinvolvement.nhs.uk, accessed 28/10/08.

National Health Service (1999) *Modern Standards and Service Models. Mental Health National Service Frameworks*, London: Department of Health.

National Health Service (2000) *The NHS Plan*, London: Department of Health.

Rethink (2003) *Just One Per Cent: The experiences of people using mental health services*, London: Rethink.

Rose, D. (2004) Telling different stories: user involvement in mental health research, *Research, Policy and Practice*, 27–35.

Royal College of Nursing: www.man.ac.uk/rcn/rs/userinvolvement, accessed 28/10/08.

Sainsbury Centre for Mental Health (2006) Choice in mental health care, *Briefing 31*, London: Sainsbury Centre for Mental Health.

Samele, C., Wallcraft, J. and Naylor, C. *et al.* (2007) *Research Priorities for Service User and Carer-Centred Mental Health services. Overview Report. Report for the National Coordinating Centre for NHS Service Delivery and Organisation R & D*, London: Sainsbury Centre for Mental Health.

Simpson, E.L., House, A.O. and Barkham, M. (2002) *A Guide to Involving Users, Ex-users and Carers in Mental Health Service Planning, Delivery or Research: A Health Technology Approach*. Leeds: Academic Unit of Psychiatry and Behavioural Sciences, University of Leeds.

Social Care Institute for Excellence (2004) *Has Service User Participation Made a Difference to Social Care Services?* London: SCIE.

Staley, K. and Minogue, V. (2006) User involvement leads to more ethically sound research. *Clinical Ethics*, **1**.

Steele R. (Ed) (2004) *Involving the Public in NHS, Public Health and Social Care Research: Briefing notes for researchers*, Second Edition, London: Involve.

Tait, L. and Lester, H. (2005) Encouraging user involvement in mental health services, *Advances in Psychiatric Treatment*, **11**, 168–175.

Tarpey, M. (2006) *Why People Get Involved in Health and Social Care Research: A working paper*, London: Involve.

Tritter, J.Q. and McCallum, A. (2006) The snakes and ladders of user involvement: moving beyond Arnstein, *Health Policy*, **76**, 156–168.

Trivedi, P. and Wykes, T. (2002) From passive subjects to equal partners, *British Journal of Psychiatry*, **181**, 468–472.

CHAPTER 12

Collaboration

Is Collaborative Research Possible?

Diana Rose

*Service User Research Enterprise (SURE), Institute of Psychiatry,
King's College London, London, UK*

Collaboration between traditional researchers and service users can occur across a range of different levels and within a variety of settings. The establishment of true collaboration and partnership is arguably the most demanding task academic and service user-researchers can strive to achieve. This chapter starts with an outline of the roots of collaborative research in England and its official position in the research scene there today. It then offers a practical example of the establishment and development of a collaborative research enterprise, and distinguishes between two practical models of collaborative research. The development, application and real-world impact of new methodologies that have been generated for user-focused collaborative research within this setting are portrayed. The second part of the chapter reflects on what it means to be a mental health user-researcher in an academic setting, on what makes this possible and productive and what the obstacles can be. Criticisms of service user-research are discussed and special consideration is paid to the critical issue of power differences and its practical sources. Finally, the current state of collaborative research in England is critically examined and a way forward is proposed.

INTRODUCTION

Leading up to collaborative research

The first user-research projects in England were user-controlled. Two user-research projects were established in NGOs in London in the 1990s. These were Strategies for Living (S4L; Faulkner and Layzell, 2000) and User-Focused Monitoring (UFM; Rose, 2001). It is

---

Handbook of Service User Involvement in Mental Health Research   Edited by Jan Wallcraft, Beate Schrank and Michaela Amering
Copyright © 2009 John Wiley & Sons, Ltd

important to state that these early efforts were carried out by people who had been active in the user movement, who wished to root their research in that movement and take their questions and priorities from it. As people who were users with research skills, they wished their efforts to contribute to the movement.

There was some dispute about methodological differences between UFM and S4L. Both drew upon user expertise in creating questionnaire or topic guides to interview other users about their experiences. In both cases, the interviewers were users trained in interviewing skills. However, the questionnaires and methods of analysis differed between the two groups. UFM was largely quantitative and S4L largely qualitative. Some heated discussions took place at conferences and most people preferred the qualitative approach. However, interestingly, there was much crossover between the results from the two projects.

S4L went on to support several local research projects. Nicholls (2003) gives a candid account of the peaks and pitfalls of this endeavour to roll out the research approach across the country with people who required training and support – as had the original S4L and UFM teams. The original researchers subsequently moved on and user involvement in these NGOs is now more policy and practically oriented although there are still user-researchers involved.

UFM now supports approximately 20 projects across England and has had effects elsewhere in Europe. However, it is no longer situated in the original NGO, projects have to secure local funding and the 'UFM Network' is largely a virtual group with face-to-face meetings on occasion. UFM as a project with a central hub no longer has funding.

User-controlled research has been diluted in mental health although in the social policy field, *Shaping Our Lives* thrives (see Beresford 2003, Chapter 13 this Handbook).

THE BEGINNINGS OF COLLABORATIVE RESEARCH

Collaborative research in England has many roots, including the influence of the user-controlled projects discussed above. Even as these projects were flourishing, in 1996 the Department of Health (DH) set up a unit called 'Consumers in NHS Research'. As its name implies, the aim was to involve consumers in NHS research. Later this unit had its remit widened to include social care and public health and it was renamed INVOLVE. INVOLVE is not specific to mental health but covers all health conditions. Nonetheless, in my view, it is heavily influenced by mental health user-researchers.

As Sweeney and Morgan explain elsewhere (Chapter 3), INVOLVE identified three levels of user involvement in research: consultation, collaboration and user-controlled research projects. All three levels were argued to be plausible forms of user involvement in research.

Later, INVOLVE had a more direct effect on research funding in England. The Department of Health decided that evidence of user involvement in research should become a condition of funding. This was put positively and if researchers did not include patients or the public in their research they had to say why. The end result of this was that funders had to specify what level of involvement there would be in their research and at what stages of the research project.

Finally, the Mental Health Research Network in England (MHRN) is a body which 'adopts' projects onto its network and supports them with activities such as recruitment of participants to large multi-site studies and with ethics and R&D applications. One of the criteria for adoption onto the network is that there should be evidence of user involvement in the projects. In addition, two user-researchers sit on the Adoption Committee. The projects adopted under this criterion will almost always involve consultation or collaboration and not user-control.

So far so good. But what does this mean in practice? Specifically, what counts as collaborative research and what are its benefits and costs?

COLLABORATIVE RESEARCH IN THE SERVICE USER ENTERPRISE (SURE)

There are many examples of user-researchers working in collaboration with mainstream researchers in England currently. However, here I will concentrate on the unit in which I work – the Service User-research Enterprise (SURE) at the Institute of Psychiatry, King's College London. This is simply because this is the work that I know best.

The Institute is the largest psychiatric research university in Europe and not known for its radicalism so this was an important step. In fact, SURE had been meeting as a 'virtual group', with some active service user involvement in research for some years. It was in 2000 that the associated mental health provider allocated some infrastructure money to SURE and thus enabled the employment of the first co-ordinator. The unit deliberately set out to be a collaboration between user-researchers and 'clinical academics'. At this point the head of SURE was a research clinical psychologist, Professor Til Wykes, who had been responsible for the virtual group referred to above. The co-ordinator was the present author who joined the unit from the UFM project described above.

SURE rapidly expanded, gaining funding for three large projects in its first year. At the end of the second year there were seven staff, including administrative staff, and most of these had experience of using mental health services. Since then the number of staff has waxed and waned depending on grant income. Currently, there are nine staff.

In 2005, I was made co-director of SURE and the world's first senior lecturer in user-led research. This ensured that the unit now had a balanced management structure as between user-researchers and clinical academics. It also meant that SURE was the first unit of its kind in Europe, employing service user-researchers and carrying out resolutely user-focused research which at the same time is collaborative. I say that SURE was the first unit of its kind in Europe. However, user-research elsewhere in Europe is blossoming. There are smaller projects elsewhere notably in the Netherlands and Germany and there has been collaboration between these projects and SURE.

TWO MODELS OF COLLABORATIVE RESEARCH

There are many models of collaborative research but two can be identified here. The first is when user-researchers and mainstream researchers work together on a single project. In that case, the two groups of researchers should bring complementary skills to the project. Alternatively, user-researchers may conduct the user led component of larger projects (Burns *et al.,* in press). Both these models have problems which will be discussed later.

New methodologies

During the course of various projects, SURE has developed new methodologies for research. These are intended to put the user at the heart of research and to adapt or challenge mainstream methods to this end. The two main methods which we have developed are, first, patient-centred systematic reviews and, second, participatory research in a mental health context. Patient-centred systematic reviews as a method evolved from SURE's first national piece of work on consumers' perspectives on ECT (Rose *et al.*, 2003; Rose *et al.*, 2004; Rose *et al.*, 2005). Our model of participatory research in a mental health context was first applied to the generation of user-focused outcome measures, for example, on continuity of care and CBT for psychosis. Papers on this model are currently under review. The two models will now be described.

Patient-centred systematic reviews

Systematic reviews are considered the highest form of scientific evidence both in psychiatry and in medicine generally. They pool the results of Randomized Controlled Trials (RCTs) which have very strict inclusion criteria if they are to be admitted to the Review. They include only trials in the peer-reviewed literature and the methodology is quantitative. From the perspective of a service user-researcher, this method has drawbacks. First, the outcome measures in trials are devised by clinicians and researchers. Second, for statistical reasons, there must be a 'primary' outcome measure which means that other measures, for example those to do with side-effects, are 'secondary'. The final way in which the voice of the user is excluded from standard systematic reviews is that there is no space for 'testimonies' about what the treatment or service actually means to those who receive it. To put it more generally, qualitative research is not permitted in mainstream models.

SURE therefore developed patient-centred systematic reviews in order to include the perspectives of those who receive treatments or services. These differ in several ways from mainstream work. First, a meta-analysis is still performed but included in this meta-analysis is the 'grey' literature. This term refers to literature which has not reached the peer-reviewed journals and we include papers and reports written by users, user groups and collaborative efforts on the treatment or service that is being investigated. Even papers from the peer-reviewed literature which are included are not RCTs. They are papers where clinicians have asked their patients what they feel about the treatment and they are, in effect, surveys or experiments. Since these papers often ask about side-effects, it becomes possible to carry out a meta-analysis not only on primary outcome measures (e.g. satisfaction with the treatment) but on secondary ones as well. In other words, we can highlight side-effects and measure their extent. Patient-centred systematic reviews also include qualitative work in order to find out what treatments and services actually mean and feel like to those who are receiving them. We analyse first-hand accounts of these experiences and call these 'testimonies'.

There are two further ways in which patient-centred systematic reviews differ from the traditional method. First, the main researchers carrying out the review will have received the treatment or service themselves thus having 'insider knowledge'. Second, for these reviews there is always a Reference Group made up mainly of people who have also received the treatment. One of the roles of this reference group is to suggest the initial coding categories for the qualitative work. However, as I have said, SURE is a collaborative unit. So we work together with non-user colleagues who have specific expertise in areas where our own knowledge might be lacking.

This model was first applied to electro-convulsive therapy (ECT) and was developed gradually from our reflections on it. The development of the model was influenced by a psychologist who had expertise in memory and a psychiatrist who had expertise in legal issues in psychiatry. However, as I will show later, this model is not acceptable to most mainstream researchers who see it as biased. However, the body that oversees medical treatment in the UK (the National Institute for Clinical Excellence or NICE) accepted our review as credible when it was developing guidelines on the use of ECT. This was the first time that user-research had made such an impact. This is very important as funders and others are now demanding evidence that user involvement in research makes a difference, that it 'adds value'. Our ECT review had a direct influence on policy and this shows that user-research can make a difference (see below).

Participatory research in a mental health context

Participatory research has a long history. It began as an approach in regeneration projects in developing countries and went on to be used in regeneration projects domestically in the UK. The driving principle of this approach is that the power relations between researcher and researched are reduced to a minimum. So, the research question comes from the community which identifies a problem and the aim of the research is to solve that problem for the community. Nevertheless, the community will engage a professional researcher to do the actual research albeit that he or she will involve the community as much as possible.

SURE has adapted this approach in developing user-focused outcome measures. We have focused on participatory models in a health context (Cornwall and Jewkes, 1995) and are mindful that it is difficult to minimise power relations in research (Mason and Boutilier, 1996). Also, in terms of the way research is funded, it is difficult for a community and associated researchers to receive funding for a project of their own. Typically, funders identify projects and then ask for tenders. This is changing in England, however. Our contribution to the model of participatory research is that the researcher is him- or herself a member of the community. In order to develop outcome measures, staff from SURE who are themselves mental health service users, work with other people with mental health problems to make sure that the outcome measures generated are true to service users' perspectives on what is important for a particular issue.

The basic method here is to hold focus groups and expert panels. These are wholly made up of service users and, as said, the researchers are service users and they disclose this. The initial measure is drawn up by the focus groups (who meet twice) and then it is taken to expert panels for refinement and amendment. We call these 'expert panels' in order to acknowledge that service users are 'experts' in their own experience and in the treatment and services they receive.

In fact, it is rather standard in measure construction in the social sciences to begin with focus groups (Oppenheim, 1992). However, traditionally members of these focus groups do not need to be part of any community to which the attitude scale or other outcome measure has relevance. They are generally recruited by Market Research Agencies and the aim is to get a representative sample of the population in terms of socio-demographic variables such as age, gender and socio-economic status. It is apparent that our method is different to this as the focus groups are made up of people with direct experience of the attribute, attitude or service to be measured and so they have a completely different role to members of focus groups in the traditional method. At the same time, we do not eschew the importance of issues such as establishing the psychometric properties of our measures. Collaborative and user-research must be rigorous.

This user-focused model has been or will be applied to four services or treatments by SURE. First, we have developed a user-focused measure of continuity of care. Second, we have developed quality standards for family doctors to use when dealing with young people with stress and other mental health problems. Thirdly, we have developed user-focused satisfaction measures for two psychological therapies: CBT for psychosis and Cognitive Rehabilitation Therapy for schizophrenia (Rose *et al.*, 2008). Indeed the last drew heavily on the method of User-Focused Monitoring mentioned earlier and served as a 'bridge' for the current author between a focus on evaluation of services and more sophisticated research. The final example of participatory research, which is ongoing, is to produce a user-defined measure of the therapeutic milieu in acute wards.

This returns me to the points made above about Randomized Controlled Trials (RCTs) and the fact that outcome measures have, until now, been produced by clinicians and researchers. It is not at all clear that these outcome measures capture a phenomenon from the point of view of service users. For example, trials of a treatment generally take the outcome measure to be one that can measure levels of symptoms. The point of the trial is to see if the intervention reduces symptom level. There may be a 'secondary' outcome on side-effects of, say, a medication. It does not occur to most researchers that service users may prefer to have some symptoms to avoid the unwanted effects of drugs.

Our measure of acute wards generated by and relevant to service users is to be part of a forthcoming RCT. This is a step forward and we will see if it is superior in capturing service user judgments of what is bad and what is good about acute wards. Of course there have been many studies on this (e.g. Sainsbury Centre for Mental Health, 2006) but, in the interests of rigorous user-research, we wish to systematically evaluate our measure. (For some more general reflections on measurement issues see also Chapter 8.)

BEING A SERVICE USER AND COLLABORATIVE RESEARCHER: PEAKS AND PITFALLS

The second half of this paper is rather more personal and reflective than it has been up until now. I am going to reflect on what it means to be a mental health user-researcher working in an established university – what makes this possible and productive? What are the obstacles and when is it impossible? There are very few references in the following sections as the discussion is rather about my own views or else issues that are talked about but not written down.

What is a user-researcher?

It is sometimes said to me that there must be many people at my place of work who use mental health services. So, they are both service users and researchers. Doesn't this make them user-researchers? In my view, no. A user-researcher is someone who insists on using their experience of using services and having mental health problems to inform their research practice. It is not enough to be both a service user and a researcher, these two attributes must be brought together to form a 'double identity'. It is akin to speaking two languages and, as any bilingual person knows, some things are impossible to translate. Linked to this, such a 'double identity' can be fragile. Professional colleagues may see you primarily as a user whereas other users may see you primarily as a researcher. This links to the issue of power to which I will return.

Criticisms of service user-research

In many cases, becoming a user-researcher is something quite personal. It means 'coming out of the closet' and re-defining one's mental distress as an asset. This appears to be the reason behind many criticisms of user-research. These are rarely written down although there are examples:

> There is a real danger that the engine of user initiatives in mental health services, although positive in principle, will accelerate out of control and drive mental health research into the sand.

>   (Tyrer, 2002, p406)

Tyrer's critique is not his alone. He is outspoken, but others concur although they may keep their comments to the spoken word.

What exactly are the criticisms? They revolve around the idea that user-research is subjective, anecdotal and carried out by people over-involved in what they are doing. Of course, such criticisms are a counter-point to how mainstream researchers conceive of what *they* are doing. That is, that their research is objective, produces universal ontological truths and that the position of the scientist is neutral. But I have yet to meet a researcher who did not have an interest, academic or personal or both, in their research question and how they pursue it. The claim that mainstream research is objective is largely a methodological one, and hangs on the conviction that RCTs are the best way of producing objective truths. I have already suggested that user-focused research needs to adapt mainstream methods if they are truly to represent the voice of the user. Otherwise, they will only represent the concerns, even the biases, of mainstream research which decides what topics are important, how to investigate them and what the important outcomes are.

To take an example, most RCTs of treatments have as their primary outcome measure the reduction of symptoms. This is what clinicians think is important. But it may not be what users think is important, or not solely so. Users may be willing to tolerate some symptoms to avoid the damaging side-effects of treatments and may wish to adopt techniques of self-management. Such an approach was developed by users in both the USA (Deegan, 1998) and the UK (Coleman, 1999). It is known as the 'recovery model' and recovery is not synonymous with 'cure'. In its radical guise, the recovery model cannot be tolerated by some psychiatrists who believe that stopping medication is a sure route to relapse. However, this model is now being taken up by other mental health professionals even if some service users regard this as a 'hijack' of a concept developed by them.

It is possible to make rational arguments about mainstream critiques of user-research. However, it should be noted that this debate is not always rational on either side. I have been in situations where the arguments of service users were summarily dismissed by very senior psychiatrists as 'biased, angry, vocal and unrepresentative'. This is especially true when there are large teams of investigators and the user-researchers are carrying out the user-led part of the study. It does not seem to me the most 'objective' way of conducting a debate.

Power

The question of power is central to the relationships that exist between user-researchers and their mainstream colleagues. This can manifest itself in many ways. First, and most simply, established academics will be likely to have a much stronger career track record than user-researchers. For example, and this is true for me, people with mental health problems are likely to experience career interruptions. Certain things matter in academic life such as publications and a record in winning funding. Some of my colleagues, younger than myself, have published more than 300 papers – I have published less than 30. Other colleagues in SURE are in this position too. Yet others are at the beginning of their careers simply because they are young. We try to develop their careers by encouraging them to do PhDs but these too can be interrupted by health problems. This discrepancy in experience and track record is one source of power differentials between user and mainstream researchers.

A more difficult and invidious way in which power operates relates back to what I said earlier about methodologies. Researchers who do Randomized Controlled Trials are prized and considered to be the most scientific of all researchers. User-researchers have a difficulty as we are not happy with the pure form of this methodology. The methods we use come further down the established 'hierarchy of evidence' (Geddes and Harrison, 1997). Indeed our focus on experience, even although we consider it expert experience, puts us at the bottom of that hierarchy. Expert experience usually means *professional* expertise and in that sense our user focus is no evidence at all. Researchers who use mainstream methods may pay some lip-service to what we do, but I see no evidence that they have really been persuaded. The power of the evidential hierarchy is another way in which mainstream researchers exercise power over user-researchers.

This argument can be pushed further although, to be fair, I think it is only implicit. Science is considered the acme of rationality. It has been seen this way for 300 years – since the Enlightenment. Indeed, reason and rationality are still influential throughout Western society. What does this mean then for the obverse of rationality – embodied in those deemed mad? It might seem that illogical people are incapable of doing anything as logical and rational as scientific endeavour. Perhaps being mad is a necessary exclusion criterion for rational thought. (Foucault, 1967)

Although never stated, I suspect that it is such a notion, or something akin to it, that lies behind the ritual criticisms that user-research is biased, anecdotal and carried out by people who are incapable of being neutral.

One can try to tease out the arguments and the practices by means of which mainstream researchers exercise power over user-researchers. One can try to be rational (!). But sometimes this power is exercised nakedly and blatantly. I have been cut off in mid-sentence by Professors. I have been refused the right to speak. Other staff in SURE have been patronised in public. It does not happen often now because in the UK user-research is on the 'agenda'. But it does still happen.

Indeed, the expression of disdain for user-research has been put to me outside the context of my workplace. A conference two years ago in London had, unusually, a specific stream devoted to user-research. The journalist tasked with writing up the conference said that the user-research stream was pure bias. A delegate to the conference said to me personally that user involvement in research was nothing but political correctness. In the face of such opinions, user-research has a long struggle ahead of it.

For a detailed discussion of aspects of power in relation to service user involvement in mental health research, see also Chapter 14.

IS COLLABORATION POSSIBLE?

When the possibility arose that I might work at the Institute of Psychiatry, the reaction of some people was very negative. These people included psychiatrists who considered themselves radical and users who would never go near what they considered conservative institutions. Comments included: 'You are going into the lion's den', 'They'll eat you for breakfast and spit you out', 'You will become one of them'. It turned out not to be like this and myself and SURE have received support from senior people within the Institute of Psychiatry. When I was promoted it proved that the people I worked with had faith in me. On the other hand, there are departments in the Institute who I am sure do not know we exist and if they did know, would probably think we shouldn't!

My previous discussion concerning power shows that collaboration between clinical researchers and user-researchers in mental health is difficult to achieve. It will usually be the case that the collaboration is unequal and not a true partnership. Creating more of a partnership has other difficulties. If user-researchers wish to form more of a partnership with their clinical colleagues then the chances are that this can only be done by surrendering some principles of user-research and accepting more of the agenda of clinical research. There can also be situations where you think a partnership has been achieved and then mid-way through a project the goalposts are changed and the user component in the research is downgraded. Another example is when users engage in research using a 'mixed methods' approach that is, combining quantitative and qualitative methods. The user-researcher is allocated the qualitative component, which indeed she or he may be happy to do, but because qualitative research does not have the status as quantitative research, the user-research work is not in true collaboration with the rest of the project.

So, is true collaboration possible at all? Some people definitely think it is not and that the only route to take is to develop user-*controlled* research. It is argued that the only way to ensure that research remains user-focused is to ensure that the entire process is controlled by service users. This approach is particularly evident in the social policy field in the UK although it is not absent from the health sector (Beresford, 2005).

It seems to me that the best we can achieve at this stage is to try to engage in research to which users and mainstream researchers bring *complementary* skills. These skills also need to have equivalent status. So the arguments I have been making about quantitative and qualitative research would not quite meet this criterion. However, to refer to our ECT project once again, here it was possible to make this happen. The design of the study was collaborative. The data collection and the organisation of the reference group were carried out by the user-researchers. The analysis included the user-researchers but also a psychologist and a psychiatrist. The psychologist (the co-director of SURE) had expertise on long-term memory loss and the psychiatrist was an expert in legal issues and coercion. This project would count for me as the most successful piece of collaborative research I have been involved with. But it was SURE's first national project and, I am afraid, this success has not been repeated.

Impacts

There is now pressure on service user-researchers to provide evidence that their research has an impact on services or 'adds value' to research itself. This pressure comes from funders, and the organization INVOLVE which I mentioned earlier is working hard to provide this evidence. However, because of our departure from mainstream methods, to evidence these impacts is difficult. Nevertheless, certain impacts can be identified. I have already mentioned that our ECT review was accepted as evidence by a national regulatory body. This led to the tightening up of procedures concerning information and consent in guidelines for changing the process whereby ECT is prescribed. Another example is the UFM project I mentioned earlier. UFM studies are now largely locally commissioned and so any impacts will be in the locality where the project takes place. The evidence is that some of these projects gather dust on a shelf. But others have made a difference. For example, the recommendations of the first UFM project provided the basis for changes in care standards. Another, an evaluation of acute wards, led to the production of leaflets for new patients albeit that this took some time.

CONCLUSION

User-research has only existed in the UK for just over 10 years. Despite its infancy, it has grown apace. This is partly because the context is right. But I would like to think that it is also because we are beginning to prove ourselves and make an impact not only on research itself but more practically. However, as I have argued in this paper, descriptively, theoretically and from a personal point of view, collaborative research is not easy to do and will take some more time to become established.

REFERENCES

Beresford, P. (2003) *User Involvement in Research: Connecting lives, experience and theory.* London: Citizen Press.

Beresford, P. (2005) Social approaches to madness and distress: user perspectives and user knowledges. In: J. Tew (Ed) *Social Perspectives in Mental Health: Developing social models to understand and work with mental distress,* London: Jessica Kingsley Publishers, pp. 33–51.

Burns, T., Catty, J., White, S. *et al.* (in press) for the ECHO Group (in press) Continuity of care in mental health: understanding and measuring a complex phenomenon, *Psychological Medicine*, not known at time of publication.

Coleman, R. (1999) *Recovery: An Alien Concept,* Gloucester: Handsell.

Cornwall, A. and Jewkes, R. (1995) What is participatory research? *Social Science and Medicine,* **41**(12), 1667–1676.

Deegan, P.E. (1988) Recovery: the lived experience of rehabilitation, *Psychosocial Rehabilitation Journal,* **11**, 11–19.

Faulkner, A. and Layzell, S. (2000) *Strategies for Living,* London: Mental Health Foundation.

Foucault, M. (1967) *Madness and Civilisation*, London: Tavistock.

Geddes, L. and Harrison, P. (1997) Closing the gap between research and practice. *British Journal of Psychiatry*, **171**, 220–225.

INVOLVE http://www.invo.org.uk, accessed 28/10/08.

Mason, R. and Boutilier, M. (1996) The challenge of genuine power sharing in participatory research: the gap between theory and practice, *Canadian Journal of Community Mental Health*, **15**(2), 145–151.

Mental Health Research Network: http://www.mhrn.info/index.html accessed 28/10/08.

Nicholls, V., Griesbaum, M., Wells, S. *et al.* (2003) *Surviving User-led Research: Reflections on Supporting User-led Research Projects*, London: Mental Health Foundation.

Oppenheim, A.[20] (1992) *Questionnaire Design, Interviewing and Attitude Measurement*, new edition, London: Printer.

Rose, D. (2001) *Users' Voices: The perspective of mental health service users on community and hospital care*, London: Sainsbury Centre for Mental Health.

Rose, D., Wykes, T., Leese, M. *et al.* (2003) Patients' perspectives on electroconvulsive therapy: systematic review, *British Medical Journal*, **326**, 1363–1366.

Rose, D., Fleischmann, P. and Wykes, T. (2004) Consumers' Perspectives on ECT: A Qualitative Analysis, *Journal of Mental Health*, **13**(3), 285–294.

Rose, D., Wykes, T., Bindman, J. and Fleischmann, P. (2005) Information, consent and perceived coercion: consumers' views on ECT, *British Journal of Psychiatry*, **186**, 54–59.

Rose, D., Wykes, T., Farrier, D. *et al.* (2008) What do clients think of cognitive remediation therapy? a consumer-led investigation of satisfaction and side effects, *American Journal of Psychiatric Rehabilitation*, **11**(2), 181–204.

Tyrer, P. (2002) Commentary: research into mental health services needs a new approach, *Psychiatric Bulletin*, **26**, 406–407.

CHAPTER 13

Control

User-Controlled Research

Peter Beresford

*Centre for Citizen Participation
at Brunel University, Middlesex, UK*

Within the context of involvement research, service user-controlled research has specific ideological underpinnings, offers distinct opportunities and faces specific difficulties. This chapter starts by exploring the history and origins of user-controlled research, comparing and contrasting it to the related movements of 'emancipatory disability research' and 'survivor research' and their associated ideas, models and theories. Definitions and practical implications related to user-controlled research and user-controlled organisations are outlined, and their associated characteristics, interests and real-world limits are described. An example is given of an established national UK user-controlled organisation which has research and development work amongst its key activities. The chapter goes on to discuss the ideologies, nature, strength and problems of user-controlled research, and its differences from other forms of involvement. Finally, the strengths and impact of user-controlled research are outlined, as are common problems and barriers from an international perspective. On this basis, proposals are made for securing the future of user-controlled research.

INTRODUCTION

Paradoxically, user-controlled research almost certainly has the longest history of any form of user involvement in research (Turner and Beresford, 2005a; Branfield *et al.*, 2006). Yet there are strong reasons to believe that it remains the most marginalised and insecure expression of such research. This contradiction perhaps highlights both the strengths and weaknesses of user-controlled research. For its exponents, it may represent the strongest and most developed expression of user involvement in research. In the broader context of research overall, however, it can expect to be treated with the greatest caution and subject to the most formidable barriers.

Handbook of Service User Involvement in Mental Health Research Edited by Jan Wallcraft, Beate Schrank and Michaela Amering
Copyright © 2009 John Wiley & Sons, Ltd

While this book and this chapter focus on user-controlled mental health research, this can best be understood in the broader context of disability research. The relationship between the mental health service user or psychiatric system survivor movement and the disabled people's movement is a complex and not always close or positive one, as we shall see. But nonetheless the best route to understanding user-controlled mental health research is through an understanding of disabled people's research. Indeed it is arguable that the links between research controlled by disabled people and that controlled by mental health service users are stronger than those between user-controlled and user-involvement mental health research. Thus this chapter will begin by tracing the modern origins of disabled people's research and then examine its similarities and differences from research controlled by mental health service users. It will then look more closely at the definition of user-controlled research and a range of key issues relating to it.

THE EMERGENCE OF EMANCIPATORY DISABILITY RESEARCH

Interest among service users and their organisations in user involvement in research originated in the disabled people's movement, which saw research as part of broader structures of oppression and discrimination in society. Disabled researchers were influenced by the 'critical social research' of feminists, Black writers and educationalists who allied themselves with oppressed groups. The disabled people's movement has highlighted the importance of changing (and equalising) the social relations of research production. Disabled people's and social care service user organisations and movements have emphasised two overlapping concerns in research and evaluation: what research is for and where control of research lies. This is reflected in the emergence of the 'emancipatory research paradigm' and related interest in 'user-controlled research'. In emancipatory research, the central purpose of research is seen as supporting the empowerment of service users and the making of broader social change (Barnes and Mercer, 1997; Oliver, 1992; Mercer, 2002; Barnes et al., 2002; Swain et al., 2004).

User involvement seems to be regarded as a necessary, but not sufficient condition for research to improve the lives of disabled people, individually and collectively. User involvement has generally been treated by disabled researchers much more as a means to undertaking helpful research rather than as an end in itself. The emphasis has been on emancipatory rather than participatory research (Mercer, 2002).

DIFFERENT APPROACHES TO INVOLVEMENT IN RESEARCH

User-controlled research needs to be seen in the broader context of user involvement in research. Three basic approaches to involvement in research can be identified. These are:

- user involvement or consultative research – where service user involvement is added by researchers to existing research paradigms and approaches
- collaborative research, where service users and researchers or their organisations jointly initiate and undertake research
- user-controlled research, where service users and their organisations initiate and run research.

Examples of all of these have now developed, although the dominant approach continues to be the first, user involvement or consultative research. For a comprehensive outline of the levels of service user involvement in research, see also Chapter 3.

DEFINING USER-CONTROLLED RESEARCH

A review of user-controlled research was commissioned and published in 2005 by Involve, the body established by government in the UK to develop public, patient and service user involvement in research and evaluation in health, public health and social care (Turner and Beresford, 2005a). While Involve's brief extends to all expressions of user involvement in research, it has also maintained a specific focus in its work on user-controlled research. Its review was based on both a survey of existing user-controlled research and feedback from service users with an interest in such research. This extended over a range of service user groups, including mental health service users. Its findings reflect the broader situation regarding user-controlled research and not only its development in the mental health context. Involve's aim in undertaking this review was not to impose a single definition of its own on 'user-controlled research', but to get a clearer idea of service users' thinking about its definition. There was considerable consensus about how user-controlled research might be defined, both among participants in the review and in the literature, as well as between the two. Of course, other stakeholders, like mainstream researchers might have other ideas to offer about user-controlled research's definition, but as yet these have not been sought in a coherent way.

Involve offers its own short definition of user-controlled research in a Public Involvement Information Pack which it has published, which draws upon the review, saying that:

> User-controlled research is research that is actively controlled, directed and managed by service users and their service user organisations. Service users decide on the issues and questions to be looked at, as well as the way the research is designed, planned and written up. The service users will run the research advisory or steering group and may also decide to carry out the research.
>
> Some service users make no distinction between the term 'user-controlled' and 'user-led' research, others feel that user-led research has a different, vaguer meaning.
>
> They see user-led research as research which is meant to be led and shaped by service users but is not necessarily controlled by them. Control in user-led research in this case will rest with some other group of non-service users who also have an interest in the research, such as the commissioners of the research, the researchers or people who provide services.
>
> (Involve, 2007)

The Involve review concluded that user-controlled research was closely linked with emancipatory disability research and 'survivor research'. It took the view that it was not always clear whether these terms demarcated different research approaches or were used interchangeably. The review essentially took them all as expressions of user-controlled research and synonymous with it generally. Thus control by service users is explicitly at the heart of the idea of user-controlled research. This control is variously seen to lie with service users generally, service users who are the research participants and also with service users' (self) organisations. Emphasis is placed on control of research not lying with non-service users.

So as might be expected, control by service users emerges as the key and defining characteristic of user-controlled research. Making change is commonly identified as the central purpose of user-controlled research, although there is also recognition that such change may not always be achieved. User-controlled research can be based on both qualitative and quantitative research methods and is also developing its own research methods. Service users see democratic accountability to service users as a key requirement for good practice in user-controlled research. This might be achieved by the research project itself being democratically constituted or it being located within a democratically constituted service user organisation.

However, while service users tend to highlight the importance of user control in all aspects and stages of user-controlled research, it is not always seen as essential that service users undertake all research tasks and activities. Where there does seem to be agreement is that other people employed in the research should be subject to the control of service users. This issue is a particular subject of discussion in relation to whether the researcher should be a service user. The Involve study indicated that there is no agreement about this. Arguments for and against using only service users as researchers are raised by service users themselves.

Much of the definition that emerged in Involve's 2005 review of user-controlled research was concerned with identifying components for good practice and characteristics associated with it. These corresponded closely with those identified by Alison Faulkner in her exploration of ethics for survivor research (Faulkner, 2004). The component most closely identified with it was a commitment to making change in line with the interests and rights of service users at individual level (empowerment) and at broader levels (political and social change).

The definition of user-controlled research offered in Involve's review, may thus be summed up as follows:

- User-controlled research is research which is actively controlled by service users and is accountable to them.
- Other terms used for user-controlled research include 'survivor research', 'user research' and 'emancipatory disability research'.
- User-controlled research can include a wide range of research methods and methodologies, including both qualitative and quantitative research.
- Service users are likely to be involved in all aspects and stages of the research, but not necessarily so. What is crucial is that they control the research.
- User-controlled research is committed to making change in line with service users' rights and needs, although there is recognition that this may not always be possible.

This is the most developed and broadly based discussion about the definition of user-controlled research known to this author and it is therefore the one on which the present discussion will be based.

However, a number of other issues might also need to be taken into account when considering the meaning of user-controlled in its real world setting.

REALITIES OF USER CONTROL IN A DISCRIMINATORY SOCIETY

A recent study of service user networking and knowledge highlights some of the complexities associated with the nature and meaning of user-controlled research and user-controlled organisations (Branfield *et al.*, 2006). Typically, a user-controlled organisation has been taken to mean one where at least a majority of those in control, through the management body or board of trustees are themselves service users. However in this study, participants felt that control should be exclusively vested in service users, who should make up the whole governing body. Otherwise, some felt that non-service user staff might take over control, or a traditional charity would present itself as user-controlled, while in fact non service users would effectively maintain control of its culture, goals and operation.

One of the findings of this project was that there was a strong perception among some service users that, in practice, not all organisations which claim to be user-controlled are actually controlled by service users. Another problem reported by service users and their organisations is that the fragility and inadequacy of their funding restricts their freedom and forces them to pursue the activities for which they can gain funding, rather than those which they would prefer to prioritise. Particular problems in maintaining user control in both organisations and projects have also been highlighted by people with learning difficulties, who can come under especial pressure from non-disabled collaborators, supporters and service providers (Taylor *et al.*, 2007).

Issues may also be raised where research projects which are themselves essentially controlled by service users are nonetheless located in organisations which themselves do not claim to be user-controlled. This has particular resonance for survivor research since many of the best known and largest research projects have actually been located in such organisations. This has, for example, been true of the original user focused monitoring project, based at the Sainsbury Centre for Mental Health (Muijen, 1998; Rose, 2001); the Strategies For Living project, based at the Mental Health Foundation (Faulkner and Nicholls, 1999; Faulkner and Layzell, 2000; Nicholls, 2001) and the SURE project (Service User Research Enterprises) based at the Institute of Psychiatry, King's College, London (SURE, 2002). Each of these has developed major innovative programmes of work in relation to user-controlled or survivor research, developing research and training, building capacity, pioneering new research methods and approaches. The SURE project particularly, undertakes and has undertaken large scale research projects and developed both qualitative and quantitative research projects. It has also developed new participatory approaches to quantitative research methodology of value and importance (SURE, 2002; see Chapter 12 this volume).

However non-service user-controlled organisations may not have the same priorities as user-controlled ones and this can affect the importance they give to user-controlled research (Lindow, 2001; Beresford, 2004). Thus both the Sainsbury Centre for Mental Health and the Mental Health Foundation decided to end the important initiatives that they had established in this area, despite the value attached to them by service users and service user researchers.

USER-CONTROLLED RESEARCH, EMANCIPATORY DISABILITY RESEARCH AND SURVIVOR RESEARCH

While as has been said, the term user-controlled research is often used as a synonym for emancipatory disability research and survivor research and while these latter two research approaches have much in common, there are also significant differences between the two and between the two movements they relate to – the disabled people's and survivors' movements. An understanding of these differences is a helpful first step towards gaining an understanding of survivor research as a form of user-controlled research.

The research developed by disabled people has a history stretching back to the late 1960s and early 1970s. The development of emancipatory disability research and the disabled people's movement are closely inter-related. To some extent disabled people's engagement in research can be seen as one of the founding activities of their movement (Campbell and Oliver, 1996; Oliver, 1996; Oliver and Barnes, 1998). The emergence of both has been closely linked to the development of two important and related ideas, models or theories. These are the 'social model of disability' and the philosophy of 'independent living'. The social model of disability distinguishes between perceived individual impairment – that is to say the loss or impaired function of a limb, sense or bodily function – and disability – which is taken to mean the societal barriers, oppressions and discriminations that may then be experienced by people with such impairments. Thus disability is no longer conceived solely as a matter of individual or personal incapacity requiring a traditional medicalised individualistic response. The social model of disability should not be oversimplified and needs to be understood as a dynamic and developing approach (Crowe, 1996; Thomas, 2007). Following from it, the philosophy of independent living challenges traditional understandings of disabled people as inherently dependent and instead posits that to live on as equal terms as possible to non disabled people, disabled people should be ensured the support they need and access to mainstream services and society. The social model of disability has become a basis for public policy and the philosophy of independent living has been adopted formally as an objective of UK government policy (Office for Disability Issues, 2008).

MENTAL HEALTH SERVICE USER/SURVIVOR RESEARCH

Research by mental health service user/survivor organisations and individual service user/ researchers developed much later than disability research. Taking 1997 as a reference point, there were hardly any large scale research projects. Much research was small scale with limited funding. Some was even unfunded. Service user/survivor researchers were generally working with very limited resources and little status or recognition. Furthermore there were relatively few such researchers and only a small number of service users/survivors with research training. (Beresford and and Wallcraft, 1997) Research has been less one of the founding influences of the survivor movement, as was the case with emancipatory disability research, but more something that has emerged later from the development of the survivor movement.

Contact between the disabled people's and survivor movements has long been limited. Mental health service users have often been reluctant to identify as disabled people and disabled people with shared experience as mental health service users, tend to be wary of identifying as such because of the stigma they associate with it (Beresford et al., 2002).

The survivor movement does not seem to have developed explicit philosophies or theories comparable to those of the social model of disability or independent living developed by the disabled people's movement. This is not to say that there has not been a set of shared values and beliefs underpinning the survivor movement. These values have focused on service users speaking and acting for themselves and seeking to challenge stigma, exclusion and the dominance of drug therapy in the psychiatric system (Campbell, 1996). The survivor movement and its associated organisations are certainly very conscious of 'the social' in their thinking and activities. Service user/survivor discourses address both material and spiritual issues; the personal as well as the political. However, this still has not led to the widespread development of any equivalent of the social model of disability. Thus while the emancipatory disability research of the disabled people's movement has been underpinned by the social model of disability and this is seen as both a defining element of it and also one of its guiding lights, there has not been such an equivalent in survivor research shaping its orientation and focus (Beresford, 2004).

This connects with another significant difference between the two movements in the UK which has impacted upon their approaches to research. While it might not be appropriate to characterise the UK disabled people's movement as 'separatist', it has certainly deliberately developed its own agenda and for a long time has placed much more emphasis on *independent* development than partnership approaches. The process adopted by the mental health service user/survivor movement has been significantly different to this. It has followed much more from a partnership model where:

- activity has mainly been concentrated in the psychiatric system;
- there have been strong pressures for mental health service users/survivors to get involved in mental health service based initiatives;
- most of the effort and energy of participating mental health service users has focused on trying to reform traditional mental health services;
- much of the involvement of mental health service users has been related to the service, policy and practice system(s) rather than agendas of their own;
- much of the funded activity of mental health service users/survivors has been in non-user-controlled voluntary and statutory organisations.

While there have been more independent survivor controlled organisations, like Survivors Speak Out and Mad Pride, these have been in a minority. Thus, while some mental health service users/survivors have taken a more radical and separatist position, developing their own initiatives rather than acting in partnership with professionals (O'Hagan, 1993), this has not been the main thrust of activity. The approach advocated by the American survivor and activist, Judi Chamberlin, doing things 'On Our Own', has been the exception, rather than the rule in the UK, for example (Chamberlin, 1988).

Thus while the user-controlled or survivor research developed by mental health service users has gained momentum and expanded in scale, with more survivor researchers gaining training and becoming established, much of it, as was observed earlier is still located in non-user-controlled settings and in volume, visibility and scope, it does not match the emancipatory disability research pioneered by the disabled people's movement.

An example of user-controlled research

As has been indicated, in the UK at least, while user-controlled research has been developing at a rapid rate in terms of scale, methodology and quality, in the context of mental health, most of the larger projects have been located in non user-controlled organisational settings.

An example which challenges this trend, with which the author is involved, is the work of Shaping Our Lives. Shaping Our Lives is an independent national service user-controlled organisation and network. It was first established in 1996 with a focus on increasing the say and involvement of service users and improving the quality of their lives and the support they receive. Research and development work are among its key activities. What distinguishes it from many other service user organisations is that it is made up of and works across a wide range of service user groups, rather than only being concerned with one. Thus it involves people with physical and sensory impairments, people with learning difficulties, mental health service users, older people, people with life limiting illnesses and conditions, young people with experience of being in state care, people living with HIV/AIDS and people with alcohol and drug problems. While most of the research projects it has been involved in undertaking have been user-controlled ones, they have not been specifically 'survivor research' projects. But they do have relevance for such research and have certainly involved mental health service users centrally.

A pattern can be seen in the research produced by Shaping Our Lives. Its research projects have ranged from small to large ones gaining significant sums of funding. The focus of its research has grown from and been developed in association with a wider range of service users, either through active consultation, or as a result of issues being raised more broadly to which it seeks to respond. As well as research projects being actively used to engage in policy discussions and developments, at both local and national levels, they have built on the findings of their predecessors. Thus there is a strategic consistency in their direction of travel, underpinned by the goals of:

- Linking research with activism
- Supporting service users to gain skills and abilities to become involved in research
- Working for the involvement of a diverse range of service user in terms both of impairment and difference expressed in relation to age, ethnicity, gender, sexuality, belief, culture and class
- Providing a democratic framework for control and accountability
- Seeking to disseminate findings broadly in accessible formats
- Identifying and pursuing appropriate follow-up action.

Areas for research have so far included the development of user-defined outcome measures; tensions between payment for involvement and existing benefit and welfare systems; the support service users receive; the development of service user networking and knowledge and enabling diverse involvement in policy and practice (Shaping Our Lives *et al.*, 2003; Turner, 1997 and 1998; Turner and Beresford, 2005b; Beresford and Branfield, 2006; Beresford *et al.*, 2005; Branfield *et al.*, 2006).

IDEOLOGIES OF INVOLVEMENT AND USER-CONTROLLED RESEARCH

We have looked at and compared the origins and value base of emancipatory disability research and survivor research and identified differences. But both, as forms of user-controlled research, can be seen to have significant differences from other forms of user-involvement research. This leads us to the ideological basis of user-controlled research and indeed ideologies underpinning user involvement more generally. An understanding of these will be helpful in gaining a better understanding of both the nature, strengths and problems of user-controlled research.

When we look more generally at user involvement – in policy, practice and planning – two distinct approaches have been identified (Hickey and Kipping, 1998; Beresford, 2005a). First is the managerialist/consumerist approach to user involvement. Framed mainly in market terms and developed by state and service systems, it has so far mainly been based on consultative models of involvement, operating as a kind of intelligence gathering/ market research activity. Second, is the democratic approach to involvement that has been developed by service users, their organisations and allies. This has been concerned with redistributing power and increasing their involvement in decision-making, so that they are able to exert more control over their own lives and can have more say in agencies, organisations and institutions which impact upon them. These are very different approaches which should not be confused with each other. It is not difficult to see similarities between these two models and the emerging strands of user involvement in research. User involvement or consultative research seems closely to reflect the managerialist/consumerist model, while service users' definitions of emancipatory/user-controlled research reflect the aspirations of a democratic approach to involvement (Beresford, 2004 and 2005).

Service user researchers, service user organisations and movements value user-involvement in research and user-controlled research as part of a process of developing their own knowledge and discourses, as a basis for change. It is to achieve such change that service users respond to calls and initiatives to get involved (Turner and Beresford, 2005a). Yet much of the user involvement on offer is based, as has been seen, on a very different model of consultation and market research. As a result, for many service users, it can feel like little more than tokenism or a 'box ticking' exercise (Stickley, 2006). This applies equally to involvement in research. On reflection, service users may see little point being involved in research whose focus, theoretical basis and objectives follow from dominant agendas. By developing user-controlled research they are least likely to find themselves co-opted into advancing such traditional agendas; a real risk when they are drawn into becoming involved in research where the focus and methods have been pre-selected by mainstream researchers or reflect government concerns and priorities.

IMPACT

There is now an increasing interest in the *impact* of user involvement in research. Both Involve and the NHS Centre for Involvement are currently undertaking projects focusing on the impact of user involvement. This widespread interest seems to be underpinned by the view that the moral and ethical arguments for equalising research relationships and including service users and their perspectives are alone not sufficient justification for involvement. Impact is a complex concept in research. Impact has been institutionalised in academic research, for example, through the UK Research Assessment Exercise (RAE), to mean how it is judged by research 'peers', particularly through the publication of 'peer review journal' articles and the number of academic citations such publications receive. Such definitions of impact are unlikely to be supportive of user-controlled research since they define impact in terms of individual researchers' competitive activity in relation to a narrow range of 'academicised' outputs (Fisher and Marsh, 2003; Gambrill, 2002, Shardlow *et al.*, 2004).

In the context of user-involvement research, impact has been taken to mean how involvement improves the quality and outcomes of research. Since the development of user-involvement research has been an ideological as well as methodological departure, a focus on research efficacy and efficiency could be seen as unduly narrow and restricted. Impact might equally be concerned with effects on policy and service users themselves. User-controlled research demands a re-conception of impact in terms of both its own values and increasing interest in the 'utility' of research; that is to say the helpful role it can play in influencing planning, policy and practice in public policy. Advocates of user-controlled research feel that it is particularly equipped to make an impact because of both its process and aims. As yet, there has been very limited evaluation of the impact of user-controlled research. However, it can be seen as having relevant strengths by:

- supporting the empowerment of service users through its commitment to developing more equal research relationships and processes
- prioritising the making of individual and broader change in its underpinning objectives
- having the support of a constituency – service users and their movements – to take forward its findings to bring about change.

STRENGTHS OF USER-CONTROLLED RESEARCH

Thus for service users and their organisations, the particular strengths they associate with user-controlled research are key to the impact they see it as having. These include:

- **The use of service user researchers and interviewers** (not restricted to user-controlled research, but particularly associated with it).

  The User Focused Monitoring project highlighted the value of having service user, rather than non-service user interviewers, in encouraging research participants to offer fuller, more frank responses (Rose, 2001). Service User Research Enterprise (SURE) at the Institute of Psychiatry is currently exploring these issues through a quantitative research study. (Find more on these examples in Chapter 12).
- **Supportive of service user agendas for research**
  A 2002 Department of Health strategic review of mental health research and development priorities showed that service users' research agendas were different from, much broader and more socially related than those of existing researchers, which were much more narrowly focused on the psychiatric system and individualized responses to mental health issues. (Department of Health, 2002) User-controlled research is based on the principle of starting from the research concerns and research questions of service users and their organisations.
- **A social perspective-based approach**
  While survivor research is not based on an equivalent of the social model of disability, it does generally challenge medicalised individual models of mental health adopting a more social perspective (Tew, 2005). This is of value for a subject of research where social and personal factors operate in complex inter-relation and where traditional medicalised research has frequently failed adequately to address all aspects of mental health issues.

THE INTERNATIONAL SETTING

This discussion builds primarily on the UK experience of user-controlled research. But just as there are now national, European, international and global organisations and networks of disabled people and mental health service users, so user-involvement research, including user-controlled research, has begun to develop internationally. Thus this discussion takes account of developments in Europe, North America, Australia/New Zealand and the majority world. Clearly, there are different local circumstances and features. There are different health and welfare systems; different balances of market, state and not-for-profit sectors; different ethnic, cultural and belief systems, which have a bearing on under-standings of and responses to mental health issues. Different countries have different policy and research contexts which offer more and less opportunities for user-controlled research. User-controlled research is at different states of development. While as yet there has been no systematic international exploration of user-controlled research, to the best knowledge of this author, we can expect that while there will be international variations, development generally is still at a relatively early stage.

SOME COMMON BARRIERS

However, what can also be identified are some common characteristics which operate internationally and which face user-controlled research with some common problems and barriers.

Globalisation

There has been a growing tendency for prevailing western models and understandings of health and welfare issues to be exported internationally and to have an increasing influence globally, affecting and replacing a wide range of indigenous approaches in the majority world. This has certainly happened in relation to mental health issues where dominant psychiatric understandings and responses have gained increasing currency. This in turn reinforces the dominance in research of traditional medicalised approaches and methodologies, to the disadvantage of alternatives like user-controlled research (Holden and Beresford, 2002; Stone, 1999; Barnes and Mercer, 2005).

The international pharmaceutical industry

Related to this is the powerful influence of the international pharmaceutical industry (Beresford, 2005b). This has both benefitted from and helped inspire and perpetuate the dominance of drug-related responses to mental health issues. It is the largest funder of psychiatric research and has had a significant influence in shaping the agenda of that research and its reliance on a narrow range of methods which tend to focus on the individual. The preoccupations of the industry seriously limit opportunities for user-controlled research to adhere to its principles of being led by service users' priorities and concerns and maintaining an holistic approach to their rights and needs. Find more on the influence of the pharmaceutical industry on the focus of research in Chapter 16.

Dominance of the medical model

While the medical model generated by psychiatry has come in for criticism from professionals, researchers and service users, there is no sign that its dominance in mental health policy or research has diminished (Pilgrim and Rogers, 1999). If anything, with the increasing 'psychiatrisation of everyday life and the growing tendency to respond to social issues in terms of individual disorder requiring drug treatment – for example, in relation to disruptive children and institutionalised older people – its influence and authority seem to be growing. This is clearly at odds with the more open agenda of user-controlled research.

TRADITIONAL RESEARCH VALUES

But perhaps the most immediate obstacle in the way of user-controlled research is the way that it can expect to be understood in the context of traditional research approaches. Two key and related elements can be identified here which disadvantage it; first, traditional hierarchies of evidence; and second, traditional positivist research values and the interpretation of user-controlled research within them as ideologically biased.

HIERARCHY OF RESEARCH METHODOLOGY

Powerful hierarchies for the production of knowledge and evidence still operate in research, not least in mental health research. These strongly disadvantage much if not all user-controlled research. The hierarchy set out in Figure 13.1 is typical. While it is that used in the government's National Services Framework for Mental Health (Department of Health, 1999), it much more widely underpins the thinking of bodies concerned with developing the evidence base for healthcare interventions. While this hierarchy, which puts the findings from much user-controlled research at the lowest level of credibility and validity, based on belief in the 'randomised control trial' (RCT) as the gold standard of research, has been criticized, it continues to predominate (Cohen *et al.*, 2004; Glasby and Beresford, 2006).

Hierarchy	Type of evidence
Type 1	At least one good systemic review, including at least one randomised controlled trial
Type 2	At least one good randomised controlled trial
Type 3	At least one well designed intervention study without randomisation
Type 4	At least one well designed observational study
Type 5	Expert opinion, including the views of service users and carers

Figure 13.1   A conventional hierarchy of evidence.

METHODOLOGICAL QUESTIONING

All user-involvement research has come in for questioning. However, research concerns about involvement based on a democratic approach are more predictable and are becoming well developed. Both approaches – managerialist/consumerist and democratic – are, of course, inherently political, but the former tends to be abstracted and treated as if it were unrelated to any broader ideology or philosophy.

User-controlled research can both expect and has been challenged as biased and lacking in rigour. Its apparent links with a democratic approach to participation highlight its ideological relations. It is seen by its advocates as a primarily political activity, rather than a neutral 'fact-finding mission'. It is concerned with improving people's lives rather than solely with generating knowledge. Fundamental questions are raised about the relation of user-controlled research with traditional positivist research values of 'objectivity', 'neutrality' and distance, even though user-controlled research, like other new paradigm research has made its own challenge to these (Beresford, 2003). Findings from such research can expect to be questioned as partial and partisan. Questions are raised about the problems which user-controlled research may pose because one sectional interest is seen to be dominant – that of service users. It is challenged in relation to criteria of 'validity' and 'reliability'. Questions are raised about who is a service user and the 'representativeness' of service users involved. All these create major barriers in the way of user-controlled research securing equal recognition and resourcing alongside other more traditional research approaches, both quantitative and qualitative.

These criticisms do not necessarily surface formally. They are more likely to be part of informal and hidden discussions. Significantly when the British Social Policy Association surveyed its members, only 24.9% thought that it was 'very important' that service users were involved appropriately in all stages of research (Becker *et al.*, 2006, p5).

All the issues identified above create major barriers for user-controlled research at both national and international levels.

WAYS FORWARD FOR USER-CONTROLLED RESEARCH

User-controlled research including survivor research, has made enormous progress in a relatively short time. There is now a growing body of such research studies. There is a growing literature both about user-controlled research as an approach and about particular projects. Accounts of user-controlled research are now finding their way into the conventionally highly valued pages of international peer reviewed journals.

At the same time, user-controlled research still comes in for questioning. There are many in the research field who are either unaware of it or doubtful of its value. It can reasonably be said that of all the approaches to user-involvement research it is the variant which has the lowest mainstream credibility and which faces the biggest barriers, not least in securing funding and support.

If the future of user-controlled research is to be secured, then a longer term strategy to achieve this is likely to be needed. It is not appropriate to prescribe such a strategy. This is something that those involved in user-controlled research will need to explore and develop. But some components are likely to be important in any such strategy. These can be expected to include:

- **Further exploration of underpinning issues for user-controlled research**
  Discussion of user-controlled research (and indeed all user-involvement research) focuses attention on a number of underpinning issues for research. These issues are truly ones which *all* research must address. There is nonetheless a need for advocates of user-controlled research to address them too. This includes exploring issues around the validity of different knowledge standpoints and knowledge claims; the ownership of knowledge and its interpretation; dominant hierarchies of credibility; the nature of the relationship between knowledge and direct experience; the meaning of 'evidence-based' and what counts as 'evidence'.

- **The systematic and coherent evaluation of user-controlled research**
  This needs to develop as part of the evaluation of user-involvement research more generally. It needs to be a process of evaluation in which service users, their organisations and user researchers are involved in fully and equally, drawing on plural perspectives.

- **Funding for user-controlled research**
  At present user-controlled research receives a tiny proportion of mental health research. A programme of monitoring the scale and proportion of research funding that it commands needs to be initiated to provide a basis for determining if and how it can be supported on equal terms with other research approaches.

- **Towards a theoretical base**
  Emancipatory disability research has been underpinned by the social model of disability and the philosophy of independent living. Survivor research does not seem to have a comparable clear theoretical or value base. It will be helpful to explore this issue and see what, if any, agreement can be reached about a theoretical basis for survivor research.

- **Including user-controlled research in research structures**
  If user-controlled research is to thrive, then while retaining its independence, it also needs to be included in mainstream research structures. This will mean supporting and monitoring the inclusion of those involved in user-controlled research in the structures, organisations and decision-making processes of research, including peer review processes for publication and the awarding of grants.

- **Building alliances**
  To maximise its strength it is important that different groups undertaking user-controlled research develop links, relationships and supportive alliances with each other. This particularly includes people with physical and sensory impairments, people with learning difficulties and mental health service users/survivors. As has been seen, disability emancipatory research and survivor research have tended to develop as separate parallel activities. Closer contact and exchange, facilitated, for example, through international disability studies organisations and events, are likely to be helpful in strengthening the position of user-controlled research overall.

REFERENCES

Barnes, C. and Mercer, G. (Eds) (1997) *Doing Disability Research,* Leeds: The Disability Press.

Barnes, C. and Mercer, G. (Eds) (2005) *The Social Model Of Disability, Europe And The Majority World,* Leeds: The Disability Press.

Barnes, C. Oliver, M. and Barton, L. (Eds) (2002) *Disability Studies Today,* Cambridge: Polity.

Becker, S., Bryman, A. and Sempik, J. (2006) *Defining 'Quality' In Social Policy Research: Views, perceptions and framework for discussion*, Lavenham: Social Policy Association.

Beresford, P. (2003) *It's Our Lives: A short theory of knowledge, distance and experience*, London: Citizen Press in association with Shaping Our Lives.

Beresford, P. (2004) Madness, Distress, Research and a Social Model. In: C. Barnes and G. Mercer (Eds) *Implementing the Social Model of Disability: Theory and research*, Leeds: Disability Press, pp 208–222.

Beresford, P. (2005a) Theory and practice of user involvement in research: making the connection with public policy and practice. In: L. Lowes and I. Hulatt (Eds) *Involving Service Users In Health And Social Care Research*, London: Routledge, pp 6–17.

Beresford, P. (2005b) Where would we be without the pharmaceutical industry? A service user's view, *Psychiatric Bullet: The Journal of psychiatric practice*, **29**(3), 84–85.

Beresford, P. and Branfield, F. (2006) Developing Inclusive Partnerships: User defined outcomes, networking and knowledge – a case study, *Health And Social Care in the Community*, **14**(5), 436–444.

Beresford, P. and and Wallcraft, J. (1997) Psychiatric system survivors and emancipatory research: issues, overlaps and differences. In: C. Barnes and G. Mercer (Eds) *Doing Disability Research*, Leeds: The Disability Press, pp 67–87.

Beresford P., Harrison, C. and Wilson, A. (2002) Mental health, service users and disability: implications for future strategies, *Policy & Politics*, **30**(3), 387–396.

Beresford, P., Shamash, 0., Forrest, V. *et al.* (2005) *Developing Social Care: Service users' vision for adult support*, (Report of a consultation on the future of adult social care), Adult Services Report 07, London, Social Care Institute for Excellence in association with Shaping Our Lives.

Branfield, F., Beresford, P., Andrews, E.J. *et al.* (2006) *Making User Involvement Work: Supporting service user networking and knowledge*, York: Joseph Rowntree Foundation.

Campbell, J. and Oliver, M. (1996) *Disability Politics: Understanding our past, changing our future*, London: Routledge.

Campbell, P. (1996) The history of the user movement in the United Kingdom. In: T. Heller, J. Reynolds, R. Gomm, R. Muston and S. Pattison (Eds) *Mental Health Matters: A reader*, Basingstoke: Macmillan, in association with the Open University, pp 218–225.

Chamberlin, J. (1988) *On Our Own: Patient controlled alternatives to the mental health system*, London: Mind.

Cohen, A.M., Stavri, P.Z. and Hersh, W.R. (2004) A categorisation and analysis of the criticism of evidence-based medicine, *International Journal of Medical Informatics*, **73**, 35–43.

Crow, L. (1996) Renewing the social model of disability, *Coalition*, July, Greater Manchester Coalition of Disabled People, Manchester, pp 5–9.

Department of Health (2002) *Report of the Service User Panel, Appendix 5, Strategic Reviews of Research And Development – Mental Health Report Appendices*, London: DH.

Department of Health (1999) *National Service Framework for Mental Health: Modern standards and service models*, London: Department of Health.

Faulkner, A. (2004) *The Ethics of Survivor Research: Guidelines for the ethical conduct of research carried out by mental health users and survivors*, Bristol: Policy Press.

Faulkner, A. and Layzell, S. (2000) *Strategies for Living: A report of user-led research into people's strategies for living with mental distress*, London: Mental Health Foundation.

Faulkner, A. and Nicholls, V. (1999) *The DIY Guide To Survivor Research*, London: Mental Health Foundation.

Fisher, M. and Marsh, P. (2003) Social work research and the 2001 Research Assessment Exercise: an initial overview, *Social Work Education*, **22**(1), 71–80.

Gambrill, E. (2002) I am not a rubber stamp: my experience as a non-UK RAE adviser. *Journal of Social Work*, **2**(2), 169–185.

Glasby, J. and Beresford, P. (2006) Who knows best?: Evidence based practice and the service user contribution, Commentary and Issues, *Critical Social Policy*, **26**(1), 268–284.

Hickey, G. and Kipping, C. (1998) Exploring the concept of user involvement in mental health through a participation continuum, *Journal of Clinical Nursing*, **7**, 83–88.

Holden, C. and Beresford, P. (2002) Globalization and disability, In: C. Barnes, M. Oliver and L. Barton (Eds) *Disability Studies Today*, Cambridge: Polity, pp 190–209.

Involve (2007) *User-Controlled Research, Jargon Buster, Public Information Pack: How to get actively involved in NHS, public health and social care research*, No 4, Eastleigh, Involve Support Unit.

Lindow, V. (2001) Survivor research. In: C. Newnes, G. Holmes and C. Dunn (Eds) (2001) *This Is Madness Too*, Ross on Wye: PCCS Books, pp. 135–146.

Mercer, G. (2002) Emancipatory disability research. In: C. Barnes, M. Oliver and L. Barton (Eds) *Disability Studies Today*, Cambridge: Polity.

Muijen, M. (1998) Users monitoring mental health services, *Q-Net*, **6**(1).

Nicholls, V. (2001) *Doing Research Ourselves, Strategies For Living*, London: Mental Health Foundation.

Office for Disability Issues (2008) *Independent Living: A cross-government strategy about independent living for disabled people*, London: The Stationery Office.

O'Hagan, M. (1993) *Stopovers On My Way Home From Mars: A Winston Churchill Fellowship report on the psychiatric survivor movement in the USA, Britain and the Netherlands*, London: Survivors Speak Out.

Oliver, M. (1996) *Understanding Disability*, Basingstoke: Macmillan.

Oliver, M. and Barnes, C. (1998) *Disabled People and Social Policy: From exclusion to inclusion*, London: Longman.

Oliver, M. (1992) Changing the social relations of research production, *Disability, Handicap and Society*, **7**, pp 101–115.

Oliver, M. and Barnes, C. (1998) *Disabled People and Social Policy: From exclusion to inclusion*, London: Longman.

Pilgrim, D. and Rogers, A. (1999) *A Sociology of Mental Health and Illness*, Second Edition, Buckingham: Open University Press.

Rose, D. (2001) *Users' Voices*, London: Sainsbury Centre for Mental Health.

Shaping Our Lives National User Network, Black User Group (West London), Ethnic Disabled Group Emerged (Manchester), Footprints, Waltham Forest Black Mental Health Service User Group (North London), Service Users' Action Forum (Wakefield) (2003) *Shaping Our Lives – From outset to outcome: What people think of the social care services they use*, York: Joseph Rowntree Foundation.

Shardlow, S., Huntington, A., Lawson, J. *et al.* (2004) *The Research Assessment Exercise (RAE) 2001 (Social Work): A Report Prepared by Salford Centre for Social Work Research for The Research Sub-Committee of the Joint University Committee/Social Work Education*. Salford: Salford Centre for Social Work Research, University of Salford. Available online at: http://www.chssc.salford.ac.uk/scswr/projects/Research%20Assessment%20Exercise%20_Exec.pdf, accessed 28/10/08.

Stickley, T. (2006) Should service user involvement be consigned to history?: a critical realist perspective. *Journal of Psychiatric and Mental Health Nursing*, **13**, pp. 570–577.

Stone, E. (Ed) (1999) *Disability and Development: Learning from action and research in the majority world*, Leeds: The Disability Press.

SURE (2002) SURE: *Service User Research Enterprise, Annual Report, 2001–2002*, SURE, Health Service Research, London: Institute of Psychiatry.

Swain, J., French, S., Barnes, C. and Thomas, C. (Eds) (2004) *Disabling Barriers – Enabling Environments*, London: Sage.

Taylor, J., Williams, V., Johnson, R. *et al.* (2007) *We Are Not Stupid*, London: Shaping Our Lives and People First Lambeth.

Tew, J. (Editor) (2005) *Social Perspectives in Mental Health: Developing social models to understand and work with mental distress*, London: Jessica Kingsley.

Turner, M. and Beresford, P. (2005a) *User-Controlled Research: Its meanings and potential, Final report*, Shaping Our Lives and the Centre for Citizen Participation, Brunel University, Eastleigh, Involve.

Turner, M. and Beresford, P. (2005b) *Contributing On Equal Terms: Service user involvement and the benefits system*, Adult Services Report 08, London: Social Care Institute for Excellence.

Turner, M. (1997) *Shaping Our Lives: Interim Report*, London: Shaping Our Lives, National Institute for Social Work.

Turner, M. (1998) *Shaping Our Lives: Project Report*, London: Shaping Our Lives, National Institute for Social Work.

CHAPTER 14

Power

Relational Power and Research Positions

Paddy McGowan, Líam Mac Gabhann, Chris Stevenson and Jim Walsh

School of Nursing, Dublin City University, Dublin, Ireland

Power is a crucial issue when service users and non service user researchers are working together. While several other chapters before have touched on this important topic, this chapter is specifically devoted to discussing in detail relevant considerations in relation to power. This chapter first outlines three different philosophical theories of relational power (power constructed in social interchanges), i.e. the work of Foucault, critical theory and social constructionism. These theories are linked to the position of service users as patients, subjects, and user researchers within these theoretical frameworks. First-person accounts from the experience of one of the authors (as a totally disempowered patient, as a service user member of an expert panel reviewing services, and finally as a researcher) are interspersed as examples of how experience of the different kinds of power help or hinder service user (involvement in) research. Finally, the authors conclude that empowerment of the mass of patients (beyond the expert user researcher) requires a sharing of the language of research at all levels and stages.

INTRODUCTION

In this chapter, we[1] take the view that power is relational, that is, power is constructed in social interchanges, including those in the research process. Power is often referred to in such terms as, 'power over', 'empowerment', 'disempowerment' or 'power struggles'. There is too little attention given to power as a concept in itself and how it has been harnessed and pervades

---

[1] We use the collective first person to write. Michael Billig (1994) has suggested that much academic writing has involved de-populating the text. In the chapter, we would be hypocritical if exposing the lack of service user voice in some research process whilst sanitizing this text of the personal.

Handbook of Service User Involvement in Mental Health Research   Edited by Jan Wallcraft, Beate Schrank and Michaela Amering
Copyright © 2009 John Wiley & Sons, Ltd

mental health systems (Ryles, 1999). When power is viewed as a 'thing' to have and to hold, it sets up polarized views and competing positions, for example, service user research versus healthcare professional research. A reconceptualisation of power as something other than 'a thing' or 'entity' to be wielded or forgone, may offer some clarity and practical wisdom as to the place of power and how it is played out in mental health research.

We present three, overlapping versions of relational power. These are derived from the work of Michel Foucault, from critical theory (Freire, 1996), and from social construction-ism (Gergen and Gergen, 2008). We expose how relational power can both disable and enable service users in the research process.

First we use Foucault to deconstruct taken-for-granted research approaches, explicitly those embedded in bioscience, with the randomised control trial being the gold standard[2]. Foucault (1981) argued that the 'sovereign' power of Church and State which wields power over individuals, was superseded with the emergence of different cultural situations, for example, population growth, and the growth of industrialism and manufacturing. The need to harness the population's implicit productivity encouraged certain concerns, such as ensuring the public health. Thus, discourses of the person, as a possible site of disease (whether physical or moral) and someone to be made/kept healthy, came into existence (Fox, 1993). In other words, the new economy of power required government as a 'form of activity [*conduct – our addition*] aiming to shape, guide or affect the conduct of some person or persons' (Gordon, 1991); the conduct of conduct. Disciplinary power became legitimated by scientific and social consensus (Foucault, 1979; 1982), knowledge about the body. And Foucault asserted that bio-power is always productive. Bio-power entails the production of objects (Foucault sometimes said 'things'), subjects (and subjectivities) and practices, all of which become the source of further legitimate knowledge and so the maintenance of unequal power relations. At an individual level bio-power involves the stripping away of people's personal self-identity and replacing it with another, e.g. 'psychiatric patient identity', through various rituals and enforced routines. At a societal level it involves legitimising the creation of these identities normalising it in social discourse and policy then regulating accordingly. Against this backdrop, or description of bio-power (later bio-psychosocial power), we explore how service user involvement in research would be enacted.

Secondly, we present a critical theory position as an emancipatory, relational power approach. Critical theory proposes that human emancipation is only achievable through explanation, praxis and normative processes. In the social world this translates into an explanation as to what is wrong with social reality, what power relationships are at play, who is in position to change it, and identifying/clarifying ways of questioning the status quo and changing this. Critical theory enables a relatively structured approach to bringing about social change that is both democratic and inclusive. It involves forms of communication between people in given social situations based on reaching a consensus about any professed truth, through critical reflection by those involved. Communication structures within the critical theory approach are designed to facilitate diverse opinions, and language has within it, universal characteristics that allow room for joint understanding and agreement. This is in contrast with the terms set out by globalization and reliance on technologies. Here, self-interest is encouraged at the cost of social cohesion whereby values are less likely to be shared. We explore how a critical theory perspective positions people who use services in mental health research.

---

[2] We appreciate that a meta-analysis of RCT's is an even higher candidate but this does not involve subjects in way that we are interested in here.

Finally, we turn to a social constructionist version of relational power as an antidote to hierarchical research. Social constructionism is part of a family or tradition of scholarship that sees human relationships as providing the origins for knowledge, meaning and understanding, as opposed to, for example, natural laws. Examples of social constructionism are found in the works of Berger and Luckman (1966), Spector and Kituse (1977), Foucault (1979, 1980), Latour (1987) and Gergen (1985; 2008). Burr's (1995) *Introduction to Social Constructionism* provides an accessible overview. In this chapter, we offer a brief outline of the three main social constructionist movements and four interlinking lines of argument as described by Gergen and Gergen (2008). The service user research contribution within a social constructionist position is defined.

In each version of relational power we illustrate the position of, and issues for, the involved service user with reference to the experience of (author of this chapter) McGowan (Boxes A, B and C) who explains how each of the different kinds of power might help (or hinder) him as a service user researcher.

FOUCAULT, BIOPOWER AND PSYCHIATRIC/MENTAL HEALTH RESEARCH

Foucault's work indicates that biopower produces objects, subjects/subjectivities and practice.

Objects

Service users have been through a process whereby they are exposed to 'the gaze' (Foucault, 1979) that is facilitated by the very structures of the clinic; for example, the waiting room, the consultation room, the CCTV camera. In relation to research, the focus is upon the internal workings of the body, the brain, synapse, receptor neurotransmitter level, although measures of behaviour are used as proxy indicators. The clinical science laboratory 'architecture' is one in which the service user is positioned as the giver of body fluid samples, or brain images, rather than a co-researcher. The artefacts of bio-psychiatry (the symptom inventories, the personality questionnaires) require only responses *from* the person in relation to their internal workings. For the service user, it is difficult to challenge the process or product of such research as it arises from a specialist knowledge base (Marsh, 2008) – the RCT, the brain imaging, the learned journal article. The language is exclusive, for example, intention to treat, random allocation and manualised treatment are not plain language research terms. The process serves to produce more knowledge for bioscience which can be *applied to* the service user, but leads, simultaneously, to the further exclusion of the service user perspective.

Subjects/subjectivities

In relation to disciplinary power, Foucault (1982, p212) noted that:

> *This form of power applies itself to immediate everyday life that categorises the individual, marks him by his own individuality, attaches him to his own identity, imposes a law of truth on him which he must recognise and which others recognise in him.*

In biopsychiatry, the above form of power is shown in the way the service user is 'subjectivised' – in other words develops a subjectivity produced by the 'truthes' of biopsychiatry. This subjectivity is one of dependence, irresponsibility, sickness, and deference to the expert practitioner (Stevenson and Cutcliffe, 2006). It is difficult for the service user, in this scenario, to have faith in his or her everyday abilities, much less in research ability which is often portrayed as exclusive and specialist. The service user's subjectivity of 'doctor knows best' is used in order to persuade involvement as a subject in research, supported by the inference that such research will assist other people in the same mental health position.

Practices

The practices that are produced through biopower involve monological episodes (Bakhtin, 1981), where the interaction is more about, for example, a professional eliciting specific answers from a service user according to his or her scripted questions, as opposed to a two way dialogue between professional and service user. For example, the person/patient/service user consults with the doctor in order to elicit the expert's help; practices aim to control symptoms and prevent relapse (Walsh *et al.*, 2008), and much store is set by the administration of medication. In relation to research, the service user is not seen as a source of interesting research questions. These are generated by the non-service user researcher. The surveillance that operates in psychiatric practice (Stevenson and Cutcliffe, 2006; Walsh *et al.*, 2008) is mirrored in the research approach. The service user is monitored for compliance with treatment regimes both within the clinic and the randomised controlled trial (RCT) and non-compliance is seen as a threat to the 'integrity' of both. In the RCT the researcher is 'blinded' to who participates in the research – the service user is invisible and becomes merely a nameless source of data.

Foucault noted that

> power and resistance are two sides of the same coin. The power implicit in one discourse is only apparent from the resistance implicit in another.
>
> (Burr, 1995, p64)

Put simply, power and resistance are connected in a circular (Foucault said 'self-conditioning'), fashion. Thus, whilst bioscience/biopsychiatry is a 'regime of truth' (Marsh, 2008) on the one hand, it is not without resistance, both in its practices and in relation to research which we discuss here. Resistance to power is possible because there are always alternative discourses available that challenge a specific 'regime of truth'. In the case of research, service users have offered 'crude' resistance to biomedical research, for example refusing to take medication in clinical trials, voting with their feet or not returning questionnaires. More subtle resistance (and for Foucault this would be more successful) has occurred, for example, through claiming compliance to medication whilst not doing so, attending therapeutic intervention sessions whilst not engaging with the work, and providing inaccurate data. In a broader context, there has been an increase in the perceived legitimacy of qualitative research, including in relation to participatory-action research, co-operative inquiry, service user-led research. The legitimacy has its source in expertise by experience. Both critical theory and social constructionism, discussed below, offer more leeway in relation to research that values the service user's perspective.

BOX A: INVASION OF THE BODY SNATCHERS

Very early into my psychiatric career in hospital I was approached by staff members from the hospital; they informed me that they would like to ask me some questions. I was given very limited information as to what the research was about. Both staff members were unknown to me. They questioned me around a range of subjects, my private life, my school history, work life and my experience of being diagnosed with mental illness. The interview lasted approximately one hour. I felt very tired and frustrated but because I was an inpatient I felt pressured into consenting. On reflection of that experience I recognise that I had no purpose in the research other than to satisfy the researchers needs; I had no voice; had no input other than to answer questions. This type of research and approach really disempowers people. It reinforced to me that I was different to the researchers. They had power over me. I was a subject to be enquired about as I was perceived to be ill. The piece of research they carried out was owned by the researchers. I had no feedback as to what the findings were. I had no evidence that the research had played any part in changing my experience or the experience of anyone else. I did not even know as to what the purpose of the research was. This type of research at the time felt very intrusive. I felt that my being had been invaded by strangers and that I was an experiment. The scientists departed never to be spoken to again and I was left to stay in my hospital ward and to wonder what it was all about.

CRITICAL THEORY AND CONSUMER-LED RESEARCH

The social reality for mental health service users is that they have been subject to treatments (led by quasi experiments) that have been degrading and extremely damaging (Frese, 2002), as told in McGowan's illustration of biopower above. From a critical theory perspective (Freire, 1996; Habermas, 1972), this is a flawed social reality. Historically, those who have dominated (psychiatry) through technological means and validity claim – and who are, therefore, in a position to change such circumstances – have failed to act or acknowledge another reality. Norms were not criticised, which left no room for social transformation. In recent times, service users have criticised the norms of biopsychiatric knowledge and how it is produced. They have questioned the overuse of technologies and the validity claims of psychiatry, and so put themselves in a position to alter the dominant social reality. For example, service users have challenged research priorities for mental health and the methodology applied to pursue their validity claim to authoritative knowledge.

Service users and self-identified problems

Service users have a multiplicity of experiences, needs, and appreciation of the problems they encounter that are directly related to their mental health (Smith, 1998). However, consistent themes appear in service user literature that point to several areas of common concern: involvement in care treatment programmes (Rose, 2003; Consumer Quality Initiative, 2007), discrimination (Repper and Perkins, 2003) and rights related issues (Olofsson and Jacobsson, 2001). Samele *et al.* (2005) in a review of service user priorities for research state that; 'Outcome measures would best reflect life goals as opposed to symptom reduction' (p19), the main concern for psychiatry.

Each area of concern identified above relates to processes of exclusion and disempowerment. Ignoring these or/and preferring to look to other areas to provide solutions (e.g. through bio-medicine) to the problems that service users encounter could be deemed biased and lead to discriminatory practice (Jarvis, 2007).

Consumer or democratic approaches?

Beresford (2002) makes a distinction between two forms of user action – Consumerist (i) and Democratic approaches (ii) (see also Chapter 13).

i. The Consumerist approach is described as a form of market research where 'improving the product' (in this case mental health services) is the ultimate goal. Here we are likely to find research processes where user participants are asked to decide on limited choices. Service users within the consumerist approach might be at risk of becoming incorporated in preserving the product (Oliver, 2002). The subjective continues to be dictated by objective measures – of efficiency, economy and effectiveness.
ii. The Democratic approach is politically and socially motivated. It is concerned about changing agencies and organisations that have direct impact on levels of inclusion, autonomy and independence. Quality of life and rights issues are the main concern of the democratic approach. The self identified problems above, we would argue, are more compatible with the democratic approach.

Research as a democratic process

Mike Oliver, a current proponent of the emancipatory research paradigm states that:

> ... the production of all knowledge needs itself to become increasingly a socially distributed process by taking much more seriously the experiential knowledge that oppressed groups produce themselves and research based upon the discourse of production will have an increasingly important role to play in this.
>
> (Oliver, 2002, p15)

Esoteric knowledge and current research techniques are developed to meet the needs of the academic and professional, which is more often than not far removed from the lived experience (Oliver, 1992). Whilst we might want to change the product, we might also do well to challenge the power relationship between the 'producers' and the potentially 'produced'. Biopower (see above), through objective and positivist research processes, has produced subjectivities of disempowerment and damaging and discriminatory practices. Moving the research focus from biological, chemical and genetic, to understanding the role of social forces in producing mental ill health (and also promoting recovery); from refining treatments to meaningfully involving the service user in the care and treatment process, would go a long way to placing service user needs at the centre of the research agenda. Of course, this is best done when the research process is guided by inclusive and democratic ideals. Power, knowledge and experience is shared, communicated and transformed into positive action.

BOX B: LEADING FROM THE FORE

Some years later when I had recovered I was asked to sit on the Expert Group Review on Mental Health Policy, a Review on Mental Health Services in Ireland which brought a new framework for the design and delivery of service provision. This review carried on from the previous document, *Planning for the Future* (Department of Health, 1984). *Planning for the Future* had no service user involvement. *Planning for the Future* clearly maintained the power of the system without question. I would argue that without service user involvement the plan was weakened and disempowering. However, it was decided that the new document would have a very proactive service user input. It was decided that service users would design and deliver a piece of research in hospitals for the long-stay community to ascertain their views on what type of changes they would like to see. The Irish Advocacy Network was commissioned to do the research as they were the service user representation involved in advocating for service users. The process involved service users from across the country. They gathered users to design the questionnaire, trained the researchers and published the research in a document called *What We Heard* (Irish Advocacy Network, 2004). This information was used to put together Chapter 3 of the new policy document *Vision for Change* (Department of Health and Children, 2006). The role of the service users was central in informing the Expert Group in the way forward. The service users involved were really upbeat about the role they played; they felt empowered and informed. The researchers also felt very good because they had worked with their peers; their voices were heard and respected. The research was owned by the service users and was not driven or restricted by anyone. This type of research really changed how the Expert Group viewed service users and the depth of knowledge and experience they possessed. It is also true to say that Chapter 3 of *Vision for Change* is the piece of the new policy which is the most advanced in implementation.

Inclusive and democratic ideals are embedded in user-led research (ULR) – research carried out by, for and with service users. ULR has attempted to challenge the legitimacy of psychiatry by constructing a knowledge base that sits outside the parameters of the positivist framework in which it operates (Faulkner and Thomas, 2002). ULR tends to emphasise the social as opposed to the biological, chemical or/and genetic, which is backed up by the global interests of pharmaceutical companies (Thomas *et al.*, 2005). (Find more on user led/controlled research in Chapter 13). Below, we use literature that is written and presented by individuals from a service user background and/or academics who are allied to, or have inspired the call for, increasingly inclusive research processes.

SOCIAL CONSTRUCTIONISM – MAKING SENSE OF POWER IN MENTAL HEALTHCARE SYSTEMS

Power can be understood as a network of social boundaries that either enable or constrain actors in society (Hayward, 1998). These networks are frequently delineated according to professional and social status in a hierarchical positioning that produces unequal power relations (Chambers, 1997), as argued above. Mental health services can be viewed as a microcosm of the social system with the social boundaries being those produced between mental health professionals, and between professionals and service users.

In this section we take a social constructionist perspective on power with two intentions:

a. to illuminate possibilities as to why service user research/involvement in research has had little impact on healthcare systems
b. to show that by increasing our understanding of how power is constructed and utilised, engaging with power can offer opportunities for increased effectiveness and impact of service user involvement in research.

First, we explain how social constructionism is embedded in three movements:

1. The *critical* movement, akin to critical social theory, refers to the ideological critique of all claims to truth in the world including empirical science, rooted in the work of Foucault and associated with human rights, such as black, gay, lesbian and anti-psychiatry movements.
2. The second *literary/rhetorical* movement demonstrates the extent to which scientific theories and explanations are more dependent on discursive conventions than on the world itself, in that it is our use of language that constructs the way we view the world.
3. The third *social* movement is associated with examining the social processes that give rise to the historical context and sociology of scientific and other forms of knowledge.

There is some disagreement between the movements but also common lines of argument across movements. Specifically, that knowledge is socially constructed through human relationships. Be it true or false, scientific or mythical, rational or irrational, knowledge becomes real only through historically and culturally situated social processes. For example, in one culture, to hear voices is to be revered and in another to hear voices is to be deemed schizophrenic. Both possibilities have consequences, bringing either an elevated or relegated position in society respectively. These social constructionist ideas are used to address both why service user research/involvement in research has had little impact on healthcare systems; and how, by increasing our understanding of how power is constructed and utilised, engaging with power can offer opportunities.

Knowledge as social construction

The dominant knowledge or truth claims in mental healthcare are underpinned by empiricism (knowledge built on observation, sensory experience and practical experimentation), and a taken-for-granted claim that mental illness can be categorised, and, consequently, diagnosed and treated with appropriately researched treatments, as argued above. This reality has its genesis in the 19th Century and has enjoyed state, international health bodies, professional and commercial sponsorship to this day. Although, other forms of knowledge are entertained, these are adjunct positions and serve only as support to the 'superior' knowledge. The dominant discourse (or regime of truth (Marsh, 2008)) is made exclusive by a specific grammar or set of language rules. Wittgenstein (1953, cited in Cronen and Lang, 1994, p18) defined grammar as the rules that allow us to '... engage in patterns of conjoint action ...'. The rules constitute a 'language game' (Wittgenstein, 1953). The person who does not know the rules of the game is precluded from playing. The power inherent in this process can be overwhelming, and those researchers (service users and others) seeking meaning in people's experiences or routes to recovery, are disadvantaged as they are seen as 'non-game players' producing lower grade understanding of mental health phenomena.

Thus, the mental health knowledge system, as constructed and perpetuated through the articulation of 'an' expert, empirically based, knowledge in practice, firmly locates the service user outside of the social networks that generate, and utilizes power. As Campbell (1996, p59) argues:

> The psychiatric system is founded on inequality. By and large, the user is at the bottom of the pile. Our unequal position is symbolized by the compulsory element in psychiatric care...

Bentall (1990, p 211) captures perhaps the genesis of this inequality in his relaying of an editorial quote from *Journal of Mental Science, 1858:*

> Insanity is purely a disease of the brain. The physician is now the responsible guardian of the lunatic and must forever remain so...

Esso Leete (1989) cited in Campbell (1998, p241) summarised the position of the service user in the psychiatric system:

> I can talk but I may not be heard, I can make suggestions but they may not be taken seriously, I can voice my thoughts, but they may be seen as delusions. I can recite experiences, but they may be interpreted as fantasies. To be a patient or even an ex-client is to be discounted.

It is against this backdrop (Rogers and Pilgrim, 2005) that service users might consider their place as researchers. In such a system, service users by default are most often useful as objects of research, as opposed to active participants in any research process (Sallah and Clark, 2005).

Adopting a social constructionist position, knowledge is political and, as such, traditional issues of truth and objectivity are replaced in the constructionist tradition by concerns with what the research brings about. The truth of the matter lies not in the objective facts, rather it lies in the implications for cultural/social life that follows acceptance of any truth claim. In accepting 'objectivity' as an indicator of truth, one must buy into the scientific paradigm (positivism) that created and utilises this tool (Rorty, 1989).

Although, competing with the system and constructing new realities has opened up avenues for service user research, there still remains the dominant institution of mental healthcare. An understanding of how power is brokered offers an opportunity for service users and healthcare professionals alike, to embrace a research approach that allows the system to continue evolving. Mental healthcare will improve by extending the social relations that enable a balancing of power relations, which will ultimately transform the hierarchical position of service users in the system. This approach is broadly referred to as Participatory Inquiry and Practice (Reason and Bradbury, 2008). It requires a commitment and participation from actors across the social networks, therefore engages with power relations from the outset. From a social constructionist perspective, the relationships that

BOX C: NOTHING ABOUT US, WITHOUT US

The Institute for Mental Health Recovery was formed by Kiaran Crowe (RIP), Diarmuid Ring and myself. We all had been involved in setting up the Irish Advocacy Network in Ireland some years earlier. The Advocacy Network had embedded itself into the framework of services and had peer advocates working in all of the hospitals and communities in the country. We decided to concentrate our efforts into working on recovery. Unlike the Advocacy Network, which was a peer-led and run organisation, we decided that the time had come to involve and work with like-minded people from different stakeholder backgrounds. We gathered a number of professionals, psychiatrists, nurses, psychologists, psychotherapists and users and carers. Together, we decided that we wanted to know what recovery was and what were the competencies required for people to work in recovery, we all of us had our own ideas but we really wanted to know the thoughts and ideas of others in the community We decided to commission an academic from Dublin City University, Richard Lakeman, to design a Delphi Study in collaboration with the institute to seek the views of groups and individuals. The Delphi Study was titled *Identifying mental health recovery competencies for workers and exemplars of recovery practice: A modified Delphi and descriptive study*. The proposal was worked up together and everybody's voice influenced the process. For me the relationship was built out of respect for me and my experience and respect for my colleagues who also had their own experiences. I felt that I had an equal input into the process which empowered me to collaborate and utilise our collective experiences. My role became more than a former service user, to being a valued member of a group with an equal part in the process. This type of involvement really empowered me and the members of the institute to work together to bring about a change in all our thinking on what recovery and its real potential really could mean to all of our practices, and the recovery pathway for people encountering emotional distress.

harness and utilize power to preserve the system take on a new role with the inclusion of new partners in that process. Where service users come together in participatory inquiry and practise with those that would normally objectify them, there is the opportunity to co-construct a different reality – one that is conducive to the preservation of difference, whilst embracing mutual possibilities for improving the system.

CONCLUSION

In this chapter, we have 'problematised' the taken-for-granted notions of 'good' research through applying Foucault's ideas about relational power. In the space created, we have further argued that other versions of relational power allow more scope for meaningful inclusion of service users. In other words, the schools of critical theory and social constructionism can be used to bridge the gap between the professional researcher and the expert user-researcher. It is very clear to us that each approach has the ability to begin to break down the barriers of power of one side or other. Yet, each is still narrowly focused on those who have the educational ability to participate[3]. The best of intentions to create inclusivity may simply mean that the largest component of these types of debates, the users who are still held firmly within psychiatric services, may become the target of more groups as tools of research rather than active, equal participants. Whether positivist/empiricist, Foucauldian, critical theory or social constructionist, knowledge may not find its way down to the masses on the ground level. What may be required is an ability to create a shared language at every stage of the research process, from design to dissemination.

REFERENCES

Bakhtin, M. (1981) *The Dialogical Imagination*, Austin, Texas: University of Texas Press.

Bentall, R.P. (1990) *Reconstructing Schizophrenia*, Routledge: London.

Beresford, P. (2002) User Involvement in Research: Liberation or Regulation? *Social Policy and society*, **1**(2), 95–105.

Berger, P. and Luckmann, T. (1966) *The Social Construction of Reality*, New York: Anchor Books.

Billig, M. (1994) 'Sod Baudrillard! Or ideology critique in Disney world.' In: H.W. Simons and M. Billig (Eds), *After Postmodernism: Reconstructing Ideology Critique*, London: Sage.

Burr, V. (1995) *An Introduction to Social Constructionism*, London: Routledge.

Campbell, P. (1996) Challenging loss of power. In: J. Read and J. Reynolds (1996) (Eds) *Speaking Our Minds: An anthology*, Macmillan: Basingstoke.

Campbell, P. (1998) Listening to Clients. In: P. Barker and B. Davidson (1998) (Eds) *Psychiatric Nursing: Ethical Strife*, Arnold: London.

Chambers, R. (1997) *Whose Reality Counts? Putting the First Last*, London: Intermediate Technology Publications.

Consumer Quality Initiatives (2007) Informed consent: strategies to improve the experience of Massachusetts mental health consumers. *Consumer Quality Initiatives*, **2**, 1–5.

Cronen, V.E. and Lang, P. (1994) Language and action: Wittgenstein and Dewey in the practice of therapy and consultation, *Human Systems*, **5**, 5–43.

Department of Health (1984) *The Psychiatric Services – Planning for the Future. Study group on the development of the Psychiatric Services*, Dublin: The Stationery Office.

Esso Leete cited in Campbell, P (1998) (1989) Listening to Clients. In: P. Barker and B. Davidson (Eds), *Psychiatric Nursing: Ethical Strife*, London: Arnold. p. 241.

Faulkner, A. and Thomas, P. (2002) User-led research and evidence based medicine. *The British Journal of Psychiatry*, **180**, 1–3.

Foucault, M. (1979) *Discipline and Punish*, Harmondsworth: Penguin.

Foucault, M. (1980) *Power/Knowledge*, New York: Pantheon.

Foucault, M. (1981) *The History of Sexuality: An Introduction* (R.Hurley trans.), Harmondsworth: Penguin.

Foucault, M. (1982) Afterword. In: H.L. Dreyfus and P. Rabinow (Eds) *Beyond Structuralism and Hermeneutics*, Brighton: Harvester.

Fox, N.J. (1993) *Postmodernism, Sociology and Health*, Buckingham: Open University Press.

Freidson, E. (1970) *Profession of Medicine*, New York: Dodd, Mead and Co.

Freire, P. (1996) *Pedagogy of The Oppressed*, (reprinted from 1972), London: Penguin Books.

Frese, F.J. (2002) Ethics in neurobiological research: One consumer/provider's perspective. In: P. Backlar and D. Cutler (Eds) *Ethics in Community Mental Healthcare*, New York: Kluwar Academic.

---

[3] Indeed, this was a debate in producing this chapter, that is, how to make social science theory accessible for a range of readers.

Gergen, K.J. (1985) The social constructionist movement in modern psychology. *American Psychologist*, **40**(3), 266–275.

Gergen, K.J. and Gergen, M.M. (2008) Social construction and research as action. In: P. Reason and H. Bradbury (2008) *Handbook of Action Research: Participatory Inquiry, and Practice*, (Second edition), London: Sage.

Goode, W.J. (1960) In: M. Morgan, M. Calnan and N. Manning (1985) *Sociological Approaches to Health and Medicine*, London: Croom Helm.

Gordon, C. (1991) Government rationality: an introduction. In: G. Burchell, C. Gordon and P. Miller (eds), *The Foucault Effect: Studies in Governmentality*, Hemel Hempstead: Harvester Wheatsheaf.

Department of Health and Children (2006) *A Vision for Change: Report of the Expert Group on Mental Health Policy*, Dublin: Stationery Office.

Habermas, J. (1972) *Knowledge and Human Interests*, London: Heinemann.

Hayward, C.R. (1998) 'De-facing Power.' *Polity*, **31**(1), 1–22.

Irish Advocacy Network (2004) *What We Heard: Report prepared on behalf of expert group on mental health policy*, Dublin: Department of Health and Children.

Jarvis, E.G. (2007) The social causes of psychosis in North American psychiatry: A review of a disappearing literature. *Canadian Journal of Psychiatry*, **52**(5), 287–293.

Latour, B. (1987) *Science in Action: How to Follow Scientists and Engineers Through Society*, Cambridge, MA: Harvard University Press.

Marsh, I. (2008) *A Critical Analysis of the Discursive Formation of Suicide as Pathological and Medical*. Unpublished PhD Thesis: University of Brighton.

Oliver, M. (1992) Changing the social relations of research production? *Disability, Handicap and Society*, **7**(2), 101–114.

Oliver, M. (2002) *Emancipatory Research: A vehicle for social transformation or policy development*. 1st Annual disability research seminar. Hosted by The National Disability Authority and The Centre for Disability Studies, University College Dublin. Available online at: http://www.leeds.ac.uk/disability-studies/archiveuk/Oliver/Mike's%20paper.pdf, accessed 28/10/08.

Olofsson, B. and Jacobsson, L. (2001) L A plea for respect: involuntarily hospitalized psychiatric patients' narratives about being subjected to coercion, *Journal of Psychiatric and Mental Health Nursing*, **8**(4), 357–366.

Parsons, T. (1968) in Eraut, M. (1994) *Developing Professional Knowledge and Competence*, London: The Falmer Press. p. 1.

Reason, P. and Bradbury, H. (2008) (Second edition) *Handbook of Action Research: Participatory Inquiry and Practice*, London: Sage.

Repper, J. and Perkins, R. (2003) *Social Inclusion and Recovery: A Model for Mental Health Practice*, London: Bailliere Tindell.

Rogers, A. and Pilgrim, D. (2005) *A Sociology of Mental Health and Illness*, Milton Keynes: Open University Press.

Rorty, R. (1989) *Contingency, Solidarity and Irony*, Cambridge: Cambridge University Press.

Rose, D. (2003) Partnership, co-ordination of care and the place of user involvement. *Journal of Mental Health*, **12**(1), 59–70.

Ryles, S.M. (1999) A concept analysis of empowerment: its relationship to mental health nursing. *Journal of Advanced Nursing*, **29**(3), 600–607.

Samele, C., Wallcraft, J., Naylor, C. *et al.* (2007) *Research Priorities for service User and Carer-Centred Mental Health Services*, Report for the National Co-ordinating Centre for NHS Service Delivery and Organisation RandD. London: Sainsbury Centre for Mental Health Available online at: http://www.scmh.org.uk/pdfs/scmh_research_priorities_overview_report.pdf, accessed 28/10/08.

Sallah, D. and Clark, M. (Eds) (2005) *Research and Development in Mental Health*, London: Elsevier, Churchill Livingstone.

Spector, M. and Kitsuse, J. (1977) *Constructing Social Problems*, CA: Cummings.

Stevenson, C. and Cutcliffe, J. (2006) Problematising special observations in psychiatry: Foucault, genealogy, discourse and power/knowledge. *Journal of Psychiatric and Mental Health Nursing*, **13**(6), 713–721.

Thomas, P., Bracken, P., Cutler, P. *et al.* (2005) Challenging the globalization of biomedical psychiatry. *Journal of Public Mental Health*, **4**(3), 23–32.

Walsh, J., Stevenson, C., Cutcliffe, J. and Zinck, K. (in press) Government and knowledge/power/resistance in mental health: creating a space for the practices of recovery by psychiatric/mental health nurses? *Nursing Inquiry*.

Wittgenstein, L. (1953) *Philosophical Investigations*, (Anscombe, G. E. M., trans.), Oxford: Basil Blackwell.

CHAPTER 15

Money

Sarah Hamilton

Senior Researcher at Rethink (severe mental illness charity)

Money is a key factor in research. In the context of service user involvement, it has specific implications for the type of involvement undertaken, its effectiveness, and the relationship between researchers and service users. This chapter discusses monetary issues in terms of payment, costs and budgeting as related to the individual service users involved, the overall project planning and funding for research with user involvement. It outlines common pitfalls associated with these issues and gives practical recommendations on how to avoid them.

Payment is a tangible way to value and reward involvement, it can be an incentive but also a real barrier for individual service users. This chapter considers the possible problems arising from various forms of payment and necessary practical considerations when planning to pay service users for their involvement. On the overall project level, it outlines the costs in terms of money as well as time that need to be considered in the budgeting stage of a project. Finally, the chapter deals with the potential influence, both positive and negative, that funding requirements can have on actual service user involvement in research. It closes with a summary of practical recommendations and important points both researchers and funders should be aware of in relation to monetary issues in service user involvement.

INTRODUCTION

Money is always an important factor in research. Access to funding will dictate what topics are researched, and the methods and resources available. Within a research team, payment can be linked to power dynamics and place a value on an individual's contribution. In this chapter, I discuss three key issues that highlight how money can influence service user involvement – both to improve and to limit it. These are: payment of service users involved, costs of user involvement, and funding for research with user involvement. I discuss how these differ for different types of involvement, for instance where service users are involved as members of the team or as consultants. I suggest some basic principles and practicalities that researchers and funding bodies should consider when planning service user involvement.

Handbook of Service User Involvement in Mental Health Research   Edited by Jan Wallcraft, Beate Schrank and Michaela Amering
Copyright © 2009 John Wiley & Sons, Ltd

This chapter draws primarily on policy guidance and service user experiences in the United Kingdom. However, many of the issues raised and suggested solutions will be relevant for readers across the globe.

PAYMENT

Where service users are involved in research projects, it is generally seen as good practice to pay them for their contribution (Involve, 2005; Department of Health and CSIP, 2006). There are a number of things to consider, however, when making decisions about the levels and structures of payment for service users.

Why pay service users for involvement in research?

Payment is generally seen as a tangible way in which to value and reward people's time, effort, skills and contribution. This is equally true of service users involved in research. Where service users are considered to make up part of the research team, it would be unreasonable and unfair to expect service users to contribute for free alongside professionals who are paid for their contributions. Payment is not the only way to value service users' involvement, but it can be an important way of doing so.

Payment can also help to address the power imbalance inherent in the collaboration between professional researchers and service users. It can reassure service users that their views will be valued, alongside those of other researchers, and that their experience is as important to the project. It may also boost their confidence in offering their opinions and in the way that they view their own role in the project.

Payment can be used to formalise the relationship between users and researchers. Involvement therefore becomes a transaction with both sides being clear about what they are offering to the project and what they expect to receive in return. Some researchers have found it valuable to establish a formal or informal agreement with service user researchers before the project starts. This can help to lay out the responsibilities on both sides. By establishing payment for a particular role and level of input, both researchers and service users can be reassured that they know what is expected from them.

Implications of paying service users for their involvement

Introducing payments into the relationship between researchers and service users may have other impacts which need to be considered and managed. Although expectations can be clarified by paying for a particular type of input, payment levels may also put some service users off, either because levels are too low, or because they imply a level of input that they are not comfortable with. It may also unreasonably raise both service users' and researchers' expectations about their contribution. Careful consideration should be given to how different roles and types of involvement are rewarded. Paying at a high rate may reasonably make service users expect a considerable level of responsibility or skills to be required. This should then be reflected in the way that they are involved.

It is also important to consider that existing relationships may be changed by payments of this kind. In research where service users are involved in evaluating or auditing their own service, it may have an impact on the therapeutic relationship that they have with that service.

There can be a danger that through paying service users their involvement is actually more limited. Budget constraints may lead to service users being included only at a few stages of the process. For example, service users may be invited to only a few meetings, instead of being involved at more frequent points. In addition, service users may only be able to be involved for a few hours in a week to prevent payment impacting on financial support received from the state. The possible impacts on social security benefits are discussed further below.

Structures for paying service users

The many different ways of involving service users in research (see also Chapter 3) are likely to require different structures for payment. Service users may be employed on a full-time or part-time basis in the same way that non-service user researchers are. In other cases, service users may be self-employed and hired as consultants. Often, involvement will be more ad hoc and payment structures will need to reflect this. Service users might be paid per interview carried out, per meeting attended, or per presentation delivered. Often it will be appropriate to pay for any time required in preparation for meetings or events as well.

Sometimes, involvement may be commissioned through a service user organisation. In this case, payment can be made directly to the organisation which will be responsible for paying the individuals involved (Department of Health and CSIP, 2006). They must then generate their own payment policy and associated guidance to distribute these payments appropriately.

In each case, care should be taken that employment law is properly adhered to as appropriate. If service users are employed directly on a full- or part-time basis, they are entitled to the same legal protection as other employees. Similarly, if service users are self-employed consultants, they are as responsible for adhering to employment law as other self-employed consultants, including registration for tax and national insurance contributions in the UK.

Where service users are paid for specific contributions they are nonetheless entitled to some of the protections that workers have under employment law. These include minimum wage, holiday entitlement and sick pay (where they are earning above the national insurance threshold in the UK).

Many service users may be on benefits or limited earnings. If service users are being paid for their time, systems should be in place to ensure that this payment is prompt and service users are not out of pocket for long. Where possible, service users should not be asked to incur expenses. Research teams can pay for travel tickets and accommodation directly so that service users do not need to be reimbursed later. Where service users do incur expenses, these should also be reimbursed as quickly as possible.

Other methods of payment have previously been used in the UK to avoid difficulties with benefits. These include making payments in store vouchers or agreeing to make donations to mental health organisations instead. There are problems with these methods however. Where they are offered in place of payment, there is a danger of appearing patronising, and it will raise questions about how far service users are being involved as equals in the research process. Also, vouchers may be considered notional earnings for the purposes of benefits, as discussed below.

Levels of payment

A national body in England, known as the Care Services Improvement Partnership (CSIP), has produced a list outlining recommended levels of pay for different types of involvement (McKenna *et al.*, 2007). These may be a useful guideline for researchers in establishing payment levels. However, projects vary considerably and a range of factors should be considered.

A principle often advocated for deciding on payment levels for service users is equality with other, non-service user, contributors (Tew *et al.*, 2004). However, there may not be a comparable role within the research team through which an equal standard of pay can be established. As with any job, payment levels will depend on levels of responsibility, the expertise and skills that they need and the amount of time that is being asked of them. These are not necessarily straightforward questions and are likely to depend on the role service users take within the project.

In some cases, service users with significant research experience and skills may be needed. This may be true where service users are carrying out skilled elements of the research. Some people have highlighted the value of 'academic consumer researchers' (see also Chapter 10). These are people who have significant research skills, qualifications or experience and who have been, or are, service users (Griffiths *et al.*, 2004). There may be strong reasons for involving people in this position. They are likely to be able to contribute to the research in more complex ways and to have the confidence and research knowledge to challenge others within the team. As with any skilled professional, someone with this level of expertise will probably require higher payment and may well be hired as a consultant or full-time researcher.

Academic researchers with experience of using services may be seen as most appropriate where the aim of user involvement is to improve the research by adding a service user perspective. However, user involvement is also often championed in terms of democratisation and emancipation. Arguably, the contribution of academic consumer researchers is limited in how far it can do this. It may be perceived by other service users as keeping the research within a small clique, rather than opening it up to broader participation.

Involvement is also seen in terms of representing other service users. This raises many issues itself as to how far such a heterogeneous group can be represented by a few individuals. However, where particular types of service user experience are sought for a research project, academic researchers may not be able to provide this type of perspective.

There is, then, a need to involve service users with a range of experiences and often basic research skill levels (e.g. through consultation, see also Chapter 11). The required skills and types of experience may be different from those required by professional researchers. They might include experience of participation in meetings or groups or contributing to forums. In some cases, it is likely that service users will not be paid at a comparative level to that of professional researchers.

It is also important to be aware that payment should not be the only reward for service users who take part in research. Research at South West Yorkshire Mental Health NHS Trust identified a range of benefits that service users felt they had received from being involved in research. These included:

- increased knowledge and research skills
- experience of research techniques
- the opportunity to speak with other service users
- pleasure and satisfaction in taking part
- feeling supported
- feeling valued and being part of a team
- increased confidence and self-esteem (Minogue *et al.*, 2005).

This should not undermine the importance of recognising service users' input through payment, but nor should payment be seen as sufficient reward for participation, to the exclusion of these other, considerable, benefits.

In all cases, it is important to be aware that service users involved in a paid capacity are protected by minimum wage legislation and pay levels must not contravene this (Department of Health and CSIP, 2006). It is also important to be aware of the possible implication for people who receive benefits.

Benefits recipients in the UK

Many service users may receive financial assistance from the state if they are not in employment. In the UK, there are three forms of this financial assistance which may be affected by paid involvement. These are:

- Incapacity Benefit – for people who are unable to work due to ill-health or disability
- Income Support – for people who are unable to work full-time and require additional income to live on
- Job Seekers Allowance – for people who are out of work but are actively seeking employment.

Benefits available and the criteria for receiving them will vary in other countries and are subject to frequent changes. Researchers should be sure that they are aware of the benefits rules that apply.

Where service users are in receipt of benefits, paid involvement in research can jeopardise this income. In the UK there has been considerable confusion about how payment for involvement should be viewed by Job Centre Plus (employment office). The 2003 report, *Contributing on Equal Terms*, by the Social Care Institute for Excellence, showed some of the problems caused by this confusion, including reduction or stopping of benefits, inability to accept full payment for the work carried out, concern about accepting reimbursement of expenses and reassessment of entitlement to Disability Living Allowance (Turner, 2004).

The reduction of benefits payments may not necessarily be a problem for service users, where the involvement is substantial, and the money received for their involvement compensates for the benefits reduction. Difficulties often arise where involvement is short term or sporadic, and service users are left with a reduced income overall.

Impacts on benefits will vary in different countries, but they are generally a concern and need to be considered carefully in determining whether people should be paid and at what level. Though governments are frequently supportive of consumer or service user participation, this is not always adequately reflected in the benefits systems.

Since 2003, the Department of Health in England has attempted to clarify the situation around benefits and employment law in 'Reward and Recognition'(Department of Health and CSIP, 2006). Nonetheless, the situation varies considerably for different service users. Some solutions, and key issues to be aware of, are laid out below. These apply specifically to the UK. It is important to check how benefits might be affected in the country where the involvement is taking place if these apply. (For additional guidance, see CSIP, 2007; Bacon and Olsen, 2003.)

Permitted earnings in the UK

People who receive benefits are limited in how much they can earn before their benefits are reduced or removed. This level is, in most cases, £20 per week. There is also a limit as to the number of hours that can be worked. In some situations it may be possible to average earnings and hours worked over a period of several weeks. For instance, someone could earn up to £80 in a four-week period and be paid at the end of this period.

Notional earnings in the UK

Even where service users do not receive payment for their contribution, it is possible for them to fall foul of the 'notional earnings' rule. This occurs where someone is offered, but declines, payment for activities. This 'notional' payment can be removed from their benefits. This should not prevent people from voluntary involvement, as long as it is not perceived that there is an available option of being paid.

One-off payments in the UK

Small one-off payments for specific activities can be made without affecting benefits. This can be done by providing the service user with a 'thank you gift' in cash. This is then treated as capital rather than earnings (Bacon and Olsen, 2003). These payments are very limited and are unlikely to be sufficient to reward for service users' involvement.

Reimbursement of expenses in the UK

Reimbursement may be seen as earnings if the service user is being paid for their involvement (though not if their involvement is voluntary). This includes travel expenses, meals and replacement care. This means that the combined payment and expenses could push service users above their permitted earnings and may then be deducted from benefits.

One way to avoid this is to provide train tickets, travel cards, hotel bookings etc directly where possible as these are not counted as earnings.

Where service user participation is unpaid, actual expenses can be reimbursed without being treated as earnings. However, if expenses are rounded up, or set expenses agreed – for example, £10 for a meeting – these may be treated as earnings.

Informing Job Centre Plus and supporting service users

It is advisable for the service user to contact Job Centre Plus before paid involvement takes place to agree on the payment methods used and to confirm that this will not affect benefits. This can help to ensure that service users are not unfairly penalised for the involvement, especially since it can be slow and costly to fix afterwards. However, many people are fearful of doing this in case they are unfairly penalised and so benefits can be a real barrier to service user involvement in research.

It is the responsibility of the service user themselves to inform Job Centre Plus of earnings and other changes in circumstance that could affect their benefits. However, researchers should ensure that service users are advised and supported in this process. Some Involvement organisations have guidance for service users which may help to explain possible implications (Scott, 2003). Researchers should also be aware that these issues can create a great deal of anxiety for service users. This may put them off becoming involved, or make them feel that they should contribute voluntarily when in fact they are entitled to be paid for their work. Again, the research team should provide information and support to service users in this position.

Costs of service user involvement

In addition to paying service users for their contribution, implementing effective user involvement in research projects carries a cost which should be properly considered before beginning a project. Inadequate resources can limit meaningful user involvement. It may be more appropriate to involve service users in a more limited way but do it well, rather than attempt to do more than resources allow. Below are a number of areas in which user involvement carries considerable cost implications.

TRAINING

Unless service users already have the required experience in research and involvement, it is likely that they will require some training in relevant areas. Training is important in providing service users with the skills and confidence to contribute meaningfully to the project. Skills development is also a considerable incentive and reward for many service users.

The amount of training required will depend on the project and the service users involved. Training may be provided within the team or by a consultant or user involvement group. Consideration should also be given to whether or not service users should be paid for attendance at training events. Though training may provide benefits to service users in itself, it may put some people off if they are expected to attend without payment. It is also important to consider fairness if non-service user researchers are paid to attend training.

Expenses

As discussed above, where possible, research teams should not ask service users to incur expenses. In many cases, it is possible to avoid this by paying in advance for travel, accommodation, food etc. Any expenses incurred through involvement should be reimbursed, whether or not the user is paid for their contribution. Care should be taken to avoid expenses being treated as earnings for benefits purposes (see above). It is important to be clear in advance about what expenses will be reimbursed. Expenses may, for instance, include paying for alternative care arrangements where service users have dependents.

SUPPORT AND SUPERVISION

It is important that service users are provided with adequate support within the project. This can take a number of forms, depending on the service users and the roles they are undertaking. Where service users are undertaking specific research activities that are new to them, they may need ongoing supervision to ensure that they are confident and able to carry them out to the expected standard.

If involvement is to be effective, service users must feel able to propose or to challenge research decisions within the project. This may be difficult in situations where service users are unfamiliar with terminology or methods used. Providing adequate research support for service users can help to remove this barrier but will often require considerable resources. Providing information in advance, or in accessible language can help service users, and other researchers, feel confident that they understand the issues.

In some projects, external support is brought in. Support from someone outside can help service users have the confidence to disagree with others within the project team without perceiving a conflict of interest. There are a number of models used to do this. Service user research groups, voluntary-sector organisations or service user consultants may be able to provide this service. Where a service user group is commissioned to facilitate user involvement, it is likely that they will provide this kind of support. Similarly, peer support from other service users in the project may be valuable but is likely to require additional resources.

However supervision and support is provided, it may take considerable time and resources to do well. Service users may face a number of emotional and practical issues which researchers should be prepared to assist with. Involvement in research can be an important part of a recovery process, and researchers may find that they are playing an important role in supporting this recovery. This can mean being available to listen and encourage service users.

Where service users have been involved specifically because they have had experiences related to those being studied, the project may be very emotional for the service users involved. As with any researchers working on an emotional subject, it is important to be able to speak with others about how this affects them (see also Faulkner, 2004).

AFTER THE PROJECT

As well as the support required during a project, researchers should consider what support may be needed after the project has been completed. Involvement can be a very significant experience for service users and relationships with others in the team can become very important to user researchers. Researchers should be careful that service users are not simply dropped at the end of a project, and at the least should remain available to them after their formal involvement has ended. It may also be appropriate to facilitate links into future projects, or groups, to allow service users to build on the experience gained through their involvement.

Time and flexibility

As well as factoring in additional costs of user involvement, researchers should be aware of the additional time that may be required if involvement is to be meaningful. Service user researchers should be empowered to influence, and sometimes to challenge the proposed research processes and activities. For this to be possible, time must be allowed for involvement at key stages. It is also important that there is sufficient flexibility in the project for user input to influence the research. Without this flexibility, service users are likely to feel that their involvement is tokenistic.

Researchers often underestimate the need for extra time when working collaboratively. In reflecting on experiences of conducting research with service users, Allam says:

> We all found that working collaboratively was much more time-consuming than expected: the training took longer than anticipated – and yet another day would have been useful; organizing interviews was a very lengthy and frustrating process, [. . .] analysis and coding took up several days of researchers' own time. We had budgeted for a payment per hour long interview, in reality this only represented a small fraction of the time that Service User and carers invested in the research. Researchers need to ensure that Service User and carers are paid realistically.
>
> (Allam, 2004)

Extra time may be needed at all stages of the research process. Researchers should also bear in mind that service users may only be able to work on a research project part-time due to other commitments, benefits issues or health. This may require that the research activities are carried out over a longer period of time than originally planned.

Though the costs of involvement can be high, the benefits to the service users, research staff and to the quality of the study can also be considerable. A number of papers have listed the benefits of involvement, though these are not always easily converted into a monetary value (Minogue *et al.*, 2005). Nonetheless, these papers show that the benefits identified by service users, carers and researchers are highly valued.

Funders and funding

Funding can be a major barrier to involving service users in research. Researchers are often influenced more by the priorities of research funders than by service users.

Furthermore, the additional costs and time outlined above require additional funding and need to be fully budgeted for when submitting funding proposals.

Internationally, key research funders are showing increased commitment to ensuring that service users are involved in the research they fund. In the USA, the National Institutes of Health (NIH) has shown this commitment through their Director's Council of Public Representatives (http://copr.nih.gov). In Australia, the National Health and Medical Research Council (NHMRC) produced its *Statement on Consumer and Community Participation in Health and Medical Research* (NHMRC, 2001) which highlights the importance of funding consumer involvement. In the UK, the Big Lottery research fund, Joseph Rowntree Foundation and Department of Health funders all ask for evidence of how beneficiary groups will be involved.

As a result of this increased commitment, involving service users has become much more mainstream in mental health research. According to the Department of Health funder Health Technology Assessment (HTA), between 2002 and 2007, 83% of their funded projects involved service users at some level (NIHR, 2007). This commitment also means that the additional costs of service user involvement should be easier to get funded. This commitment to service user involvement offers a range of benefits and opportunities, though it has also provoked concerns for some advocates of service user involvement.

Opportunities

Commitment from many of the large-scale research funders means that user involvement is forced to become more mainstream. Service users are involved in a wide range of large-scale projects, rather than being limited to a specialist field of research. As well as mainstreaming user involvement, it also legitimises it. This public recognition that user involvement is vital to quality research can help to redress the power imbalance between service users and professional researchers.

Funders are also more willing to accept the additional costs necessary to carry out user involvement in research. Guidance from funders such as the Big Lottery encourages applicants to plan and budget for user-involvement activities when applying for funding.

Funders' insistence on user involvement can encourage researchers to think of new and innovative ways to include service users in complex research studies. This can help to move away from the limited methods of involvement through consultation or data collection.

Since user involvement must be evidenced in funding applications, early involvement of service users may be encouraged. This facilitates involvement in the early, critical stages of research design so that service users are not simply invited to input after the important research decisions are signed and sealed. There are, however, difficulties with this. Where funding deadlines are tight, opportunities for user involvement will be very limited. Similarly, researchers may struggle to find resources for adequate involvement prior to a project being funded.

Concerns

This embrace of service user involvement by funders has not been without critique, however. Some researchers have expressed concern about a funder-imposed requirement to involve service users (Beresford, 2003). Key among these concerns is that service user involvement will become a tick-box activity, where a minimum level of involvement is included because it is required. This could lead to poorly managed involvement, tokenism and even harm to the service users or the project. It has also been known for researchers to describe involvement on funder application forms but not put in place the structures to enact these plans once grants are awarded. Few funders monitor the quality of service user involvement, and thus a culture of tokenism can flourish.

Though funders may insist on user involvement wherever possible, they do not necessarily define what is viewed as meaningful involvement. The HTA figure of 83% of projects involving service users, includes 'consultation with user groups, membership of trial steering committees and involvement in protocol development' (HTA, 2007). It does not, however, provide a view on how well service users are involved. Consultation can easily be tokenistic, especially where required by a third party, rather than justified on its own merits. Alternatively, much may be promised in a research proposal, but may not be followed through in the project itself. If promises of involvement are not delivered, service users may justifiably feel that there is insufficient commitment to their involvement.

Funders' requirements could also encourage inappropriate types of involvement. Involvement for involvement's sake may put service users and researchers in a difficult position. For example, inviting untrained service users to a meeting in which complex research methodologies or science are discussed, without supporting the person fully, is likely to be disheartening or patronising to a service user and is unlikely to produce any benefits to the research. Key to productive service user involvement is clear role planning and defining expectations for all involved.

Beresford also argues that this approach tends to ignore the complex and controversial nature of service user involvement (Beresford, 2003). Involvement does pose challenges to research principles and practice which should be properly considered and worked out, rather than glossed over. It could mean changing the way a project is carried out or how a topic is investigated. Requiring service user involvement may discourage a critical view of involvement that is necessary to developing effective methods of involving service users.

Involving service users in funding decisions

Increasingly key funders internationally are involving service users in decisions about what research to fund (O'Donnell and Entwistle, 2004). Among these are the UK Department of Health funding bodies, and Australia's National Health and Medical Research Council (NHMRC, 2004). Research in 2004 showed that of 69 UK funding organisations surveyed, 42 tried to involve service users in their work in some way (O'Donnell and Entwistle, 2004).

Involving service users in making decisions about research priorities and individual research proposals is intended to ensure that research is relevant to the people it is supposed to benefit. Some funders have also suggested that service user involvement improves the quality and legitimacy of their decision-making processes. It can also be valuable in evaluating the effectiveness of proposed user involvement in funding applications reviewed.

The HTA published a report of research examining their own commissioning practices involving service users. It highlighted the difficulties of involving service users in commissioning processes. These include finding appropriate service users or members of the public to involve, organisational structures becoming barriers to involvement, and avoiding tokenism (Oliver *et al.*, 2006).

CONCLUSION

This chapter has looked at three key areas in which money plays an important role in service user involvement – payment, costs and funding. The issue of money cannot be separated from the other issues discussed in this book. It has implications for the type of involvement undertaken, its effectiveness, and the relationships between researchers and service users.

Payment of service users widens accessibility, empowers and values service users and helps to establish clear agreements about responsibilities and expectations. Payment should not, however, be the only reward for service users involved in research. Decisions about how much to pay and what structures to use will depend on the research project. In all cases, however, care must be taken that service users are never financially disadvantaged through their involvement. This means taking care around the implications for benefits recipients, and ensuring that actual expenses are fully reimbursed.

The costs of service user involvement can be a barrier to effective collaboration. Enabling service users to be fully involved carries a cost in both resources and time. Researchers need to be aware of these costs in advance of a project as they will influence the level of involvement possible, and the level of funds required. Researchers should not try to do involvement 'on the cheap' as this is likely to lead to tokenism, to undermine and discourage the service users involved and can leave people vulnerable if adequate training and support are not provided.

Researchers should be aware of the expectations of funders in requiring user involvement in proposed projects. Care should be taken, however, that this does not lead to tokenism, or an uncritical approach to involvement. Funders also have a responsibility to ensure that user involvement is genuine and well considered. Part of making this assessment, and funding decisions more generally, should require the involvement of service users in funding bodies.

Recommendations

1. Service users should be paid for their involvement in research. The amount of payment will vary but should not be tokenistic.
2. Service users should be promptly reimbursed for any expenses incurred through their involvement.
3. Care should be taken to ensure that the method and structure of payment is appropriate to the level and type of involvement, and that it adheres to employment law.
4. Researchers should be aware of how payment may affect the receipt of benefits and financial support. Service users *must* be informed about any possible impacts, and encouraged to speak to the relevant benefits agency before taking part. Researchers should provide support in this process.
5. Researchers and funders should be aware of the financial and time costs of conducting genuine service user involvement and should factor these in to the budget and timeframe of the project.

6. Funders should carefully evaluate plans for involvement in research proposals and, as far as possible, avoid tokenistic involvement. They should also monitor involvement to ensure that it is carried out as proposed.
7. Researchers should be careful that in meeting funders' requirements they are not introducing tokenistic involvement. They should also be careful that proposed involvement is realistic and followed through.
8. Funders should involve service users in their funding decisions, and ensure that their contribution is valued fully. This may require changes in the system for reviewing proposals.

REFERENCES

Allam, S. (2004) Our experience of collaborative research: service users, carers and researchers work together to evaluate an assertive outreach service, *Journal of Psychiatric and Mental Health Nursing*, **11**(3), 368–373.

Bacon, J. and Olsen, K. (2003) *Doing the Right Thing: Outlining the DWP's approach to ethical and legal issues in social research*, London: Department for Work and Pensions.

Beresford, P. (2003) 'User Involvement in Research: Connecting Lives, Experience and Theory', Making Research Count Conference, University of Warwick. Available online at: http://www2. warwick.ac.uk/fac/soc/shss/mrc/userinvolvement/beresford/], accessed 28/10/08.

Department of Health and CSIP (2006) *Reward and Recognition: The principles and practice of service user payment and reimbursement in health and social care – A guide for service providers service users and carers*, London: DH/CSIP.

Entwistle, V. *et al.* (1998) Lay perspectives: advantages for health research, *British Medical Journal*, **316**, 463–466.

Faulkner, A. (2004) *The Ethics of Survivor Research: Guidelines for the ethical conduct of research carried out by mental health service users and survivors*, Bristol: Policy Press.

Griffiths, K., Jorm, A. and Christensen, H. (2004) Academic consumer researchers: a bridge between consumers and researchers, *Australian and New Zealand Journal of Psychiatry*, **38**, 191–196.

Involve (2005) *A guide to paying members of the public who are actively involved in research*, Available online at: http://www.invo.org.uk/pdfs/PaymentGuide_amended%20241105.pdf, accessed 28/10/08.

McKenna, R. *et al.* (2007) *Valuing Involvement: Making a Real Difference Strengthening Service User and Carer Involvement in NIMHE and CSIP: Payment and Reimbursement Policy Guidance*, London: CSIP/NIMHE.

Minogue, V., Boness, J., Brown, A. and Girdlestone, J. (2005) The impact of service user involvement in research, *International Journal of Health Care Quality Assurance Inc Leadership Health Services*, **18**(2–3), 103–112.

National Health and Medical Research Council (2001) *Statement on Consumer and Community Participation in Health and Medical Research*. Available online at: http://www.nhmrc.gov.au/publications/synopses/r22syn.htm, accessed 28/10/08.

National Health and Medical Research Council (2004) *A Model Framework for Consumer and Community Participation in Health and Medical Research*, London: NHMRC.

National Institute for Health Research (2007) *NIHR, Health Technology Assessment Programme Annual Report*, 2007, London: NIHR.

O'Donnell, M. and Entwistle, V. (2004) Consumer involvement in decisions about what health-related research is funded, *Health Policy*, **70**(3), 281–290.

Oliver, S., Armes, D. Gyte, G. (2006) *Evaluation on public influence of the NHS Health Technology Assessment Programme*, London: Social Science Research Unit, Institute of Education, University of London.

Ryan, T. and Bamber, C. (2002) A survey of policy and practice on expenses and other payments to mental health service users and carers participating in service development, *Journal of Mental Health*, **11(6)**, 635–644.

Scott, J. (2003) *A Fair Day's Pay: A Guide to Benefits service user involvement and payments*, London: Mental Health Foundation.

Tew, J., Gell, C. and Foster, S. (2004) *Learning from Experience: involving service users and carers in mental health education and training*, York: Mental Health in Higher Education/NIMHE West Midlands/Trent WDC.

Turner, M. (2004) *Contributing on Equal Terms*, Shaping Our Lives National User Network.

CHAPTER 16

Politics

Politics of Research in Mental Health

Daniel B. Fisher
Executive Director, National Empowerment Center, USA

This chapter provides a critical discussion of the influence of culture, politics, and the drugs industry on the agenda for mental health research. The author recounts his own life journey, as a biochemist who was diagnosed with schizophrenia and recovered. Starting with a reflection on and critique of the prevailing focus on biological research in mental health from the background of the author's own life experiences, the chapter discusses the political influence of mainstream US culture on diagnosis, on the ranking of evidence, and on public education. It goes on to outline the influence of pharmaceutical companies on the politics of research and publication serving mainly as marketing strategies. Finally, the chapter proposes ways to change the cultural underpinnings of research and education in mental health, with the involvement of service users being an important means of doing so.

INTRODUCTION

In this chapter, I will describe ways that our culture and the drugs industry have narrowed our research lens and agenda to a dangerous degree. An old saying describes this: 'The one who pays the piper calls the tune.' We are overly reliant on the drugs industry to fund our research. This funding is centred on finding new medications and reinforces a view that our behaviour is mainly the product of our brain. This recent preoccupation with brain chemistry, as the primary subject of research into human behaviour and thought is reducing our humanity and our broader understanding of ourselves in this world. Our life cannot be dissected in a laboratory. I will also describe how the mental health consumer/survivor movement has been broadening the research agenda to include the whole person in their whole community. This broader view of consumers as persons in the community is based on

Handbook of Service User Involvement in Mental Health Research Edited by Jan Wallcraft, Beate Schrank and Michaela Amering
Copyright © 2009 John Wiley & Sons, Ltd

our research into what has helped us recover from the life interrupting experiences labelled mental illness. This movement is also advocating for newer participatory research approaches.

From a personal side, research has always been of great interest to me. My father carried out research on penicillin that indirectly saved my life. I myself spent the first nine years of my working life as a biochemical researcher. I have never stopped being a researcher in the broadest sense of searching for knowledge.

> Research [according to Wikipedia] is a human activity based on intellectual investigation and is aimed at discovering, interpreting, and revising human knowledge on different aspects of the world.

In this broad sense, research is an integral part of living for all humans. It is the daily activity we engage in to stay attuned to reality and to learn more about the world we live in. I left the formal laboratory when I felt betrayed by its narrow scope. In fact, I had to leave the laboratory to regain my sanity, because I had become convinced that I was the chemicals I was studying. I had become trapped in the monologue of a single version of reality. I decided I needed to broaden my enquiries to encompass life in the community and I needed to include my own life as a subject of research. My enlightenment, which I have described as recovery from schizophrenia, was from my personal research into my life. My recovery was also greatly aided by others who helped me to break out of the narrow monologue into dialogue with a variety of persons who had been on a similar journey. Their personal research created a peer-reviewed climate, which deepened my knowledge of myself and my relationships in the world.

This is a topic I have been concerned about for many years. An editorial I wrote for the Washington Post (Fisher, 2001) neatly summarizes concerns that are as relevant today as they were seven years ago:

> I have recovered from schizophrenia. If that statement surprises you – if you think schizophrenia is a lifelong brain disease that cannot be escaped – you have been misled by a cultural misapprehension that needlessly imprisons millions under the label of mental illness.
>
> In the last 20 years, the pharmaceutical industry has become the major force behind the belief that mental illness is a brain disorder and that its victims need to take medications for the rest of their lives. It's a clever sales strategy: If people believe mental illness is purely biological, they will only treat it with a pill.
>
> Drug companies have virtually bought the psychiatric profession. Their profits fund the research, the journals and the departments of psychiatry. Not surprisingly, many researchers have concluded that medication alone is best for the treatment for mental illness. Despite recent convincing research showing the usefulness of psychotherapy in treating schizophrenia, psychiatric trainees are still told 'you can't talk to a disease'. This is why psychiatrists today spend more time prescribing drugs than getting to know the people taking them.
>
> I, too, used to believe in the biological model of mental illness. Thirty-one years ago, as a PhD biochemist with the National Institute of Mental Health, I researched and wrote papers on neurotransmitters such as serotonin and dopamine. Then I was diagnosed with schizophrenia – and my experience taught me that our feelings and dreams cannot be analyzed under a microscope.
>
> Despite what many people assume when they hear about my recovery, that original diagnosis was no mistake: a board of six Navy psychiatrists confirmed it after my four-month

inpatient stay at Bethesda Naval Hospital. Being branded a schizophrenic devastated me. My life seemed over. Six years later, however, I had defied everyone's expectations and recovered. The most important elements in my recovery were a therapist who believed in me, the support of my family, steadfast friends and meaningful work. And I had a new goal: I wanted to become a psychiatrist. My therapist validated that dream, saying, 'I will go to your graduation'. (When I received my degree from George Washington University Medical School in 1976, he was there.) Drugs were a tool I used during crises, but I have been completely off medication for 25 years.

I am not an anomaly. Thousands of others have recovered, but are afraid to disclose their past due to the stigma of mental illness. The definitive Vermont Longitudinal Study, led by Courtenay Harding, followed 269 patients diagnosed in the late 1950s with severe schizophrenia (Harding et al., 1987). Three decades later, Harding found that two-thirds of them were living and functioning independently; and of those, half were completely recovered and medication-free.

The Swiss psychiatrist Manfred Bleuler – whose father, Eugene, coined the term schizophrenia in 1908 – obtained similar results (Bleuler, 1974). His father had mistakenly concluded that people did not recover from schizophrenia – because he rarely saw his patients after discharge. Our own research at the National Empowerment Center (NEC), funded by the federal Center for Mental Health Services, shows that the most important factor in recovery from mental illness is people who believe in patients and give them hope: Medications are a less important factor.

But that is not how psychiatrists are being taught; recently I was reminded of how tightly training is controlled. I contacted a colleague at a major West Coast medical school to see if he could get me an invitation to conduct one of their teaching rounds. He apologetically told me that he couldn't: Since he had published a critique of the biological model of mental illness, demonstrating that people could recover from schizophrenia without medication, he himself was no longer allowed to speak to the residents in training – even though he was on the faculty.

The pharmaceutical industry also controls the public's education. Who can avoid the TV image of the phobic man who needs Paxil to socialize? Industry-funded research and experts have a huge impact on media coverage. Finally, the drug companies have taken advantage of well-intentioned advocacy groups who support the biological model of mental illness – and they give those groups much-needed financial support.

Schizophrenia is more often due to a loss of dreams than a loss of dopamine. At the NEC[1], we try to reach out across the chasm of chaos. I know there are many people who feel they have done all they can, have struggled against mental illness to no avail, and we understand their pain. Yet we believe that recovery is eventually possible for everyone – although it can take a long time to undo the negative messages of past treatments. We can offer hope from first-hand experience.

Addressing the needs of people with mental illness will require a large-scale retraining of mental health workers, decision-makers, families and the public. There will need to be more research into the ways that people recover. There will need to be more jobs, housing, peer support and self-help, for these are the pathways to self-determination and independence. And there needs to be a cultural shift toward people rather than pills to alleviate this form of human suffering.

---

[1] NEC or the National Empowerment Center is consumer/survivor-run training, education, research, and advocacy centre located in Lawrence, Mass. The Center is funded by the US government, private foundations, and sales of products. The Center has researched the conditions leading to recovery and, since its founding in 1992, has advocated for a recovery-based, consumer/survivor-driven system of care and supports.

POLITICS OF DIAGNOSIS

This is a related topic because much of research as well as treatment are based on diagnostic categories. So let us ask, 'how scientific are diagnostic categories?' In 1851, Dr. Samuel Cartwright (cited in Jackson, 2005), a prominent Louisiana physician and one of the leading authorities in his time on the medical care of 'Negroes',[2] identified a mental disorder peculiar to slaves: drapetomania, or the disease causing Negroes to run away. It was noted as a condition,

> unknown to our medical authorities, although its diagnostic symptom, the absconding from service, is well known to our planters and overseers.

Dr. Cartwright observed,

> The cause in most cases, that induces the Negro to run away from service, is such a disease of the mind as in any other species of alienation, and much more curable, as a general rule.

Cartwright was so helpful as to identify preventive measures for dealing with potential cases of drapetomania. Slaves showing incipient drapetomania, reflected in sulky and dissatisfied behavior should be whipped-strictly as a therapeutic early intervention. Planter and overseers were encouraged to utilize whipping as the primary intervention once the disease had progressed to the stage of actually running away. Overall, Cartwright suggested that Negroes should be kept in a submissive state and treated like children, with

> ...care, kindness, attention and humanity, to prevent and cure them from running away.
>
> (Jackson, 2005)

Another dramatic illustration of the political basis of diagnosis is the case of homosexuality. Until 1973, homosexuality was considered a form of mental illness. Then in 1973 the American Psychiatric Association (APA) declassified it as mental illness. This was not due to a medical breakthrough but instead was due to the political pressure of the gay and lesbian movement whose protests forced the APA to remove from its definitions, homosexuality as a form of mental illness. The decision was partly based on arguments before the APA nomenclature committee by gay and lesbian advocates. But the final decision to declassify homosexuality as an illness was based on a vote by the entire APA membership (Conrad and Schneider, 1992).

The standardization of psychiatric diagnoses into stricter categories has also narrowed inquiry into the cultural context of behaviour. In a very short period of time, mental illnesses were transformed from broad, etiologically defined entities that were continuous with normality to standardized symptom-based, categorical diseases. The third edition of the American Psychiatric Association's Diagnostic and Statistical Manual of Mental Disorders (DSM-III) was responsible for this change. This standardization was the product of many factors, including:

- professional politics within the mental health community
- increased government involvement in mental health research and policymaking

---

[2] Term used in his notes to describe Black African Americans.

- mounting pressure on psychiatrists from health insurers to demonstrate the effectiveness of their practices, and
- the necessity of pharmaceutical companies to market their products to treat specific diseases. (Mayes and Horowitz, 2005).

POLITICS OF THERAPY

There have been numerous attempts to make psychotherapy more attuned to the culture of the client. However, these attempts generally fail because they do not understand that the primary function of psychotherapy, especially in a public setting, is to reinforce the cultural values of the most powerful class in society. This point was illustrated by a study, conducted in 1938, of the ideals of psychotherapy. The study showed that the ideals of the mental hygiene movement (name for the mental health system at that time) at that time coincided with the ideals of the dominant class: proper Bostonians. Those ideals were individualism, self-reliance, enhancement of wealth and social status, and rationalism. Not surprisingly the mental hygiene movement, and the society, was run by proper Bostonian administrators and psychiatrists (Davis, 1938).

Another illustration of the influence of politics on therapy is the question of whether psychotherapy is helpful in people's recovery from schizophrenia. There had been several case studies in the 1950s and 60s (Green, 1964) indicating that psychotherapy could be useful for persons with schizophrenia. Then a study carried out at a prestigious Harvard teaching hospital showed there was little advantage to adding psychotherapy to medication (Grinspoon *et al.*, 1968). The pharmaceutical industry widely disseminated these results, and by the time I entered my residency in 1976, psychotherapy for schizophrenic consumers was being discouraged. Ever since the release of the Harvard study it has been increasingly difficult to get insurance companies to fund psychotherapy visits, while medication visits face few limitations. However, another in-depth study of psychotherapy with consumers labelled with schizophrenia by Dr. Bertram Karons in the late 1970s showed that psychotherapy can be very useful (Karons and VandenBos, 1981). Dr. Karons cited the reason for the discrepancy was related to the selection of therapists. In the Harvard study, 'senior therapists' were used. Unfortunately these therapists actually had minimal experience working over lengthy time periods with consumers with schizophrenia, as they had spent more of their time carrying out supervision and seeing less disturbed consumers. In contrast, the Karon study used only therapists experienced in providing psychotherapy to persons labelled with schizophrenia. More recent studies have upheld the efficacy of psychotherapy with schizophrenia (Eells, 2000).

POLITICS OF EVIDENCE

Another area where political considerations have played a large role is the question of evidence-based practice (EBP). This mantra has been increasingly used by those supporting traditional treatment strategies. First the medical community defines randomized, double blind studies as the gold standard of evidence. This criteria favour drug trials over all other types of research. It is never possible to carry out double blind studies in community-based, consumer-run programs in the same manner as defined by the criteria.

The frustration of the consumer/survivor movement with this restrictive approach to evidence was expressed at the last meeting of the New Freedom Commission on Mental Health. During public testimony, one of the advocates, Laurie Ahern, in describing her own recovery from mental illness, said, look at us, look at those of us who have recovered, 'we are the evidence!'

The proponents of EBP's say that the newer, community-based and consumer-run alternatives to traditional clinical services are not supported by evidence. In point of fact, the use of hospitalization is not an EBP. Dr. Loren Mosher's important research in the 1970s showed that small, home-like settings based on an interpersonal philosophy produced better outcomes than hospitalization (a lower relapse rate and fewer side-effects from medication). Dr. Mosher called these two pilot-study homes Soteria Houses. There was much less reliance on medication and the staff had less professional training. He was head of schizophrenia research at National Institute for Mental Health (NIMH) at the time he conducted the research. Instead of being rewarded for this groundbreaking research, Dr. Mosher was removed from his position at NIMH. He spent the last 25 years of his life crusading for the adoption of this model. He was saddened to see that the hospital lobby, drugs industry, and psychiatric profession are too invested in the medicalisation of behavioural problems to accept the evidence of his research (Mosher et al., 2006).

Another example of the rejection of evidence not fitting the needs of the drugs industry is the case of St. John's Wort. Twenty-two European research studies have shown that St. John's Wort is as efficacious as tricyclic or SSRI antidepressants in cases of moderate depression (Kim et al., 1999). Recently, I have recommended St. John's Wort to several consumers who wanted an anti-depressant with fewer side-effects. In two instances, they complained to our medical director that they wanted to get the real anti-depressants that were advertised on TV. I was discouraged from recommending St. John's Wort because it lacked a research base. I pointed out to our medical director that there were 22 European studies confirming the use of St. John's Wort. Of particular note is a recent large scale German study, funded by the German government, confirmed the finding that St. John's Wort was equivalent in effectiveness to Prozac in cases of moderate depression, and had far fewer side-effects. The authors of the study concluded that St. John's Wort should be the first line of somatic therapy recommended for persons with moderate depression (Schrader, 2000). The Medical Director said that the studies did not count because they were carried out in Europe. In contrast, he pointed out that the one US study of St. John's Wort showed no significant difference between it and the placebo. I pointed out that the SSRI in the study (sertraline) showed no better result than the placebo also. In fact the article concludes, 'the overall response to sertraline on the primary measures was not superior to that of placebo, an outcome which is not uncommon in trials of approved anti-depressants. In fact, this apparent lack of efficacy occurs in up to 35 percent of trials of anti-depressants' (Davidson, 2002).

POLITICS OF PUBLIC EDUCATION

At this point the majority of public education is carried out by the pharmaceutical companies in the form of direct-to-consumers advertising (DTCA). Pharmaceutical companies justify the high mark-up of their medications by saying they need to spend the money on research and development. In fact, a new study (Gagnon and Lexchin, 2008) has shown that these companies spend far more of their revenues on advertising than they do on research. The researchers' estimate is based on the systematic collection of data directly from the industry and doctors during 2004, which shows the US pharmaceutical industry spent 24.4% of the sales dollar on promotion, versus 13.4% for research and development, as a percentage of US domestic sales of US$235.4 billion. That means that in 2004, the last year such data was available, the pharmaceutical companies spent 57 billion dollars on advertising and medical education.

Does all the money spent by pharmaceutical companies improve patient education? The FDA showed that most consumers do not even read the summaries of medications effects and side-effects (Aiken, 2002). Researchers have concluded that DTCA is intrinsically misleading and does not allow consumers to make informed choices. This issue stems from the motivation of the companies, which is to sell their product, not inform the public of the options available. A medication manufacturer is not going to inform the public that in cases of moderate depression exercise is as effective, and has fewer side-effects, as medication. One researcher has concluded:

> that there is an unmistakable conflict of interest for drug manufacturers when 'educating' patients about therapeutic alternatives. The incentives for exaggeration and persuasion are great, and the patients' ability to verify promotional claims is limited by lack of technical expertise and access to unbiased information sources. He goes on to state that economic theory and historical experience indicate that the marketplace for ideas created by consumer-directed drug advertisements will inevitably be unbalanced and biased.

(Morgan, 2001)

POLITICS OF RESEARCH AND PUBLICATION: INFLUENCE OF THE PHARMACEUTICAL COMPANIES

When several dozen consumer/survivor leaders were polled concerning the topics they particularly wanted covered, they cited the following issues involving the influence of drug companies:

- showing that the drug companies have a vested interest in the brain disease model of mental illness
- studying the amount of money the drug companies pay to get the evidence-based results they want
- the conflict of interest in allowing the drugs companies to dominate mental health research: the impropriety of allowing those who profit from the research to define what counts as evidence and to be selective in their publication of results of their research.

From my experience the following is a list of the ways that the pharmaceutical industry influences research results and dissemination of those results to practitioners and the public.

Ways in which the drugs industry influences research

- The pharmaceutical companies claim that the SSRIs act by selectively increasing serotonin, but the scientific evidence does not support this theory (Lacasse and Leo, 2005).
- The drugs industry suppresses evidence of dangerous side-effects: example of Zyprexa and diabetes (Berenson, 2006 and see below).
- The administrative overhead from drug trials, along with speakers' fees, and consultations, fund many of the most prestigious research universities.
- Research is carried out, with positive results published for new populations, which expands the sales of medications (see below).
- Publication of articles focused on medications is ensured because journals are heavily subsidized by the drugs industry. (I receive an average of 15 free psychiatric publications per month. Nearly half their pages advertise medications. In addition, they often carry free continuing medical education (CME) credits, which are required for renewal of my license. All the CMEs are focused on medication.)
- Congress is lobbied by the drugs industry ensuring a very high percentage of NIMH funding is devoted to a study of the brain, which often favours the development of more medications (a notable exception was the CATIE study funded by NIMH. It showed that the older psychotropic medication, Perphenazine, was as effective as several of the newer, more expensive, atypical antipsychotic medications (NIMH, 2006).
- The direct TV advertising to the general public of the efficacy of medications, without giving the 'true' information – the full picture – further influences the public to pressure the politicians to fund more biochemical research and influences the public to believe that emotional problems are primarily due to chemical imbalances, which should be treated primarily by medications (see below).
- The drugs industry also influences the definition of highest value of research, the gold standard, is the randomized, double blind study, which highly favours drug research (Mosher *et al.*, 2004)

In order to gain tenure and status within academia, one needs to publish or perish. These publications need to appear in the peer-reviewed journals, which are subsidized by the drugs companies. Many of these points are illustrated by the case of Parke-Davis's promotion of the off-label use[3] of gabapentin or Neurontin. The following study was carried out through a careful analysis of Court documents available to the public from United States ex. rel David Franklin vs. Pfizer, Inc., and Parke-Davis, Division of Warner-Lambert Company, mostly from 1994–1998 (Steinman *et al.*, 2006)

Research and publications on gabapentin served as key elements in the marketing strategy for the drug (US, 2001a). For some clinical uses, such as monotherapy for epilepsy, research was used to support the company's attempt to obtain FDA approval for a new

---

[3] 'off-label use' is the promotion of prescribing of a medication for a use not approved by the US Food and Drug Administration (FDA). This can be legally carried out when the medication has been previously approved by the FDA for another use. For instance, gabapentin was approved by the FDA for use with persons with seizure disorders. It could then be prescribed for off-label usage for persons with bipolar disorder, without approval of that usage by the FDA.

'on-label' indication. However, in other cases Parke-Davis employed a 'publication strategy,' the goal of which was to use research not as a means to gain FDA approval for new indications but 'to disseminate the information as widely as possible through the world's medical literature' (US, 2001b), generating excitement in the market and stimulating off-label prescribing despite the lack of FDA approval. This strategy focused primarily on expanding gabapentin use in neuropathic pain and bipolar disorders, for which detailed decision analyses projected the greatest revenue potential.

The success of this strategy depended in part on publications being favourable to gabapentin. Management expressed concern that negative results could harm promotional efforts, and several documents indicate the intention to publish and publicize results only if they reflected favourably on gabapentin. As stated in a marketing assessment,

The results of the recommended exploratory trials in neuropathic pain, if positive, will be publicized in medical congresses and published.

(US, 2001c)

Similarly, in discussing 2 nearly identical trials that yielded conflicting results on gabapentin as seizure monotherapy, the 'core marketing team' concluded that

the results of [the negative trial] will not be published

(US, 2001d).

Beyond publishing its own clinical trials, Parke-Davis expanded the literature on gabapentin by contracting with medical education companies to develop review papers, original articles, and letters to the editor about gabapentin for $13,375 to $18,000 per article, including a $1000 honorarium for the physician or pharmacist author. For example, one 'grant request' from a medical education company to Parke-Davis proposed a series of 12 articles, each with a pre-specified topic, target journal, title, and list of potential authors (to be 'chosen at the discretion of Parke-Davis') (US, 2001e). This proposal noted that

all articles submitted will include a consistent message ... with particular interest in proper dosing and titration as well as emerging [off-label] uses

mirroring Parke-Davis promotional goals for the drug (US, 2001e). In several instances the medical education company offered substantial assistance in the development of manuscripts, reporting in a status report that

at [the author's] request, we did an extensive literature search and submitted selected articles to him for reference ... We have offered him help in identifying and collecting his appropriate cases, analyzing data, writing a manuscript, or whatever he needs.

(US, 2001f)

Another study of drugs industry collusion with medical researchers is the case of a psychiatrist researcher at Brown University. Ed Silverman of Pharmalot is a psychiatrist who was the lead author of an infamous study published in 2001 in the *Journal of the American Academy of Child and Adolescent Psychiatry* claiming that Paxil, which is known as Seroxat in the UK, was 'generally well tolerated and effective for major depression in adolescents'. Known as study 329, the findings were used to widely promote the drug, which became a huge seller.

However, the study was later held in disrepute after it was learned the results didn't tell the whole story. In fact, 329 was one of three studies cited by former New York Attorney General Eliot Spitzer, who filed a suit charging Glaxo with 'repeated and persistent fraud,' alleging the drugmaker had promoted positive findings, but hadn't publicized unfavourable data.

As it turns out, study 329, which already had a negative history that included ghostwriting charges, were worse than imagined. A recent study in the International Journal of Risk & Safety of Medicine disclosed that, after sifting through some 10,000 documents that surfaced during Paxil litigation, highly selective reporting was used to skew the results favourably.

You can read more about the psychiatrist in the recent book about Paxil, *Side-effects*, by Alison Bass (Silverman, 2008).

Pharmaceutical companies fail to disclose serious side-effects and the FDA does not adequately ensure that such reports are made public. The case of Zyprexa illustrates this point. As early as 1999, scientists at Lilly knew that Zyprexa caused great weight gain and hyperglycemia. In 2000, a group of diabetes doctors, that Lilly had retained to consider potential links between Zyprexa and diabetes, warned the company that 'unless we come clean on this, it could get much more serious than we might anticipate,' according to an e-mail message from one Lilly manager several years later (Berenson, 2006).

In fact Lilly did not 'come clean' on this information and as a result has already paid out US$1.2 billion in settling claims against the company. Lawsuits keep proliferating: in a recent lawsuit by the state of Connecticut, Attorney General Richard Blumenthal cited the following illegal practices carried out by the manufacture (Blumenthal, 2008):

- **Peer-selling enterprise:** Lilly compensated medical marketing firms and several physicians who routinely promoted Zyprexa to peer physicians in venues nationwide. Physicians who attended 'educational' events were deceived into thinking that the events were independent of Eli Lilly. Conspiring physicians concealed information about the efficacy of Zyprexa in off-label uses and dangerous side-effects, as well as the doctors' financial ties with Eli Lilly.
- **The role of pharmacies:** Eli Lilly targeted pharmacies, particularly those that serviced long-term care facilities. Typically, an Eli Lilly sales representative and a pharmacy would agree that the pharmacy formally request funding from Eli Lilly in order to present an 'educational program' – for example, a programme on the treatment of dementia.

  Both the pharmacy and the Eli Lilly representative would agree that the program include a presentation by a doctor – handpicked by Eli Lilly – who would promote off-label use of Zyprexa for dementia. The Eli Lilly sales representative would file a formal request funds from Eli Lilly for an educational grant. Eli Lilly would issue a cheque to the pharmacy and the pharmacy would issue a cheque to the doctor, concealing compensation from Lilly to the physician.
- **Publication enterprise:** Eli Lilly created a 'Publication Enterprise' that hired writers to create articles, and then paid specialists to 'author' the articles. The articles only included favourable results of Eli Lilly's own internal trials, and suppressed unfavourable results, including a clinical trial that failed to show Zyprexa's efficacy for bipolar disorder.
- **Public payer enterprise:** Eli Lilly captured the Medicaid and Medicare markets by paying officials in various states, paying them substantial sums of money to spread

falsehoods regarding the efficacy, safety and side-effects of Zyprexa and to promote off-label use. Eli Lilly targeted those who oversaw treatment for people with serious mental illness, including patients in mental hospitals and clinics who are on Medicaid – among the largest users of anti-psychotic drugs. Lilly also influenced prescribing physicians to over-medicate senior citizens in nursing homes and adolescents in detention centres with anti-psychotics.

The US Senate Finance Committee has been investigating the Head of the Department of Psychiatry at Stanford University, who holds stock worth US$6,000,000 in the drug company Corcept Therapeutics. The company has the patent on an abortion drug, mifepristoine, that his team is investigating as a possible anti-depressant with NIMH funding (Pharmalot, June 25, 2008).

NEED FOR RECOVERY RESEARCH

The National Empowerment Center has been carrying out qualitative research into the nature of recovery for several years. This research has resulted in a new paradigm for the nature of mental illness and of recovery. We call it the Empowerment Paradigm of Recovery and Development (as shown in Figure 16.1) (Fisher, 2008). In order to carry out research on the nature of recovery it is important to have a theory on how mental illness develops and what factors assist in recovery. Our research resulted in 13 principles of recovery (Ahern and Fisher, 2001). Other studies have supported these principles of hope, and empowerment (Ralph, 2000). Most of these principles were born out in the 10 components of recovery that were agreed upon by 110 mental health stakeholders convened by SAMHSA in Dec., 2004 (SAMHSA, 2005). In another aspect of politics, the NIMH warned SAMHSA that they should not release their 10 components of recovery. They said

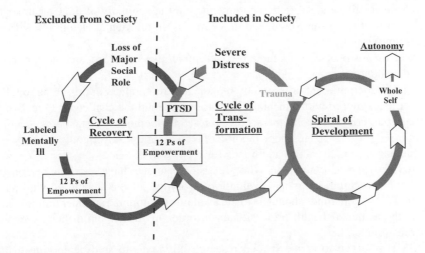

Figure 16.1   Empowerment paradigm of development and recovery © 2006 National Empowerment Center.

that persons with mental illness can never become self-directed and therefore releasing these components would be an embarrassment (personal communication from a government official). In fact, these components have greatly assisted consumer advocacy at the state and federal levels.

HOW TO IMPROVE RESEARCH AND EDUCATION IN MENTAL HEALTH

One of the best ways to improve research is to ask consumers what they feel would be best. When I asked consumer/survivor leaders what could be done to improve mental health research, they made the following recommendations:

1. More emphasis on recovery narratives and lived experience of recovery.
2. Studies of the ways the psychosocial philosophy of causation and treatment enables the person to be an expert in their recovery.
3. Consumer/survivor involvement in all aspects of research:
   - consumer/survivors should be paid and trained to conduct research
   - 'If people living with mental health challenges are not active participants in setting research priorities, framing research questions, working as researchers, and critiquing other researchers then we will continue to be defined by others. Many therapeutic approaches and supports are not funded because experts say they are not evidence based. We need to take greater ownership in participating in the research process.'
   - All publicly-funded research should ensure that the research is informed by consumer/survivors and the results should be evaluated on the basis of whether they lead to peoples' recovery.
   - Funding agencies should include qualitative and participatory research designs into their funding streams, looking into areas such as housing, education, jobs, nutrition and purpose
        Some of these ideas were recommended in the summary of the Consumer Issues Subcommittee of the New Freedom Commission on Mental Health (New Freedom Commission, (2003):
   - Involve consumers and promote recovery in all aspects of research design, conduct, and evaluation.
        The Subcommittee urges policy makers and researchers in this arena to talk with people diagnosed with a mental illness to learn about the challenges to recovery that they face. For many consumers, current research methods and standards – which are intended to advance our understanding of mental illness and effective services – pose challenges to their values and hopes for recovery.
   - Providers and administrators who are also consumers have a unique perspective to offer on research design and evaluation involving persons diagnosed with a mental illness. As such, funds should be made available to support a summer training institute for these mental health professionals in order to further build their research and evaluation skills.
   - NIMH is urged to create special research initiatives to study emerging evidence-based practices such as peer-support programs and to develop and measure service-

satisfaction and outcomes that reflect recovery principles, and other service outcomes important to mental health consumers (e.g. healing, personhood, well-being, or effects of coercion).

- The Subcommittee recommends that NIMH offer incentives to researchers to encourage research on recovery from mental illness.
- The Subcommittee recommends that CMHS continue to support the development of a core set of system level indicators that measure critical elements and processes of recovery, and that CMHS integrate these items into a multi-state 'report card' of mental health performance measures.

Another aspect of political influence on setting the agenda for mental health has been the selective publication of subcommittee reports of the New Freedom Commission. The full papers on less controversial reports such as acute care and evidence-based practice were published. However, the papers on the two topics I chaired, Consumer Issues and Rights and Engagement, were never published.

In addition, there is a need for unbiased research and education about the actions and side-effects of medications. These studies and education should follow the other New Zealand recommendation (Toop, 2003):

> That the Government establishes an independent medicine and health information service free of commercial interest.

There needs to be an end to DTCA. The US is one of only two countries with DTCA. The other country, New Zealand is under considerable pressure to end DTCA. The US and New Zealand should follow the recommendation of the New Zealand study of DTCA (Toop, 2003):

> That the New Zealand government introduce regulations and/or legislation to prohibit the advertising of prescription medicines directly to the public, through print and broadcast media or any other means.

Summary of recommendations to improve research and education in mental health

1. End direct-to-consumer advertising by the pharmaceutical companies.
2. Government-funding of unbiased research into the actions of medications and their side-effects such as carried out in the CATIE study (NIMH, 2006).
3. Involve mental health consumers in all aspects of research using a participatory-action research approach.
4. Significant investment into researching recovery from cultural, social, and community aspects which would include research into peer support and alternatives to hospitalization.
5. Strengthen the regulatory functions of the FDA and its equivalent in all industrialized countries to ensure research studies, publication of results, and training of professionals are carried out in an unbiased fashion.

CONCLUSION

Though I have focused on the inordinate influence of the pharmaceutical companies on the definition of mental health issues, and on their treatment, there is the much broader issue to consider: why has the American public allowed this state of affairs to occur? The US must face the much deeper issue of identifying our cultural values. Though it is beyond the scope of this paper, the extreme individualism, and its attendant fragmentation of community cohesion, leaves our population vulnerable to simplistic, individual, materially-based solutions. We have as a people lost sight of the experience of social connections which informs most other countries. Our vastly successful material production has robbed us of our humanity and allowed us to see ourselves and others as machines to be serviced like our cars. We can hope that the consumer movement in mental health and other sectors of our society will wake the population from this chemically-induced trance before we have polluted our bodies and our environment beyond repair. We can hope for a green revolution not only in our environment but in our relations with each other and the world. Only then will we start to see the world as a healthy planet.

REFERENCES

Ahearn, L. and Fisher, D. (2001) Recovery at your own PACE. *Journal of Psychosocial Nursing*, **39**, 22–32.

Aiken, K.J. (2002) *Direct-To-Consumer Advertising Of Prescription Drugs: Preliminary Patient Survey Results*, Rockville, MD: Division of Drug Marketing, Advertising and Communications, Food, and Drug Administration.

Berenson, A. (2006) 'Eli Lilly Said to Play Down Risk of Top Pill'. *Washington Post*, Dec. 17.

Bleuler, M. (1974) The long-term course of the schizophrenic psychoses, *Psychological Medicine*, **4**, 244–254.

Blumenthal, R. (2008) 'Blumenthal Sues Eli Lilly For Illegally Marketing Antipsychotic Drug Zyprexa For Unapproved Uses', Press release by the State of Connecticut. Available online at: www.ct.gov/ag/cwp/view.asp?A=2341&Q=411630, accessed 28/10/08.

Charlton, B.G. (2006) Why are doctors still prescribing neuroleptics? *Quarterly Journal, Medicine*, **99**, 417–420.

Conrad, P. and Schneider, J. (1992) *Deviance and Medicalization: From Badness to Sickness*. Philadelphia, PA: Temple University Press.

Davidson, J. (2002) Hypericum Depression Trial Study Group. Effect of Hypericum perforatum (St. John's Wort) in major depressive disorder: a randomized, controlled trial. *Journal of the American Medical Association*, **287**, 1807–1814.

Davis, K. (1938) Mental hygiene and class structure. *Psychiatry*, **1**, 55–65.

Eells, T. (2000) Psychotherapy of schizophrenia. *Journal of Psychotherapy Practice and Research*, **9**, 250–254.

Fisher, D. (2001) 'We've Been Misled by the Drugs industry', Outlook Section, *Washington Post*, August, 19, p 3.

Fisher, D. (2008) Promoting Recovery. In: T. Stickley and T. Basset (Eds) *Learning About Mental Health Practice*, Chichester: John Wiley & Sons Ltd.

Gagnon, M. and Lexchin, J. (2008) The cost of pushing pills: a new estimate of pharmaceutical promotion expenditures in the United States. *PLoS Medicine*, January 3, an online journal published by the Public Library of Science.

Green, H. (1964) *I Never Promised You a Rose Garden*. Henry Holt Publisher, New York, New York.

Grinspoon, L., Ewalt, J. and Shader, R. (1968) Psychotherapy and pharmacotherapy in chronic schizophrenia. *American Journal of Psychiatry*, **124**, 1645–1652.

Harding, C. *et al.* (1987) The Vermont longitudinal study of persons with severe mental illness, I. Methodology, study sample, and overall status 32 years later. *American Journal of Psychiatry*, **144**, 718–728.

Jackson, V. (2005) *In Our Own Voices: African American Stories of Oppression, Survival and Recovery in the Mental Health System*, pp 1–36, p 4–8. Available online at: http://www. mindfreedom.org/kb/mental-health-abuse/Racism/InOurOwnVoice, accessed 28/10/08.

Karons, B. and VandenBos, G. (1981) *Psychotherapy of Schizophrenia: The treatment of choice*, New York: Aronson.

Kim, H.L., Streltzer, J. and Goebert, D. (1999) St. John's Wort for depression: a meta-analysis of well-defined clinical, trials. *Journal of Nervous Mental Disorders*, **187**, 532–539.

Lacasse, J. and Leo, X. (2005) Serotonin and Depression: A Disconnect between the Advertisements and the Scientific Literature. *PLoS Medicine*, **2**(12), pp 1211–1216.

Morgan, S. (2001) *An assessment of the health system impacts of direct to consumer advertising of prescriptions medicines (DTCA), Volume V. Predicting the welfare and cost consequences of direct to consumer prescription drug advertising*, Vancouver: Centre for Health Services and Policy Research, University of British, Columbia.

Mosher, L., Gosden, R. and Beder, S. (2004) Drug companies and schizophrenia, In: J. Read, L. Mosher and R. Bentall (Eds) *Models of Madness: Psychological, Social and Biological Approaches to Schizophrenia*, New York: Brunner-Routledge, pp. 115–130.

Mosher, L., Hendrix, V. and Fort, D. (2006) *Soteria: Through Madness to Deliverance*. Available online from Xlibris at www.xlibris.com.

Mayes, R. and Horwitz, A.V. (2005) DSM-III and the revolution in the classification of mental illness. *Journal of Historical Behavioral Science*, **41**(3), 249–267.

New Freedom Commission, (2003). New Freedom Commission For Mental Health, 2003, SAMHSA, Rockville, MD, www.mentalhealthcommission.gov.

National Institute of Mental Health (2006) *Clinical Antipsychotic Trials of Intervention Effectiveness (CATIE): NIMH Study to Guide Treatment Choices for Schizophrenia*. Available online at: www. nimh.nih.gov/health/trials/practical/catie/index.shtml, accessed 28/10/08.

Pharmalot (2008) 'Senate Targets Stanford Psychiatrist over Conflicts', June 25, 2008.

Ralph, R. (2000) *Review of recovery literature: A synthesis of a sample of recovery literature 2000*, Alexandria, VA: National Technical Assistance Center for State Mental Health Planning (NTAC), National Association for State Mental Health Program Directors (NASMHPD).

SAMHSA (2003) *Achieving the Promise*. Rockville, MD: New Freedom Mental Health Commission, www.mentalhealthcommission.gov

SAMHSA (2005) *National Consensus Statement on Mental Health*. Available online at: http:// mentalhealth.samhsa.gov/publications/allpubs/sma05-4129/, accessed 28/10/08.

Schrader, E. (2000) Equivalence of a St. John's wort extract (Ze 117) and fluoxetine: a randomized, controlled study in mild-moderate depression. *International Clinical Psychopharmacology*, **15**(2), 61–68.

Silverman, E. (2008) Grassley targets Brown's Keller over grants *Pharmalot*, July 14. Available online at: www.pharmalot.com/2008/07/grassley-targets-browns-keller-over-grants/, accessed 28/10/08.

Steinman, M., Bero, L., Chren, M. and Landefeld, C. (2006) Narrative review: the promotion of gabapentin: an analysis of internal industry documents. *Annals of Internal Medicine*, **145**(4), 284–293.

Toop, L., Richardes, D., Dowell, T. *et al.* (2003) *Direct to Consumer Advertising of Prescription Drugs in New Zealand: FOR HEALTH OR FOR PROFIT? Report to the Minister of Health supporting the case for a ban on DTCA*, New Zealand Departments of General Practice, Christchurch, Dunedin, Wellington and Auckland Schools of Medicine.

United States ex rel. Franklin v. Parke-Davis

United States ex rel. Franklin v. Parke-Davis (2001a) 147 F. Supp.2d 39 Exhibit 40. Neurontin Northeast CBU [customer business unit] 1997: X001884-X001900.

United States ex rel. Franklin v. Parke-Davis, (2001b) 147 F. Supp.2d 39 Exhibit 21. [Interoffice memorandum from Atul Pande to John Boris, re: 'Gabapentin Approvals', and handwritten response]; 28 March 1995: X029227.

United States ex rel. Franklin v. Parke-Davis, (2001c) 147 F. Supp.2d 39 Exhibit 31. [Parke-Davis memo from John Boris to 'Distribution' re: 'Marketing Assessment – Neurontin in Migraine,' and cover letter]; 31 July 1996: V082736-V082761.

United States ex rel. Franklin v. Parke-Davis, (2001d) 147 F. Supp.2d 39 Exhibit 120. Neurontin 14th Core Marketing Team Meeting [agenda, conclusions, action items]; 8–9 April 1997:V047116-V047129.

United States ex rel. Franklin v. Parke-Davis, (2001e) 147 F. Supp.2d 39 (Exhibit 181. Grant request – Scientific Article Series in Support of Epilepsy Education [from Medical Education Systems, Inc]; 12 December 1996: X005719-X005723.

United States ex rel. Franklin v. Parke-Davis, (2001f) 147 F. Supp.2d 39 Exhibit 64. [Letter from Jacki Gordon (AMM/Adelphi, Ltd) to Phil Magistro (Parke-Davis), re: development of manuscripts for Parke-Davis Northeast Customer Business Unit]; 8 November 1996: X005.

Winters, K. (2007) *GID Reform Advocates*, Available online at: www.gidreforms.org, accessed.

CHAPTER 17

Good Practice Guidance

Beate Schrank
*Medical University of Vienna, Department of Psychiatry
and Psychotherapy, Vienna, Austria*
Jan Wallcraft
Service user Researcher and Consultant, Worcester, UK

This chapter summarises and supplements the recommendations made for good practice in service user involvement in mental health research throughout this book. It is aimed at researchers who are planning to involve service users in their projects or who seek to improve existing involvement. It is also aimed at service users in order to help them figure out what they can expect from their involvement, and at funding bodies to help them assess the adequacy of service user involvement outlined in research proposals. Hence, these recommendations mainly apply to research projects with various levels of collaboration between traditional researchers and service user researchers. For recommendations on conducting user-controlled research, please refer to Turner and Beresford (2005).

The following list of recommendations cites from this book Faulkner (Chapter 2), Sweeney and Morgan (Chapter 3), Delman and Lincoln (Chapter 10), Minogue (Chapter 11), and Hamilton (Chapter 15), as well as Faulkner (2004), the SURGE (Service User Research Group for England) Good Practice Guidance (SURGE, 2005) and SURGE 'Project Good Practice Support Exercise' (2006).

For more in-depth advice on good practice in specific areas of service user involvement, please refer to the respective chapters in this book.

GOOD PRACTICE IN SERVICE USER INVOLVEMENT IN MENTAL HEALTH – AN OVERVIEW

Laying the foundations

- Be aware of and honest about what you expect from service user involvement.
- Carefully consider the level of involvement you aim for at each specific stage of your research project.
- Be aware of additional resources needed to take into account the time and money required to involve people fully.

Handbook of Service User Involvement in Mental Health Research Edited by Jan Wallcraft, Beate Schrank and Michaela Amering
Copyright © 2009 John Wiley & Sons, Ltd

- Specifically consider planning for:
  - flexibility and periods of absence
  - adequate support for service users: practical, emotional and research related
  - training in relevant knowledge and skills for both service users and researchers.
- Particularly in large institutions, communicate well in advance with the Finance department and Human Resources department about your intention to involve or employ mental health service users in research – in order to facilitate the process and pre-empt any difficulties that may arise.

Capacity-building

- Explore the local community and identify local service user groups:
  - refer to mental health voluntary sector organisations for this information
  - identify existing experience within the Trust and/or research institution of carrying out collaborative research, in order to build on this experience and any associated contacts.
- Build collaborative relationships over time in order to build up trust as well as expertise. Attempting to recruit service user participants at the last minute when a research bid needs to be submitted can be damaging to both parties.
  - remain in contact with service users and researchers who have completed collaborative projects
  - keep a record of people within your organisation who have relevant experience and expertise in this field so that this can be built on.
- Ensure that a budget to develop collaborative relationships can be identified, e.g. to pay people's expenses, for preliminary training and support, and so on.
- Be prepared to offer and receive relevant training that will help to build everyone's capacity for successful collaborative research.

Identifying research priorities

- Consult with local service users and user groups about their priorities for research and seek to find some areas of common interest with current national, trust or institutional research priorities.
- Inform service users about your priorities and research currently being carried out within your department.
- Ensure that existing Research Interest Groups are consulting with and including service users in the development of research topics.

Undertaking research

Consulting with service users

- Consultation should take place as early in the research process as possible.
- Always involve more than one service user in a consultation.

- Ensure that adequate, accessible and jargon-free information is provided in due time before the consultation.
- Provide payment of fees and travel expenses on the day of the consultation.
- Consult with people with integrity: be clear about how their views will be taken on board.
- Offer preliminary training where necessary.
- Offer mentoring and support.

Planning and starting a project

- Involve service users from the start of a project.
- Plan resources in advance to take into account the time and money required to involve people fully.
- Prepare to connect to a public benefits counsellor/Job Centre Plus (UK) to clarify payment issues.
- Plan for flexibility, support, training and periods of absence.
- Researchers need to communicate well in advance with:
  - Finance department
  - Human Resources department
  - Occupational Health team.

Supporting and maintaining a project

- Provide adequate support for service users: practical, emotional and research related.
- Make sure that support for personally delicate issues is provided by a person outside the research team.
- Provide training in relevant knowledge and skills for both service users and researchers.
- Communicate clearly and regularly with service users, particularly if they are not attending the work place on a regular basis.
- Be prepared to be flexible and to negotiate about the research process in an atmosphere of collaboration, sensitivity and respect.

Employment of service user researchers

- Develop a clear and realistic job description, highlighting the essential job functions and minimal qualifications necessary.
- Distribute the job notice widely; include user groups and diverse community groups.
- Interview job applicants in teams including at least one service user.
- Be clear and realistic about the amount of control over the research-project that the person to be employed will have.
- Communicate in clear language, and be aware that people with different backgrounds may understand things differently.
- Provide for a possibility for regular open discussion, formal and personal support, and for supervision.

- Make clear arrangements about who to talk to and where to turn in case of personal problems. This should be separate from the workplace.
- Discuss openly the possibility of the service user researcher becoming ill or unable to work and make clear arrangements in case of this happening.
- Provide for sufficient training opportunities (the advancement of professional skills is one major reason for service users to accept a position in a research institution in the first place).
- Provide for opportunities to meet up with other service user researchers and share common experiences (working in an academic environment may lead to a feeling of alienation among service user researchers).

Dissemination and implementation

- Dissemination to service user audiences in accessible formats must form part of any dissemination strategy. Implementation is a priority for many service users:
  - if possible, it should be built in from the start of a project through adequate budgeting and through the involvement of local stakeholders
  - if implementation is not likely, then this needs to be clearly communicated to the service users involved.
- Ensure that service users are informed about any publications that result from the research in which they have been involved.
- Endings need to be given due consideration: find a way to mark the ending of a project and a way to enable service users and researchers to reflect upon their experience and the learning they have gained through collaborating.

Payment and budgeting

Payment

- Service users should be paid for their involvement in research. The amount of payment will vary but should be adequate to their role and task.
- Promptly reimburse service users for any expenses incurred through their involvement.
- Ensure that the method and structure of payment is appropriate to the level and type of involvement, and that it adheres to employment law.
- Be aware of how payment may affect the receipt of benefits and financial support.
- Service users *must* be informed about any possible impacts, and encouraged to speak to the relevant benefits agency before taking part. Researchers should provide support in this process.

Budgeting

- Be aware of the financial and time costs of conducting genuine service user involvement and factor these in to the budget and timeframe of the project.

Checklist for funding/budget planning

Payment of fees and travel and care expenses to user-researchers
Fees for research participants
Enough funding to include more service user interviewers, consultants or researchers than the project needs, to cover for periods of absence
Support for service users (maybe an additional support worker or alternative)
External supervision
Physical resources, such as space and communication technology to enable service users to take an equal part in the project
Training for service users and for staff (as appropriate)
Time/venue/refreshments to meet with each other for mutual/peer support
Dissemination and feedback to participants: in different formats relevant to your project (e.g. language, accessible written and oral presentations)
Insurance – liability

REFERENCES

Delman, J. and Lincoln, A. (2009) Service Users as Paid Researchers. In: J. Wallcraft, B. Schrank and M. Amering (Eds) *Handbook of Service user Involvement in Mental Health Research*, Chichester: Wiley-Blackwell, (Chapter 10 of this book).

Faulkner, A. (2009) Principles and Motives. In: J. Wallcraft, B. Schrank and M. Amering (Eds) *Handbook of Service user Involvement in Mental Health Research*, Chichester: Wiley-Blackwell, (Chapter 2 of this book).

Faulkner A. (2004) *The Ethics of Survivor Research: Guidelines for the ethical conduct of research carried out by mental health service users and survivors*, Bristol: Policy Press.

Hamilton, S. (2009) Money. In: J. Wallcraft, B. Schrank and M. Amering (Eds) *Handbook of Service user Involvement in Mental Health Research*, Chichester: Wiley-Blackwell, (Chapter 15 of this book).

Minogue V. (2009) Consultation. In: J. Wallcraft, B. Schrank and M. Amering (Eds) *Handbook of Service user Involvement in Mental Health Research*, Chichester: Wiley-Blackwell, (Chapter 11 of this book).

SURGE (Service User Research Group for England): *Guidance for Good Practice Service user involvement in the UK Mental Health Research Network* (2005) Available online at: http://www.mhrn.info/index/ppi/service user-involvement/good-practice-guidance/mainColumnParagraphs/0/text_files/file/SURGE%20Guidance%20for%20Good%20Practice%2006%5B1%5D.pdf, accessed 25/10/08.

SURGE (2006) *Project Good Practice Support Exercise, Service user involvement in MHRN adopted projects*. Report of a survey conducted in 2006. Available online at: http://www.mhrn.info/index/library/surge-docs/mainColumnParagraphs/01/document/Final%20Report%20-%20Project%20Good%20Practice%20Support%20Exercise.pdf, accessed 25/10/08.

Sweeney, A. and Morgan, L. (2009) Levels and Stages. In: J. Wallcraft, B. Schrank and M. Amering (Eds) *Handbook of Service user Involvement in Mental Health Research*, Chichester: Wiley-Blackwell, (Chapter 3 of this book).

Turner, M. and Beresford, P. (2005) *User Controlled Research – Its meanings and potential, Shaping Our Lives and the Centre for Citizen Participation, Brunel University*. Download from www.shapingourlives.org.uk.

Index

Note: Italic page numbers denote tables and figures. Abbreviations used: SURs for service user researchers; DoH for Department of Health

3 Keys to a Shared Approach in Mental Health Assessment 55, 56
10 Essential Shared Capabilities, training programme 44–5

academic user researchers 9
  experiences and perspectives of 62, 67–70
  pitfalls and pratfalls of 69–70
advocacy groups, Boston 79–84
Advocacy Network, Ireland 205, 208
advocacy and research 83–4
agency
  reclamation of 74–6
  Sen's capabilities framework 76–9
Allam, S. 19, 20
American Psychiatric Association (APA) 55, 108, 230
Andreasen, N. 47, 106–7
antidepressants, lack of efficacy 232
Arnstein, S.R., ladder of participation 27, 155–6
assessment, values-based practice 54–6
Asylums (Goffman) 73–4
Australia, initiatives in 125–6, 222
awareness of values, raising 42–3, 44, 45, 53, 56

Beeforth, M. 124
Belenky, M. F. 116
Bellack, A. S. 106
benefits of service user involvement 18–20, 91, 93, 96, 140–2, 159–63, 217, 221
Benefits system, UK 18–20, 215–16, 217–19, 224, 246

Beresford, P. 8, 26, 30, 124, 140, 155, 204, 223
Bertaux-Wiame, I. 117–18
biopower, Foucault 201–2
Bleuler, M. 229
Blumenthal, R. 236
Boote, J. 28
Braithwaite, T. 35
Branfield, F. 140
budgeting
  additional resources 147–8, 150
  good practice guidance 246–7

Campbell, J. 4, 47, 101–2, 103, 119, 207
Campbell-Orde, T. 107
Campbell, P. 47–8
Canada, initiatives in 4, 92, 123
'capabilities' framework 76–7
capacity building 73–85, 244
Care Services Improvement Partnership (CSIP)
  3 Keys to a Shared Approach 55
  payment levels in the UK 216
Carpenter, J. 107
Cartwright, Dr. Samuel 230
Castells, M. 75
challenges to service user involvement 20–2, 142–3
Chamberlin, J. 107, 115, 187
civil rights movement 94
Clark, C. C. 141
coercion
  human subjects/ethics 94
  scale measuring 105

collaboration   169
  beginnings of collaborative research
     170–1
  differing experiences of   61–2
     academic perspective   62, 67–70
     being a user-researcher   174–7
     survivor perspective   62–7
  first projects in England   169–70
  level of involvement   29–30
  recommendations for   71
  SURE (Service User Research Enterprise)
     171–3
     participatory research   173–4
     patient-centred systematic reviews
        172–3
Collins, K.   156
Columbo, A.   47, 51
communication
  clarity of   145
  skills of SURs   43, 44
  see also voice of service users
community-based participatory research
     (CBPR)   73–84
community-based peer support   121–3
community-based treatment, effectiveness
     of   232
community mental health services, evaluation
     of   123–4
compulsory treatment   52–4
concept-mapping, focus groups   121
concerns
  about evidence-based practice   100
  about funders' requirements   222–3
  about power of drug companies   228–9
  of service users   121
consultation   153–4
  benefits of   159, 162–3
  definitions of   154–5
  effectiveness of   163–5
  examples
     peer review panels   162–3
     service user research group   164
  good practice guidance   244–5
  levels of   155–6, 157
  points of 160–2
  research process   158, 158–9
Consumer Operated Service Program (COSP)
     multi-site research initiative   103–6,
     122–3, 128–31
consumer-run organisations, longitudinal study
     of   123

consumer/survivor/ex-patient (c/s/x), origin of
     term   8
consumerist approach   30, 65, 155, 189, 204
Contributing on Equal Terms (Social Care
     Institute for Excellence)   217
contribution, level of involvement   29, 34
control, level of involvement   27, 30, 32–3
  see also user-controlled research
Coping with Coming off Psychiatric Drugs
     (Mind)   5
COSP Multisite Research Initiative   103–6,
     122–3
  Consumer Advisory Panel (CAP)   128–31
costs of service user involvement   219
  payment of service users   214–19
  support and supervision   220
  training and expenses   219–20
  see also funding
critical movement   206
critical theory   200, 203–5

data collection   32, 128–9
Davidson, L.   48, 54, 57
de-institutionalization   75–6
Delman, J.   144
Delphi Study   208
democratic approach   65, 155, 184, 189, 193,
     204–5
demonstration projects   6–7, 62, 68, 122
diagnosis, political basis of   230–1
direct-to-consumers advertising
     (DTCA)   232–3, 239
Disability Discrimination Act (1995)   14
disabled people's movement   182, 186–7
disciplinary power   201–2
discrimination   45, 103, 185
dissemination stage of research process   20,
     33, 141, 142, 162, 246
diversity
  of service users   14, 15, 80–2, 163
  of values, respect for   38, 45
drapetomania   230
drug companies
  advertising of drugs   232–3
  barrier to user-controlled research   191–2
  influence of   233–7
  rejection of evidence   232
Druss, B. G.   102
Druzich, N. M.   101
Dumont, J.   121, 122
Dworkin, R.J.   2

education
    about side-effects of drugs   232–3, 239
    of senior researchers about lives of
        SURs   141.2
    of service user researchers   146
electro-convulsive therapy (ECT)
    collaborative study   177–8
    first-person account   3
    patient-centred systematic reviews   172, 173
Eli Lilly (pharmaceutical company), illegal
        practices   236–7
emancipatory disability research   182, 185–7
employment
    hiring of SURs   81, 140–3, 146–8, 245–6
    motivation for future   17, 96
empowerment   120
    paradigm of recovery and
        development   237–8
    participatory research enabling   94, 95, 96
    World Bank definition of   84
Estroff, S.   126–7
ethical issues   35
    ethical conduct in research   94–5
    and values-based practice   51–4, 57
Ethics of Survivor Research, The
        (Faulkner)   15
Evans, C.   26
Evidence-Based Medicine: How to Practice
        and Teach EBM (Sackett)   54
evidence-based practice   47–50
    concerns about   100
    political issues   231–2
experts by experience   9
    research roles of   63–7

Fairweather Lodge, social engineering
        project   68
Faulkner, A.   15, 17, 20, 22, 42, 53, 145, 184
financial assistance to service users   18,
        214–19, 224
first-person research   6, 9, 89–90, 118
Fisher, D.   5, 7, 50, 114
focus groups   92, 121, 122, 173–4
Foucault, M.   200, 201–2
'framework of values' approach   52–4
Frank, L.R.   3, 6
Freire, P.   95
funding   16, 100, 150, 194
    checklist for planning   247
    concerns about funder requirements   222–3
    difficulty obtaining   69, 143, 173, 185, 186

by drugs industry   103, 227, 234, 236
    involving users in decisions   223–4
    opportunities provided by   222
    preparation of bids for   161
    priorities of funders   221–2
    recommendations   224–5
    in the UK   159, 170–1
    in the US   70, 101, 121

gabapentin, marketing of   234–5
Gergen, K. J.   201
Gergen, M. M.   201
Glaxo, fraud charge   236
globalisation, barrier to user-controlled
        research   191
Goffman, E.   73–4
gold standard of research evidence   192, 200,
        231–2
good practice guidance   148–50, 243–7
government policy   5–6
    and direct to consumer advertising (DTCA),
        NZ   239
    for mandatory user involvement, UK   7
    quality assurance, UK   123
    Values Framework, England   46–7
government reform
    Involve, UK   5, 183–4
    political agendas   69–70
    research priorities, US   101
government support
    lack of funding, UK   69
    for peer-run services, US   68, 121
'grey' literature   6, 172
Griffiths, K.   126
Guidance for Service-user Involvement in the Mental
        Health Research Network (SURGE)   14
Guiding Principles, Code of Practice MHA
        (1983)   46, 52–4

Hall, B.   95
Hanley, B.   27
Harding,, C.   229
Health Employer Data Information Set
        (HEDIS)   102
Hempel, C.   37–8
Hill House Project, Ohio   3–4, 119
hiring SURs   81, 144, 146, 148, 245–6
historical perspectives   1–5, 118–19
Hoff, P.   50
homosexuality as an illness, declassification
        of   230

hooks, bell   126
Hopper, K.   50
hospitalization, reducing agency   74–5
Human Rights Act   52
human rights issues, avoidance of unethical
    research   94–5

ideological basis of involvement   188–9
IGPB (Instituut voor Gebruikersparticipatie en
    Beleid)   125
impact of user involvement   189–90
  pressure to provide evidence of   178
inclusion, sense of belonging of SURs   144–5
individual research   3, 6
individuality of SURs   147
'insider' research   4–5
Institute for Mental Health Recovery   208
Institute of Psychiatry, collaborating
    with   177–8
instruments for measuring recovery-promoting
    environments   107–9
international variations in user-controlled
    research   191–2
interpersonal difficulties, negotiating   22
Introduction to Social Constructionism
    (Burr)   201
INVOLVE   5, 163–4, 170, 178
  impact of user involvement   189–90
  involvement levels   27–30, *32–3*, 34–5
  involvement stages   31, *32–3*, 34
  INVONET network   18
  providing evidence of user
    involvement   170–1
  review of user-controlled research   183–4
Irish Advocacy Network   205, 208
Ison, R.   156

Jones, K.   122

Karons, B.   231
Khandelwal, S.   101
King, C.   50
Knowing Our Own Minds (Faulkner)   125
knowledge
  imbalance between researchers and service
    users   142–3
  as social construction   206–8
  values-based practice   43, 44

'ladder of participation'   27, 155–6
language issues   7–9, 26–7, 80, 201

Leete, E.   207
Leff, H. S.   107
legislation   7, 52
Leibrich, J.   6
'level playing field' approach   48
levels and stages   25–6
  involvement levels   27–8
    collaboration   29–30
    consultation   28
    contribution   29
    control   30
    examples of   32–3
  involvement stages   31–4
  terminology issues   26–7
Liberman, R. P.   106, 107–8
Lilly, pharmaceutical company, illegal
    practices   236–7
Lindow, V.   3
literary/rhetorical movement   206
lives of service users, improving   93–4
  by guiding research questions   95–6
  human rights protection in research   94–5
Luhrmann, T. M.   74
Lynch, M. M.   101

Martin, E.   127–8
McCallum, A.   156
McGowan, P.   201, 203
medical model   2, 7, 8, 114, 192
Mental Health Act (1983), guiding principles in
    Code of Practice   46
mental health assessment, values-based practice
    in   54–6
Mental Health Foundation   20, 50, 125, 185
*Mental Health Recovery: What Helps and What
    Hinders?* (Onken)   122
Mental Health Task Force User Group   124
mental illnesses, reasons for first-person
    perspective   89–90
methods   113–15
  future directions   131–2
  voice of service users   115–18
MHARN (mental health and addiction-recovery
    needs), Boston, US   80–3
Mills, C. W.   132
Minogue, V.   7
Misztal, B.   117
models, discourses and worldviews   8
money   18, 213–14
  payment of service users   214–19
  spent on drug advertising   233

support after the project 221–4
support and supervision 220
training 219–20
see also funding
Morgan, L. 170
Mosher, Dr. L., Soteria Houses 232
motives and incentives 15–16
  for researchers 16–17
  for service users 17–18

narratives 6, 9, 54
  accounts of recovery 116–18
  interpretation of 126–8
  of life stories 119, 125
  value of 54, 125
National Empowerment Center 237–8
National Institute for Health Research (NIHR) 159
National Institute for Mental Health in England
    (NIMHE) 46
  best practice in assessment 55
  NIMHE Values Framework 45, 47
National Institute of Mental Health (NIMH), US
  rejection of evidence-based practice 232
  research priorities of 101
Netherlands, initiatives in 125
New Freedom Commission on Mental
    Health 106, 113–14, 232, 238, 239
New NHS: Modern, Dependable, The (DoH) 123
Nicholls, V. 170
non-profit organisations, support from 5, 123–4
'normalisation talk' 127

O'Hagan, M. 3
'off-label use' of gabapentin 234–5
Oliver, M. 204
outcome measures 19, 32
  definitions of recovery 106–7, 114
  divergent views on 100–3, 203–4

Parke-Davis, promotion of off-label user of
    gabapentin 234–5
participation 73–4
  'capabilities' framework 76–7
  participatory research 6, 95, 173–4
  practical questions 79–84
  in public mental health 77–9
  reclaiming agency 74–6
participatory-action research projects 4, 6,
    91–3, 123
partnership
  dealing with power differences 82–3

model of user/survivor movement 187
  in research 71
  user and mainstream researchers 177
  and values-based practice 50
patient-centred systematic reviews 172–3
Paxil (Seroxat), litigation 235–6
payment of service users 148,
    214–19, 246
Peer Outcomes Protocol (POP) Project 122
peer review panels 162–3
peer-run services, US 121–2
'peer specialists' 9
Pembroke, L. 6
personal commitment of SURs 144
pharmaceutical corporations, major source of
    research funding 103
pharmaceutical industry
  barrier to user-controlled research 191–2
  direct-to-consumers advertising
    (DTCA) 232–3
  influence of 233–7
pilot projects 6–7, 81, 122
Planning for the Future (DoH) 206
planning and starting a project 245
politics 227–30
  of diagnosis 230–1
  of evidence 231–2
  need for recovery research 237–8
  of public education 232–3
  of research and publication 233–7
  of therapy 231
  ways of improving research nad
    education 238–9
positivist research values 37–8, 193
poverty, stigma of 76–7
power 199–201
  critical theory 203–5
  dealing with differences 82–3, 176–7
  Foucault's biopower 201–2
  and resistance 202
  social constructionism 201, 205–8
Powers, R. 83
principles and motives 13–14
  benefits 18–20
  challenges 20–2
  laying the foundations 22–3
  motives and incentives 15–16
    for researchers 16–17
    for service users 17–18
  negotiating difference 22
  underlying principles 14–15

problems of service users, self-identified   203–4
psychiatric system
  dominance of drug therapy in   187, 192,
    228–9, 232
  position of service user in   207
  training controlled by drug companies   229
psychotherapy, political influences   231
public education, politics of   232–3, 239
publication of research
  academic researchers   142
  selective   239
  strategies used by drug companies   233–6
purposes and goals   87–9
  impact on service user lives   93–6
  improving quality of research   89–93

quality assurance   102, 123
quality of life
  two perspectives of   77, 78
  Well-Being Project   102, 119

Ralph, R. O.   108–9
Ramon, S.   19
randomized controlled trials (RCTs)   172,
    174, 175, 192, 202
  COSP Multisite Research Initiative   122–3,
    128–31
  evidenced-based practice (EBP)   231–2
Rawls, J.   77
reasoning skills   43, 44
recovery
  definitions of
    clinical outcomes/criteria   106–7
    by consumers   107
  empowerment paradigm of   237–8
  factors promoting   107–8
  measurement instruments   107
  movement, civil rights   94
  'recovery model'   175
  US research project   122
  Well-Being Project   96
recruitment of SURs   81, 146, 160, 161
relational power   199–200
  critical theory   200, 203–5
  Faucault's ideas   200, 201–2
  social constructionist version of   201,
    205–8
research   228
  influence of drug companies on   233–7
  power exerted by mainstream   176–7
  priorities

divergent views on   41–2, 100–3
identification of   126, 160, 244
involving service users in decisions
    about   223–4
quality, relevance and utility,
    improving   89–90
  by involving users in existing
    approaches   90–1
  by involving users in new
    approaches   91–3
questions, users defining   95–6
recommendations for improving   238–9
types of   5–7
value-ladenness of   38
Research and Development for a First Class
    Service (DoH)   16
Research Governance Framework for Health
    and Social Care (DoH)   16
Researching Persons With Mental Illness
    (Dworkin)   2
'resistance identities'   75
Rheinharz, S.   116
Ridgway, P. A.   100–1, 118
Roberts, G.   52
roles in research partnerships   61–70
  necessary conditions   71
Rose, D.   7, 19, 29

Sackett, D.L.   38, 54
Sadler, J. Z.   54
Sainsbury Centre for Mental Health   123–4,
    185
Samele, C.   203–4
SAMHSA (Substance Abuse and Mental Health
    Services Administration)   103–4, 237–8
Sartori, G.   4
schizophrenia
  Cognitive Rehabilitation Therapy for   174
  efficacy of psychotherapy for   231
  participatory-action research project   92
  recovery from, personal account   228–9
Schneider, B.   92
Schraiber, R.   103
scientific knowledge/research
  hierarchy of evidence   192
  traditional positivist values   37–8, 192
  value-ladenness of   55, 56
Scott, A.   103, 115
Second Opinion Society (SOS), Canada   4
Sen, A.   74, 76–7, 78–9
service-satisfaction teams, user-led   90–1

Service User Research Enterprise *see* SURE
Service User Research Group England *see*
    SURGE
service user researchers (SURs), definition
    of 9
service users as paid researchers 138–40
  benefit system as barrier to 217–19
  benefits of 140–2
  challenges to 142–3
  good practice guidance 148–50
  nine key principles for 143–8
Shaping Our Lives, user-controlled
    research 188
Share Your Bounty, demonstration project
    68
Shimrat, I. 6
Side-effects (Bass) 236
side-effects of drugs 232, 233
  failure of drug companies to disclose
    236–7
  need for unbiased research 239
  patient-centred systematic reviews 172
Silverman, E. 235–6
Simpson, E. L. 154
skills areas of values-based practice 42–5
Smith, Adam 77
social constructionism 201, 205–8
social model of disability 8, 186–7, 190
social movement 206
St. John's Wort, efficacy of 232
*Statement on Consumer and Community
    Participation in Health and Medical
    Research* (NHMRC) 125–6, 222
stigma of mental illness 74, 103, 127, 186–7,
    229
Strategies for Living (S4L) program 125, 170
suicidality, lived experience of 9
supervision for SURs 149
support for service user researchers 147, 245
  after the project 221–4
  during the project 220
SURE (Service User Research Enterprise)
    171, 185
  participatory research 173–4
  patient-centred systematic reviews 172–3
SURGE (Service User Group England)
  benefits of user involvement 18–22
  suggestions for researchers 22–3
  underlying principles 14–15
'survivor', evolution of term 8
survivor movement 2–3, 186–7

survivor research, underlying principles of 14
survivor researchers
  perspectives of 62–3
  research roles 63–7
Susko, M. A. 6
Sweeney, A. 170
systematic reviews, patient-centred 172–3

Tarpey, M. 156
Telford, R. 17, 26, 27–8
terminology issues 7–9, 26–7, 80
time, underestimation of 221
topics for research 99–100
  consumer-operated services program multi-
    site research initiative 103–6
  divergent views on priorities and
    outcomes 100–3
  recovery 106–9
Townend, M. 35
traditional research values
  hierarchy of evidence 192
  positivist values 193
training
  control of psychiatric 229
  'Experts by Experience' courses 125
  of SURs 21, 146, 149, 219–20
  in values-based practice 43–5
transformative research, problems
    encountered 69–70
TREE program, Netherlands 125
Tritter, J. Q. 156
Trivedi, P. 19, 30
Turner, M. 30

usefulness of SURs 65–6
user-controlled research 181–2
  approaches to involvement in
    research 182–3
  barriers to 191–2
    international 191–2
    traditional research values 192–3
  definition in INVOLVE review 183–4
  disability research 182
  emancipatory disability and survivor
    research 185–6
  example of 187–8
  future directions in 193–4
  ideologies of involvement 188–9
  impact of 189–90
  mental health service user/survivor
    research 186–7

user-controlled research (*Continued*)
  problems maintaining control   185
  strengths of   190
User-Focused Monitoring (UFM)   124, 169–70
user-led research (ULR)   30, 124, 183, 205
  see also user-controlled research
user research
  criticisms of   175–6
  first projects in England   169–70
user-researchers   174–5
  power exerted over by mainstream
    researchers   176–7

values-based practice   37–8
  defining values   38, *39*
  key points   *57*
  outline of   38–9
  practical examples of   51
    ethical issues   51–4
    mental health assessment   54–6
  and service user involvement   42
    evidence-based practice   47–50
    the four skills areas   42–5
    partnership, importance of   50
    policy framework   46–7
  ten key pointers   39–42
Van Tosh, L.   6, 121
'Vicki Scale', perceived coercion   105
Vision for Change (Department of Health and
  Children)   205

voice of service users   95, 113–15
  challenges and rewards of   128–31
  defining voice   115–18
  from perspective of professionals
    126–8
  future practice   131–2
  historical perspective   118–26
voluntary sector support   5
  dissemination stage of research   20
  for service user research   123–4
Vouri, H.   123

Wallcraft, J.   3, 8, 124–5
Webb, D.   6, 9
welfare recipients in the UK   217–18
well-being   76–8
Well-Being Project, California   4, 6, 96, 102,
  119–20
What We Heard (Irish Advocacy
  Network)   205
Whose Values? (Woodbridge and Fulford)   42,
  43–5, 49
Wittgenstein, L.   206–7
Woodbridge, K.   43
Woolf, Lord   52
World Bank, definition of empowerment   84
Wyatt, K.   145
Wykes, T.   19, 30, 171

Zyprexa, litigation case   236–7

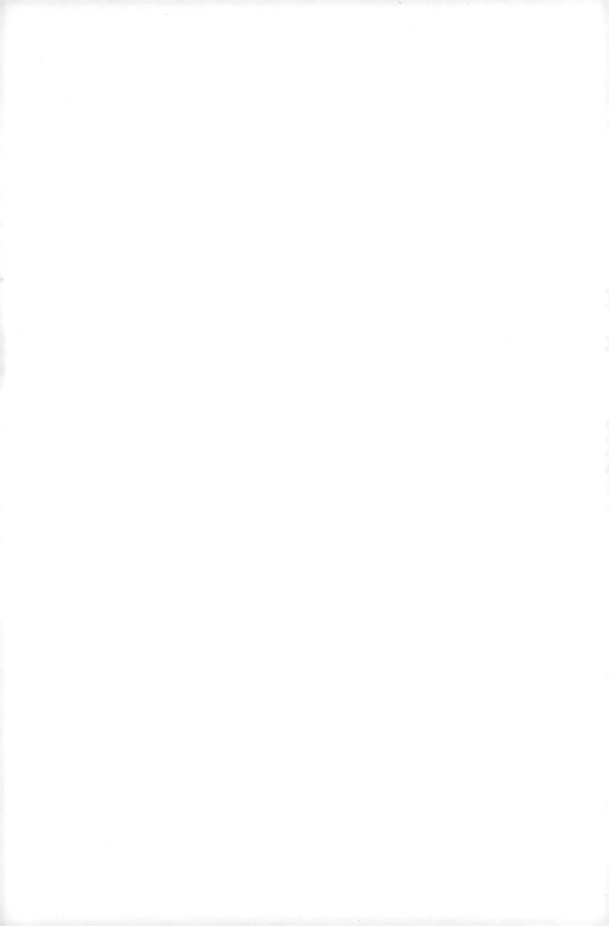